Foot Ankle Deformity in the Child

Editor

MAURIZIO DE PELLEGRIN

FOOT AND ANKLE CLINICS

www.foot.theclinics.com

Consulting Editor
Cesar de Cesar Netto

December 2021 • Volume 26 • Number 4

ELSEVIER

1600 John F. Kennedy Boulevard • Suite 1800 • Philadelphia, Pennsylvania, 19103-2899

http://www.theclinics.com

FOOT AND ANKLE CLINICS Volume 26, Number 4
December 2021 ISSN 1083-7515, ISBN-978-0-323-83574-9

Editor: Lauren Boyle
Developmental Editor: Arlene B. Campos

Foot and Ankle Clinics (ISSN 1083-7515) is published quarterly by Elsevier, Inc., 360 Park Avenue South, New York, NY 10010-1710. Months of issue are March, June, September, and December. Periodicals postage paid at New York, NY, and additional mailing offices. Subscription price per year is $344.00 (US individuals), $741.00 (US institutions), $100.00 (US students), $371.00 (Canadian individuals), $778.00 (Canadian institutions), $100.00 (Canadian students), $479.00 (international individuals), $778.00 (international institutions), and $215.00 (international students). To receive student/resident rate, orders must be accompanied by name of affiliated institution, date of term, and the *signature* of program/residency coordinator on institution letterhead. Orders will be billed at individual rate until proof of status is received. Foreign air speed delivery is included in all *Clinics* subscription prices. All prices are subject to change without notice. **POSTMASTER:** Send address changes to *Foot and Ankle Clinics*, Elsevier Health Sciences Division, Subscription Customer Service, 3251 Riverport Lane, Maryland Heights, MO 63043. **Customer Service: 1-800-654-2452 (US and Canada). From outside of the United States and Canada, call 314-447-8871. Fax: 314-447-8029. E-mail: JournalsCustomerService-usa@elsevier.com (for print support); JournalsOnlineSupport-usa@elsevier.com (for online support).**

Reprints. For copies of 100 or more, of articles in this publication, please contact the Commercial Reprints Department, Elsevier Inc., 360 Park Avenue South, New York, NY 10010-1710. Tel.: 212-633-3874; Fax: 212-633-3820; E-mail: reprints@elsevier.com.

Contributors

CONSULTING EDITOR

CESAR DE CESAR NETTO, MD, PhD
Orthopaedic Foot and Ankle Surgeon, Director of the UIOWA Orthopedic Functional Imaging Research Laboratory, Assistant Professor, Department of Orthopaedic and Rehabilitation, University of Iowa, Carver College of Medicine, Iowa City, Iowa, USA

EDITOR

MAURIZIO DE PELLEGRIN, MD
Head, Pediatric Orthopedic and Traumatology Unit, San Raffaele Hospital, Milan, Italy

AUTHORS

MARYSE BOUCHARD, MD, MSc
Assistant Professor, Division of Orthopaedic Surgery, The Hospital for Sick Children, Department of Surgery, Division of Orthopaedic Surgery, The University of Toronto, Toronto, Canada

DOMENICO ANDREA CAMPANACCI, MD
Director, Department of Orthopaedic Oncology and Reconstructive Surgery, Careggi University Hospital, Firenze, Italy

EMILY O. CIDAMBI, MD
Staff Surgeon, Department of Orthopaedics, Rady Children's Hospital, Clinical Assistant Professor of Orthopaedic Surgery, UC San Diego Medical School, San Diego, California, USA

MAURIZIO DE PELLEGRIN, MD
Head, Pediatric Orthopedic and Traumatology Unit, San Raffaele Hospital, Milan, Italy

LEONARD DOEDERLEIN, MD
Orthopaedic Hospital Aukammklinik, Wiesbaden, Germany

DAVI P. HAJE, MD
Centro Clinico Orthopectus e IGESDF, Brasília-DF, Brasil

JOHANNES HAMEL
Professor, Schoen Klinik Muenchen Harlaching, Munich, Germany

ANJA C. HELMERS, MD, PhD
Head of Department of Paediatric Orthopaedic, EWK Spandau, Berlin, Germany

ALEXANDER KIRIENKO, MD
External Fixation Unit, Humanitas Clinical and Research Center IRCCS, Rozzano, Milan, Italy

HUBERT O. KLAUSER, MD
Orthopaedic Surgeon, General Surgeon, Hand Surgeon, Certified Foot Surgeon, Medical Director, HAND- UND FUSSZENTRUM BERLIN, Berlin, Germany

SHUYUAN LI, MD, PhD
Department of Orthopaedic Surgery, University of Colorado; International Program Director, Steps2Walk, Denver, Colorado, USA

SUSAN T. MAHAN, MD, MPH
Staff Surgeon, Department of Orthopaedics and Sports Medicine, Boston Children's Hospital, Assistant Professor of Orthopaedic Surgery, Harvard Medical School, Boston, Massachusetts, USA

EMILIANO MALAGOLI, MD
External Fixation Unit, Humanitas Clinical and Research Center IRCCS, Rozzano, Milan, Italy

FREEMAN MILLER, MD
Emeritus, Department of Orthopedics, Nemours/Alfred I. duPont Hospital for Children, Wilmington, Delaware, USA

DÉSIRÉE MOHARAMZADEH, MD
Orthopedic and Traumatology Unit, San Raffaele Hospital, Milan, Italy

MARK S. MYERSON, MD
Professor of Orthopedic Surgery, University of Colorado; Executive Director and Founder, Steps2Walk, Denver, Colorado, USA

CHRISTOF RADLER, MD
Associate Professor, Department of Pediatric Orthopaedics and Adult Foot and Ankle Surgery, Head of the Pediatric Orthopaedic Team, Orthopaedic Hospital Speising GmbH, Vienna, Austria

TAYLER DECLAN ROSS, MB BCh BAO
Division of Orthopaedic Surgery, The University of Toronto, Toronto, Canada

GUIDO SCOCCIANTI, MD
Consultant, Department of Orthopaedic Oncology and Reconstructive Surgery, Careggi University Hospital, Firenze, Italy

JULIEANNE P. SEES, DO
Associate Professor, Department of Orthopedics, Thomas Jefferson University, Philadelphia, Pennsylvania, USA

THOMAS WIRTH, MD, PhD
Department of Orthopaedics, Olgahospital, Klinikum Stuttgart, Stuttgart, Germany

Editorial Advisory Board

Contents

involve not only the foot but also the ankle are necessary to analyze the location and size of the coalitions, determining the presence of arthritis in the involved or adjacent joints, and if there are any deformities including a ball-and-socket ankle, which is frequently associated with complex tarsal coalitions.

FOOT AND ANKLE CLINICS

FORTHCOMING ISSUES

March 2022
Alternatives to Ankle Joint Replacement
Woo-Chun Lee, *Editor*

June 2022
Managing Complications of Foot and Ankle Surgery
Scott Ellis, *Editor*

September 2022
Managing Challenging Deformities with Arthrodesis of the Foot and Ankle
Manuel Monteagudo, *Editor*

RECENT ISSUES

September 2021
Controversies in Managing the Progressive Collapsing Foot Deformity (PCFD)
Cesar de Cesar Netto, *Editor*

June 2021
Deltoid-Spring Ligament Complex and Medial Ankle Instability
Gastón Slullitel and Roxa Ruiz, *Editors*

March 2021
Advances in the Treatment of Athletic Injury
Mark S. Myerson, *Editor*

RELATED SERIES

Orthopedic Clinics
Clinics in Sports Medicine
Physical Medicine and Rehabilitation Clinics

Foreword
Getting My Feet Wet!

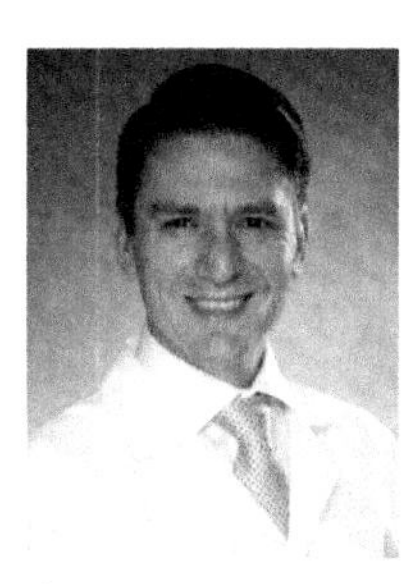

Cesar de Cesar Netto, MD, PhD
Consulting Editor

Dear Foot and Ankle Community Friends,

As I get more and more involved with the *Foot and Ankle Clinics of North America* editorial process, I also get more and more excited about the future of the journal and some innovations it is hoped we will soon bring to your attention. The intention is to keep and intensify the international presence of article authorship and guest editors for the specific issues. I'm also bringing on board three extensively published and internationally respected associate editors, representatives of different continents, to support and enlighten the choice of topics to be covered as well as increase and expand our network with innovative expert surgeons and researchers around the globe. Names will be announced and presented to our audience soon on our Web site.

I'm also thrilled to announce that we have been working on a quarterly audio/video *Foot and Ankle Clinics of North America* podcast ("Foot Talk Show") where we will be hosting and interviewing protagonists and leaders in the Foot and Ankle Surgery Community. Our first guest could not be other than Dr Mark Myerson, previous Editor-in-Chief of *Foot and Ankle Clinics of North America* for the last 25 years! Dr Federico Usuelli and Dr Mark Easley will be joining me for the interview. We will also have some last-minute surprise participants in what we are planning to be a very informal, joyful, and interactive event. We will provide more details soon on our Web site and social media.

I genuinely hope you will enjoy this journal's current issue led by Dr Maurizio De Pellegrin on Pediatric Foot and Ankle Deformities. Dr De Pellegrin brilliantly led a rock-star roster of pediatric foot and ankle specialists. The resultant work will significantly contribute to our understanding of the most recent updates and innovations to optimize the assessment and treatment of pediatric foot and ankle pathologic conditions.

I want to keep the doors of our journal open to the International Foot and Ankle Community. Multiple heads think better than one. Please feel free to contact me by

Foot Ankle Clin N Am 26 (2021) xiii–xiv
https://doi.org/10.1016/j.fcl.2021.10.001
1083-7515/21/© 2021 Published by Elsevier Inc.

e-mail if you have ideas, experience, expertise, or innovative approaches in specific subjects or techniques. You can reach me at cesar-netto@uiowa.edu.

I am looking forward to interacting more with you all!

Stay safe!

Cesar de Cesar Netto, MD, PhD
Department of Orthopaedics and Rehabilitation
University of Iowa
Iowa City, IA, USA

E-mail address:
cesar-netto@uiowa.edu

Preface

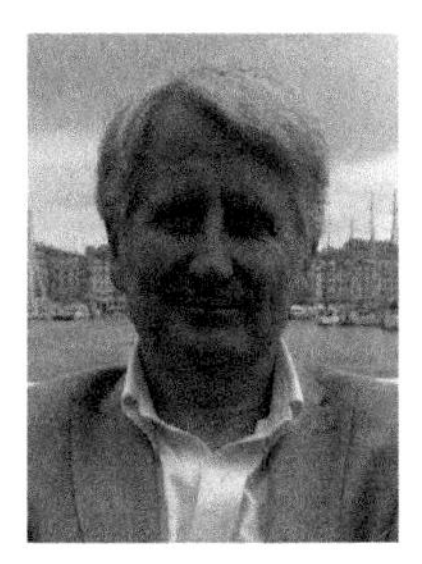

Maurizio De Pellegrin, MD
Editor

When Mark Myerson offered me to guest edit an issue dedicated to the child's foot, I felt honored, and I accepted with pleasure and enthusiasm. As a member of many Pediatric Orthopedic and Foot societies, I thought of keeping abreast of the hot topics and of the less discussed pathologic conditions but with an important clinical relevance.

The authors invited to collaborate on this issue are recognized experts of the topics, and I gratefully thank my colleagues for participating. The issues proposed, on which authors have given as much information as possible in order to have a state-of-the-art review with clear key points, are of absolute interest. On some topics, much has already been written, such as flatfoot and clubfoot. On the contrary, new topics, with few references in literature, have been described, like brachymetatarsia and maligned and benign foot tumors in children. For the "classic topic", we chose new aspects such as the neglected clubfoot, very common and current in the developing countries and mainly treated in humanitarian programs. The recurrent clubfoot and the overcorrected clubfoot were also considered. For the flexible flatfoot, we wanted to get the point up-to-date on performing the surgical techniques, like subtalar arthroereisis, and bony procedures, such as osteotomies, as well. For rare foot diseases, we proposed a synthesis of strategies in which the reader could learn the peculiar aspects. The same is valid for known topics, like coalitions, hallux valgus, and congenital vertical talus, in which giving useful algorithms could help define the surgical approach in children. For foot disorders in cerebral palsy and in other neurologic diseases, we asked experts to make an updated review.

We hope the reader of this *Foot and Ankle Clinics of North America* issue will find not only helpful information but also hints for future topics that are always in evolution like imaging, surgical techniques, and evaluation systems.

Foot Ankle Clin N Am 26 (2021) xv–xvi
https://doi.org/10.1016/j.fcl.2021.08.001

Thanks to all the staff at Elsevier for their support, especially Arlene Campos.

Maurizio De Pellegrin, MD
Pediatric Orthopedic and Traumatology Unit
San Raffaele Hospital
Via Olgettina, 60
Milano 20132, Italy

E-mail address:
depellegrin.maurizio@hsr.it

The Treatment of Recurrent Congenital Clubfoot

Christof Radler, MD

KEYWORDS

• Clubfoot • Recurrent clubfoot • Ponseti • Tendon transfer • Achilles lengthening

KEY POINTS

- Despite the widespread use of the Ponseti method high rates of clubfoot recurrence are still reported.
- There is little consensus on treatment of recurrence, which ranges from neglect to open joint surgery.
- This review reflects the literature and describes the treatment of recurrent congenital clubfoot within the realm of the Ponseti method.
- Indications, surgical procedures, and their variations are discussed.

Treatment of congenital clubfoot has changed in the last decades with the introduction and dissemination of the Ponseti method of clubfoot treatment. Most pediatric orthopedic centers in North America[1] and around the world[2] use the Ponseti method for treatment of congenital clubfoot in newborns. Nevertheless, high numbers of recurrences are reported and open release surgery within the first 3 to 4 years of life is still performed frequently.[3–5] These facts highlight the necessity to look at the reasons for clubfoot recurrence, prevention of clubfoot recurrence, and the treatment of recurrent congenital clubfoot within the realm of the Ponseti method.

EARLY RELAPSE VERSUS RESIDUAL DEFORMITY/NONCOMPLIANCE VERSUS FAILURE TO ENABLE COMPLIANCE

Especially in the first year of life it is often difficult to differentiate between clubfoot recurrence and clubfoot residual when evaluating clubfoot treated elsewhere. In early recurrence before the age of 2 years it is usually believed that noncompliance with bracing is the most common reason for relapse. However, in daily practice this scenario is more complex.

1. Sometimes feet that are deemed recurrent are not fully corrected after removal of the last cast after tendo Achilles tenotomy, lacking abduction/subtalar derotation and/or dorsiflexion. Those feet are then forced into foot abduction braces;

Department of Pediatric Orthopaedics and Adult Foot and Ankle Surgery, Orthopaedic Hospital Speising GmbH, Speisinger Strasse 109, Vienna A-1130, Austria
E-mail address: christof.radler@oss.at

Foot Ankle Clin N Am 26 (2021) 619–637
https://doi.org/10.1016/j.fcl.2021.07.001 foot.theclinics.com
1083-7515/21/

sometimes into insufficient models, sometimes into too big shoes. Parents report the feet slipping out of the shoes and/or skin problems that make bracing nearly impossible despite best efforts. Many of those parents are deemed noncompliant, the feet atypical or resistant, and surgery is recommended. Luckily, those feet can still be corrected well when the Ponseti method is applied in the right way. In the difficult and atypical clubfoot,[6] which should be less than 3% to 5% of an institution's caseload, bracing is more difficult. In some of those cases dorsiflexion can only be achieved to about 5° despite expert casting and tenotomy. Additionally, abduction in the last cast must often be limited to about 30° to 40° to avoid a transverse midfoot break.[6] However, especially in those cases it must be ensured that the brace fits and that the patient is seen regularly even within weeks to make sure that the foot is placed and fixed well within the shoe. If bracing is successful almost all of these feet develop into well-corrected clubfeet and increase the dorsiflexion within a couple of months. Despite the success in initial correction higher rates of relapse have been reported for atypical/complex clubfoot.[7,8]

2. True early recurrence is extremely rare in the author's opinion. It does require noncompliance with the brace, and especially in the first years of life almost all parents try their respective, relative best to achieve bracing. The few parents who do struggle need extra guidance and counseling.[9] As pediatric orthopedic surgeons dealing with children and parents all the time, we should be used to handling parents doubts, fears, and difficulties that can arise from specific family situations or difficult social and financial backgrounds. Nevertheless, we should be compassionate and persuasive enough, making them understand the need for bracing and to make them understand that there is no Plan B. This means to emphasize that surgery, no brace, or an ankle foot orthosis-type brace, especially in the first years of life, are simply not an option.

Treatment of early recurrence of an initially well-corrected clubfoot is considerably easy and not different than initial Ponseti casting. Usually, two to three casts are enough to again achieve abduction of the calcaneus from underneath the talus. If dorsiflexion is less than 10°, a repeat percutaneous tendo Achilles tenotomy is performed.

In the same way recurrent residual clubfeet or "atypical" clubfeet treated elsewhere are approached. However, casting is made more difficult by iatrogenic problems, such as a very high rising calcaneus caused by cast slipping, massive cavus, shortening of the first ray, and frontal midfoot break, which is often combined in feet described as atypical. Additionally, rocker-bottom deformity (sagittal midfoot break) and skin defects/ulcerations from the brace/casts is encountered. In those cases, a long experience with Ponseti casting is essential to being able to correct the foot well enough to be suitable for bracing. The shortening of the first ray usually corrects well with sufficient casting focusing on stretching out the planter surface and applying the first cast in mild supination. Residual cavus usually corrects through casting and bracing and later after walking-age with weight bearing.

An important factor in treatment of recurrence is detection and diagnosis of recurrence. This emphasizes the need for regular follow-up. Follow-up during the bracing period should be done at least twice per year and more frequently in families that seem to struggle with bracing (**Table 1**).

LATE RECURRENCE: A RECURRING PATTERN

Late recurrence is usually seen after the braces have been stopped, which should not be before the age of 4 to 5 years. If recurrence is seen before that age, it is usually because bracing has been stopped too early because of difficulties with bracing or

Table 1
Typical secondary treatment indications within the first 2 years of life and their respective clinical signs

Not Fully Corrected Feet/ Residual Deformity	Atypical/Complex Feet with Residual Deformity	True Early Recurrence
Limited dorsiflexion	Residual equinus	Loss of dorsiflexion
Insufficient abduction/subtalar correction	Midfoot break in the anteroposterior plane with hyperabduction in the Chopart/Lisfranc joints	Loss of abduction
Pseudocorrection/midfoot break with hindfoot still in equinus	Plantarized/pantarflexed and shortened first ray and cavus	Bracing problems as a result of the above

because of wrong treatment recommendations. Another reason for relapses in the age group 2 to 4 years is the use of other-than foot abduction braces (eg, unilateral braces, hinged braces, local traditional braces, local high-technology braces). Multiple studies have shown that braces that are not foot abduction braces are not sufficient in preventing relapse.[10,11]

Early signs of relapse are usually supination and adduction in the gait pattern, in the beginning most noticeable during swing phase in the gait cycle. In a three-dimensional (3D) gait analysis of clubfoot treated with the Ponseti method supination and adduction was found in most children to a certain extent, in many subclinical only detected by 3D gait analysis.[12] It seems that there are two common pathways or reasons for this supination and adduction: one poor peroneal muscle/evertor activity and the other loss of dorsiflexion. The weakness and fibrosis of the calf muscles seem to include to some extent the peroneal muscles. Muscle imbalance has been reported in 66% of idiopathic clubfoot based on pathologic electrophysiologic findings[13] and poor evertor muscle activity was found to be associated with recurrence.[14,15] Weakness of the evertor muscles leads to a strong tibialis anterior muscle and thereby to supination and adduction. This is clinically detected and seen clearly when asking the child to stand on the heel or asking them to actively dorsiflex against resistance in sitting position. However, in many children supination and adduction is triggered by loss of dorsiflexion. Shortening of the soleus muscle leads to supination and adduction. One of the reasons is that the eversion power of the peroneal muscles is stronger when the foot is in more dorsiflexion. If active dorsiflexion decreases, the power of the evertor muscles also decreases. A second reason is the biomechanics of the subtalar joint, which makes the calcaneus move in a complex patter: while the calcaneus dorsiflexes, it abducts and everts; less dorsiflexion mean less eversion.[16]

Loss of dorsiflexion can result from stopping the brace or insufficient time in brace per night. After the brace has been stopped dorsiflexion can decline during growth spurts. The fibrotic muscles and tendons found in clubfoot can grow and stretch less than normal muscle. Therefore, a regular stretching regime should be recommended when the brace is stopped or at least when the patient is old enough to perform active stretching of the calf muscles.

Another reason for loss of dorsiflexion, sometimes seen around the age of 3 to 4 years, is a loss of flexibility in the midfoot, which can unmask a rocker-bottom deformity/pseudocorrection. This emphasizes the importance of the percutaneous Achilles tendon tenotomy in completing the correction and preventing rocker-bottom deformity/pseudocorrection.[17]

TREATMENT OF LATE RECURRENCE

Detailed Examination: Not all Recurrent Clubfeet Are the Same

A thorough clinical assessment is necessary to decide which treatment steps and surgical procedures are necessary. Clinical examination must include measurement of passive and active dorsiflexion with the patient lying on the examination table with the knee extended. The use of a small wooden board/block as used to evaluate leg length discrepancy and a goniometer allows for reproducible measurements. Additionally, the flexibility of the subtalar joint and the amount of abduction and eversion possible must be evaluated. Midfoot deformity, such as cavus, or midfoot hypermobility needs to be assessed.

Femoral torsion and tibial torsion can largely influence the gait pattern and the torsional profile should be assessed clinically.[18] Decreased tibial torsion as the reason for in-toeing and reduced foot progression angle is rare in clubfoot. At the same time assessment of tibial torsion is more difficult in cases where the fibula has moved more posterior as a result of treatment.[19] In those cases tibial torsion can seem normal or even excessive while the flexion extension axis in the ankle joint is in fact reduced. This is assessed by MRI where scans are performed at the level of femoral head and neck, distal femur, proximal tibia, and distal tibia, and finally overlapped to measure torsion. Careful evaluation of the distal tibia versus ankle mortice and position of the talar dome must be performed to find the right axes to measure torsion. Note that the talar neck is deviated medial, so only the first cuts of the talar dome, which can be small because of talar flattening (flat-top talus), should be assessed.

Finally gait analysis must be performed. Although 3D gait analysis is helpful to assess even subtle changes, especially when including a foot model,[12] clinical assessment is sufficient in most cases. Another enlightening option is to use the slow-motion video function of a smartphone. With good knowledge of gait analysis, the slow-motion video is used to define heel position at initial contact, detect initial contact at the lateral midfoot in more severe recurrence, the amount of adduction and supination during swing, possible hyperextension of the knee joint at the end of the stance phase to compensate loss of dorsiflexion, and of course foot progression angle. Looking at reduced foot progression angle the position of the knees should be noted. If the knees are externally rotated it might be a sign of compensation of foot adduction; if the knees are turned in it might be the result of increased femoral antetorsion, which might explain decreased foot progression angle in the presence of a well corrected and well-balanced clubfoot.

Casting

If the subtalar joint is not well corrected and flexible with decreased eversion and abduction casting is necessary before any other steps are performed independent of the age of the child and has been shown to be effective to treat recurrence even as a stand-alone procedure.[20] In cases without any previous open surgery two to three casts are usually sufficient to achieve subtalar correction and abduction. If prior open joint surgery was performed or in rigid cases it might take up to four to six casts to achieve correction.[21] Generally, above the knee casts are recommended. However, in severe recurrence needing more casting the first casts can be applied also as molded below-the-knee casts and still achieve good correction. For the last or last two casts the author prefers above-the-knee casts to achieve full abduction and stretching of the medial structures.

Achilles Lengthening

If dorsiflexion is less than 5° to 10° an Achilles tendon lengthening needs to be included into the treatment plan, more readily if a tibialis anterior tendon transfer is planned. If there is clinical or radiologic evidence for a rocker-bottom deformity with the calcaneus in equinus and much of the dorsflexion resulting from the midfoot deformity/midfoot motion, Achilles tendon lengthening can be necessary in feet with clinical dorsiflexion well greater than 10°.

The author prefers a percutaneous three step-cut Hoke Achilles tendon lengthening.[22] Although there is a concern that a percutaneous Achilles lengthening might not achieve sufficient correction in the presence of scarring from previous percutaneous Achilles tendon tenotomy,[23] other authors found that the addition of posterior capsulotomy to Achilles tenotomy does not improve dorsiflexion.[24]

Open Achilles tendon lengthening does not lengthen the tendon more compared with percutaneous lengthening. Of course, adhesions cannot be addressed in a percutaneous technique. Nevertheless, the author believes in Ponseti's credo: "the scar is the disease." Releasing all the soft tissues around the Achilles tendon might improve dorsiflexion during surgery, but a decrease of dorsiflexion is usually found in follow-up because of scarring and new adhesions. This additional scar and adhesions will not grow and stretch during the growth spurts to come and will again limit and decrease dorsiflexion. The same seems to be true for adding a capsulotomy, which might increase dorsiflexion especially during surgery even in the presence of a flat top talus. However, this dorsiflexion again usually does not pertain over time.

The author presented unpublished preliminary data on the effect of a percutaneous three step-cut Hoke Achilles tendon lengthening on dorsiflexion in recurrent clubfoot during the "Ponseti @ 20" Precourse of the 29th Annual Baltimore Limb Deformity Course in 2019. A total of 41 patients with 60 clubfeet, only five initially treated and followed in the authors institution, were evaluated. All had undergone previous casting and percutaneous tendo Achilles tenotomy, seven feet had additional previous posteromedial release, and two feet previous open tendo Achilles lengthening. At a mean age of 5.6 years all feet had a tibialis anterior tendon transfer and a percutaneous three step-cut Hoke Achilles tendon lengthening with 23 feet having additional percutaneous plantar fasciotomy and 16 feet casting before surgery. The passive dorsiflexion was measured supine with knee extended with wooden board and handheld goniometer preoperatively and minimum and 3 to 15 months after the procedure. Dorsiflexion increased from preoperative average of 7° (−15° to 18°) to a postoperative average of 22° (14°–30°) with an increase of 15° on the average (4°–30°). Even feet with a preoperative dorsiflexion of 5° or less ($n = 18$) increased from an average of 0° (−15° to 5°) to a postoperative average dorsiflexion of 19° (14°–25°). These data confirmed the clinical experience that percutaneous three step-cut Hoke Achilles tendon lengthening is sufficient to correct loss of dorsiflexion in recurrent clubfoot.

The percutaneous three step-cut Hoke Achilles tendon lengthening is a technically simple procedure; however, it needs to be done carefully to avoid injury to the medial neurovascular bundle or the peroneal artery; this is especially true if a previous open Achilles lengthening or other open surgery has been performed. The calcaneus must be well palpated, and the most distal cut should be marked. It should be as distal as possible at the same time making sure not to cut into the cartilaginous attachment of the tendon. In the second step the most proximal cut is marked where the tendon can still be felt well, before turning into the aponeurosis. The third cut is marked between those prior two cuts (**Figs. 1** and **2**). Cutting is performed from distal to proximal in half medial half lateral and again half medial direction (**Fig. 3**). Especially if there was no prior open surgery to the Achilles tendon a marked increase of dorsiflexion is felt with the tendon being structurally intact, which is well palpated (**Fig. 4**). Sometimes flat top talus might limit excessive dorsiflexion. In those cases, the tension of the tendon is felt with the foot in maximum dorsiflexion. With only limited increase of

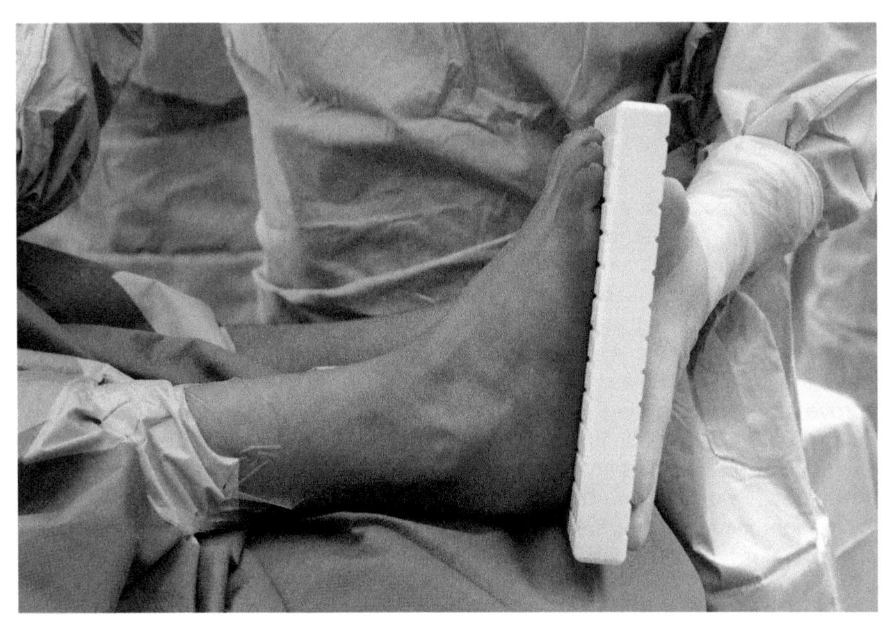

Fig. 1. Clubfoot recurrence with approximately 5° of equinus.

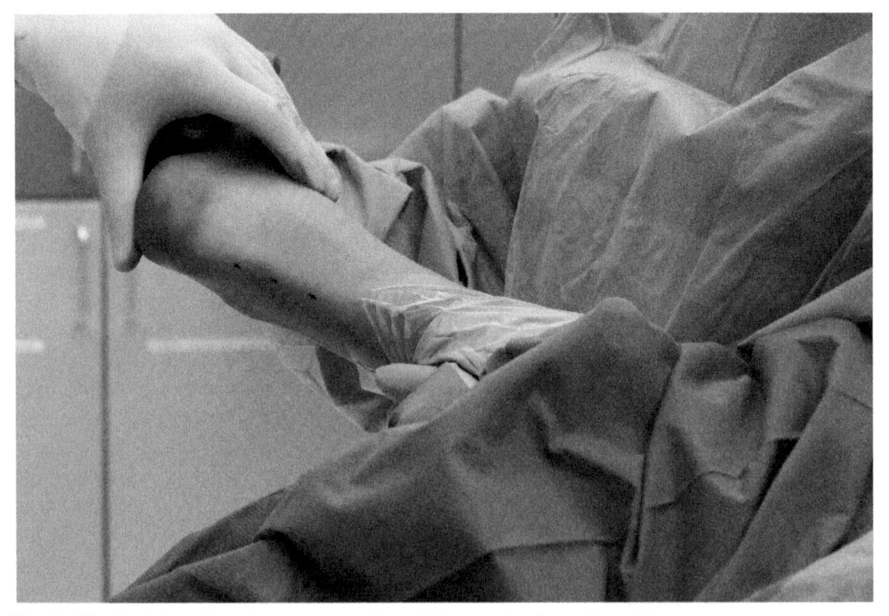

Fig. 2. The incisions for the step-cuts should be marked on the skin.

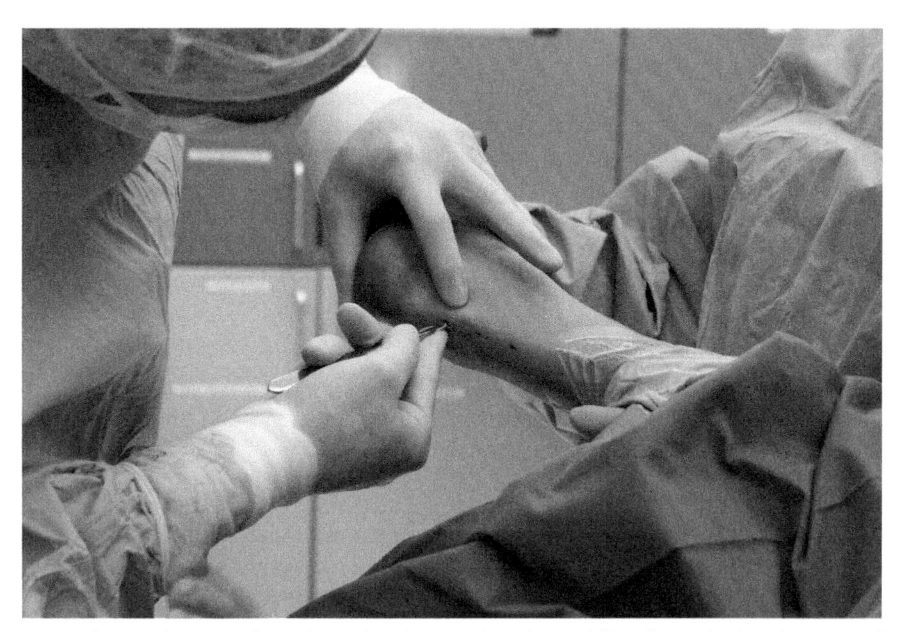

Fig. 3. The tendon must be palpated and pierced in the middle. The scalpel is then turned, and half of the tendon is cut carefully.

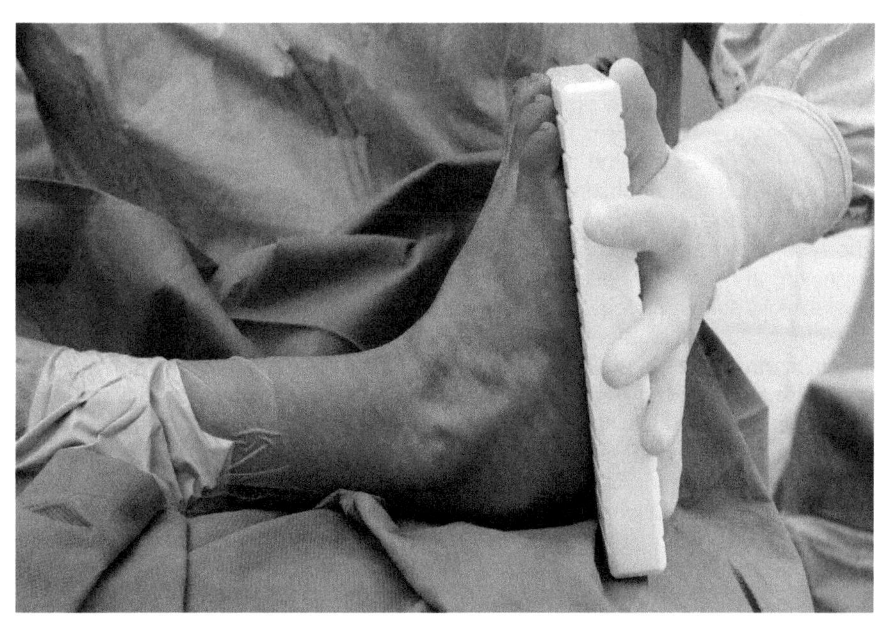

Fig. 4. After Hoke Achilles tendon lengthening dorsiflexion has increased to approximately 8°. Further dorsiflexion is expected after the postoperative cast, when the soft tissue and capsule have been stretched further.

dorsiflexion at the time of the procedure, when tightness of the capsule might be suspected, dorsiflexion increases in the time in the cast and even after cast removal through stretching and/or bracing. Especially if the preoperative dorsiflexion was around 0 to equinus and in children younger than the age of 8 years temporary bracing after Achilles lengthening seems to further improve and keep the dorsiflexion. An ankle foot orthosis or an abduction dorsiflexion mechanism brace is used. There is a concern of increasing talar flattening using abduction dorsiflexion mechanism braces or other dynamic braces or ankle foot orthosis.[25] Although, clear evidence to back this observation is missing, this risk should be considered, especially in the age group younger than 4 years of age.

Tibialis Anterior Tendon Transfer

Tibialis anterior tendon transfer is an important part of the Ponseti method and is a powerful tool to correct recurrence with good mid-term[26–28] and long-term[29] results reported. A study using 3D gait analysis including the Oxford foot model showed normalization of the main components of clubfoot recurrence after tibialis anterior tendon transfer in a cohort treated with the Ponseti method.[30] It has been shown that relapse increases with age[3] and with it the rate of tibialis anterior tendon transfer, which also has been shown to increase and peak at age 4 to 6 years.[31] Despite good long-term results[29] recurrence after tibialis anterior tendon transfer has been reported, with young age[32] and neuromuscular deficits[33] being risk factors for a second recurrence.

The indication for tibialis anterior tendon transfer is increased supination and adduction in gait. Although it is sometimes difficult and debatable how much supination and/or adduction can be accepted, heel varus at initial contact is a clear marker that should prompt action. Again, limited dorsiflexion must be taken into consideration. Some clubfeet might improve the adduction- and supination-gait pattern through tendo Achilles lengthening only. However, in the author's experience this is a small group and it seems difficult to take the risk of needing to add a tibialis anterior tendon transfer in a second step, if Achilles lengthening turns out not to be enough.

A concern in tibialis anterior tendon transfer is the risk of overcorrection. Overcorrection may occur in three scenarios. First, the risk of overcorrection but also the risk of a second recurrence is higher when tibialis anterior tendon transfer is done at a very young age. Before the age of 3 to 4 years it is usually sufficient to recast and go back to foot abduction bracing. Rarely, when the brace acceptance is already bad and the brace has not been used for a long time, it seems unrealistic and fruitless to hope for good brace compliance, although a cast for 2 to 3 weeks is sometimes convincing. In those few cases an anterior tibialis tendon transfer before the age of 4 years might still be necessary. The second group of clubfeet that are more prone to overcorrection are clubfeet that had previous open joint surgery or postero-medial release. In those feet the posterior tibial tendon might have been overlengthened during surgery and a full transfer of the tibialis anterior tendon might result in flat foot position. The third group of feet that need to be approached carefully, are clubfeet presenting a flexible midfoot. Although this group has been found to have less risk of recurrence,[34] they might still present with supination and adduction. However, a full transfer might again lead to overcorrection and flat foot. In these three cases scenarios the indication for a full transfer must be made cautiously, or in rare cases, a split tibialis anterior tendon transfer might be the better option (**Table 2**).

Tibialis Anterior Tendon Transfer: Surgical Technique

Tibialis anterior tendon transfer is done in supine position on a radiolucent table without a tourniquet. The use of a tourniquet might increase swelling and

Table 2
Treatment options for late recurrence and their typical indications

Casting	Achilles Lengthening	Tibialis Anterior Tendon Transfer
Insufficient abduction/ subtalar correction	Dorsiflexion <5°	Adduction/supination in walking
Adduction/supination in walking	Dorsiflexion <10° if tibialis anterior tendon transfer is performed simultaneously	Heel varus at initial contact
Bracing problems as a result of the above	Pseudocorrection/midfoot-break with hindfoot equinus	Supination with heel stand

postoperative pain and possible problems in the cast. A 1.5- to 2-cm incision is made on the dorsal medial side of the foot after palpating the tibialis anterior tendon. The tendon sheet is opened, and the tendon should be followed distally to its insertion. Meticulous hemostasis is performed throughout the surgery. I usually use the rectangle clamp to lift off the tendon and detach it from the origin using the scalpel (**Fig. 5**). Care must be taken not to cut into the cartilage at the insertion and not to injure the growth plate of the first metatarsal. A holding suture (Vicryl 0) is used at that point to secure the tendon and free the tendon from possible adhesions to proximal, taking care not to split the extensor retinaculum. Sometimes and especially in severe or syndromic cases the tendon might show a lot of adhesions to the tendon sheet and/or to the extensor digitorum longus, which must be cut carefully. Contrary to the originally described technique, which involves creating a subcutaneous tunnel to lateral for

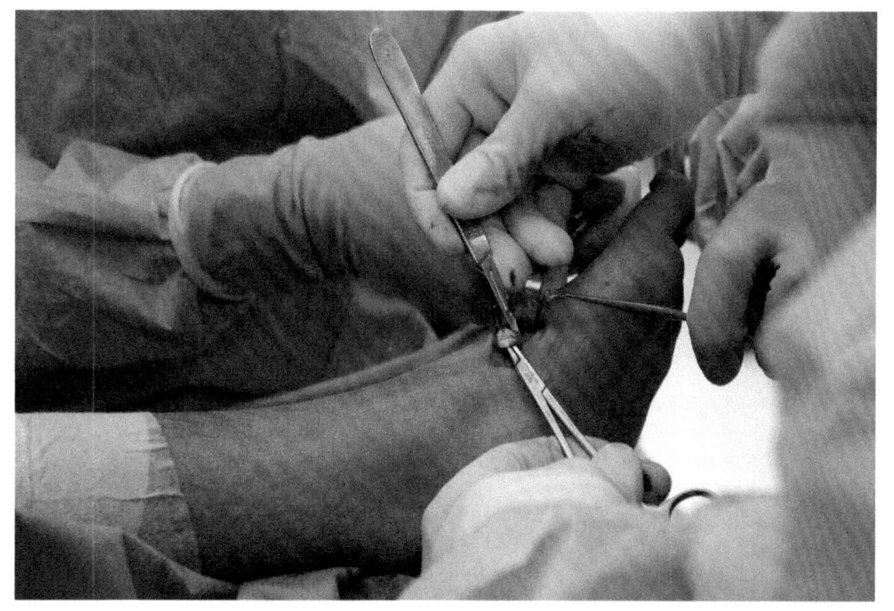

Fig. 5. The tendon is elevated with a small rectangle clamp and detached as distal as possible.

passing the tendon to the new position, a three-incision anterior tibial tendon transfer, routed proximally, is preferred by the author. Therefore, another 1.5-cm incision proximal to the ankle joint and proximal to the retinaculum is done. The tendon sheet is incised, and the tendon is pulled from distal to proximal (**Fig. 6**). At that point, the tendon is augmented with an anchoring suture (Vicryl 0 or 1) that is achieved quickly using a whip-stitch technique[35] with a straight Keith needle (Aspen Surgical Products, Caledonia, MI) (**Fig. 7**). The tendon diameter is measured with a 0.5-mm incremental sizing block (Arthrex, Naples, FL).

At that point, a fluoroscopy is used to place a 1.6-mm Kirschner wire into the middle of the lateral cuneiform (**Fig. 8**). The Kirschner wire is then drilled through the bone to exit at the sole of the foot. It should be aimed toward the middle of the foot with an inclination of approximately 22° to the plantar surface in the frontal plane and 4° in the sagittal plane to minimize the risk of nerve damage.[36] The skin incision at the Kirschner wire is usually proximal to the third web space and close to the superficial peroneal nerve, which needs to be protected (**Fig. 9**). The extensor digitorum longus tendons and the extensor digitorum brevis muscle and its tendons are spread and retracted. The wire is now overdrilled with a cannulated drill equal in diameter to the diameter of the tendon (**Fig. 10**). A 4-mm drill is the right size in most cases for the age group 4 to 6 years.

Now the tendon needs to be pulled down to its new insertion. Therefore, a long tendon passer is used and is placed under the retinaculum and into the tendon sheet of the extensor tendons (**Fig. 11**). The tendon is pulled down distally and the sutures are inserted into a straight Keith needle. The Keith needle is brought down to the planter aspect and out of the sole of the foot and through a foam sponge and a suture button (Smith and Nephew, Memphis, TN). The two arms of the suture need to be

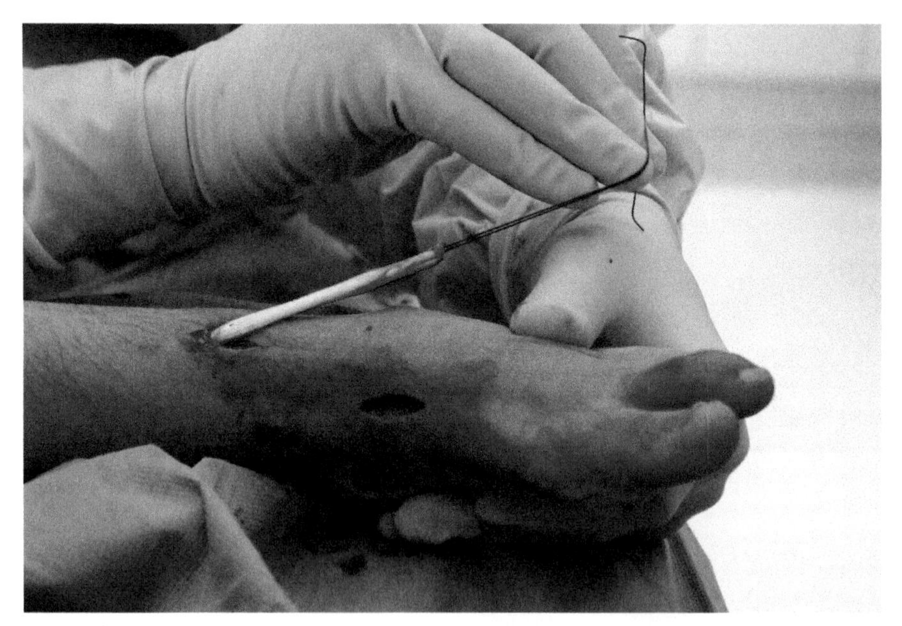

Fig. 6. After incision of the tendon sheet, the tendon is luxated with a rectangle clamp. If all adhesions were separated well from the tendon, the tendon is pulled from distal to proximal without major resistance.

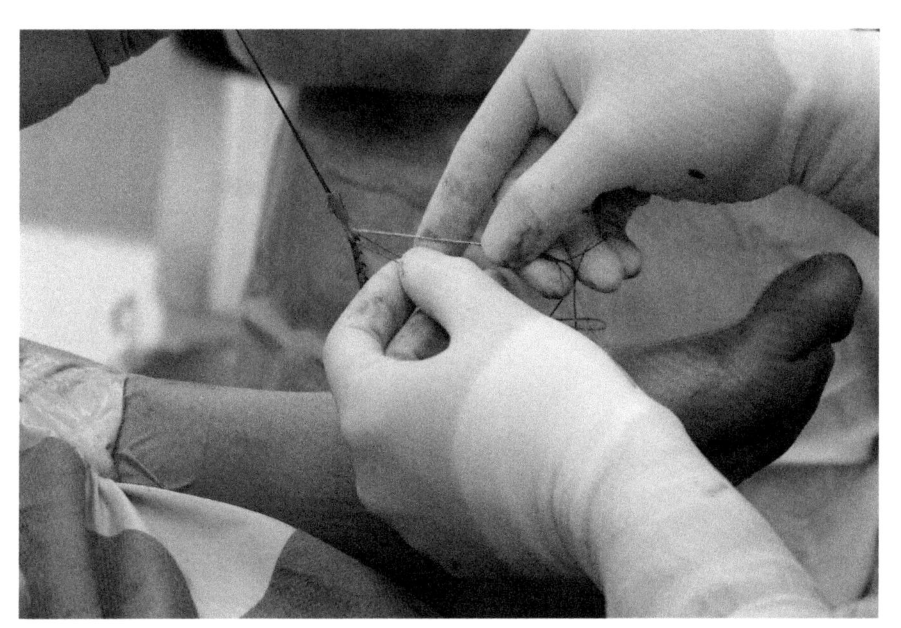

Fig. 7. The tendon is held with a small mosquito clamp, a special tendon clamp, or a holding suture while the whip-stitch suture is applied. Care should be taken that the stiches are closer at the end of the tendon, so that the tendon does not fan out when being inserted into the drill tunnel.

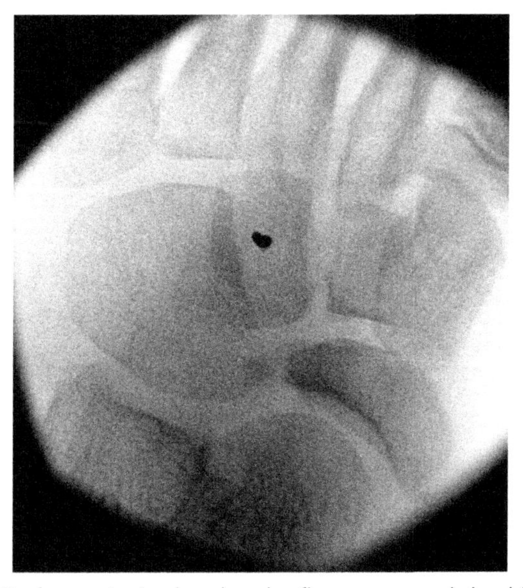

Fig. 8. A 1.6-mm Kirschner wire is placed under fluoroscopy and should be exactly in the middle of the ossific nucleus of the lateral cuneiform bone.

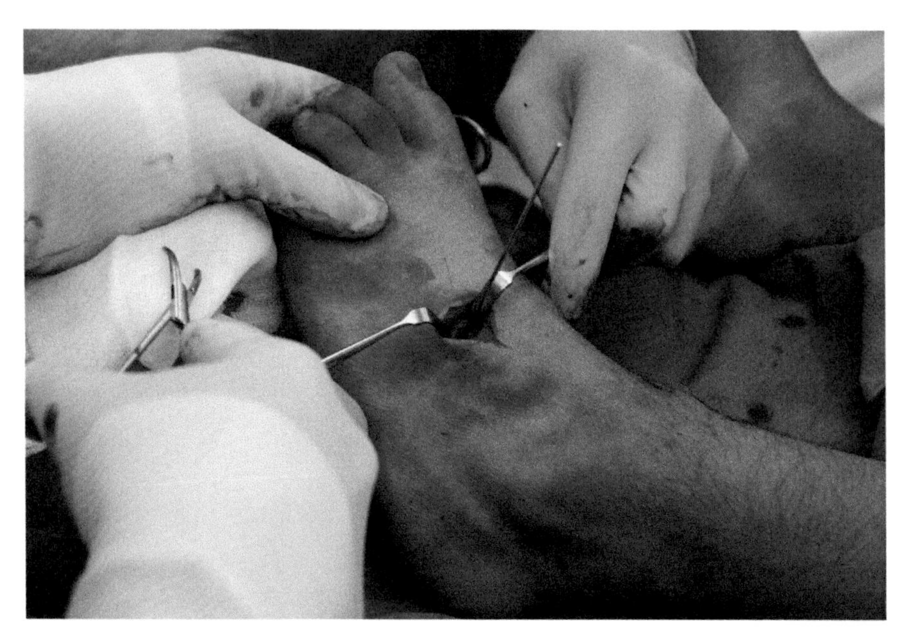

Fig. 9. The fascia of the extensor tendons is incised and the fibers of the short muscles of the foot are retracted.

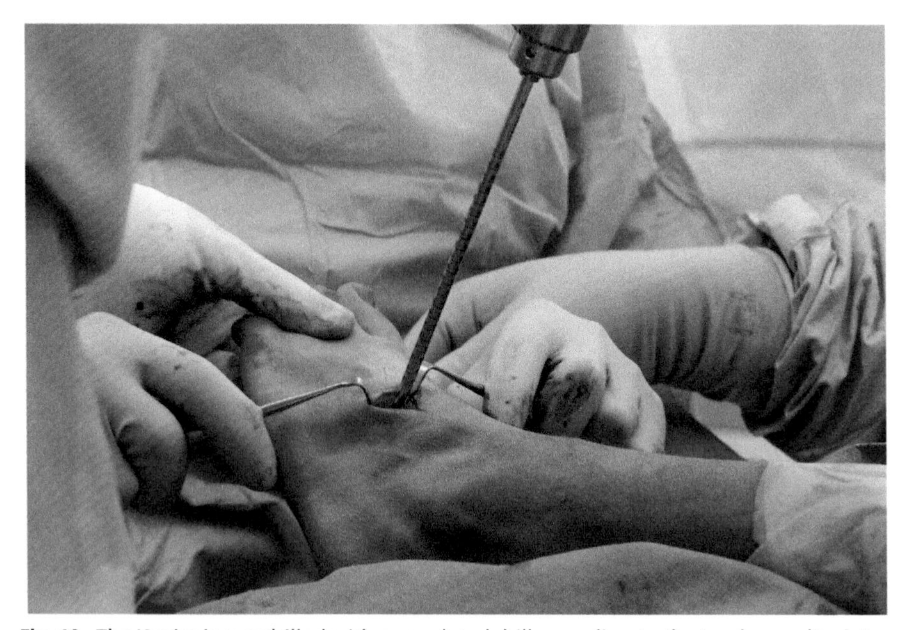

Fig. 10. The K-wire is overdrilled with a canulated drill according to the tendon and/or interference screw diameter.

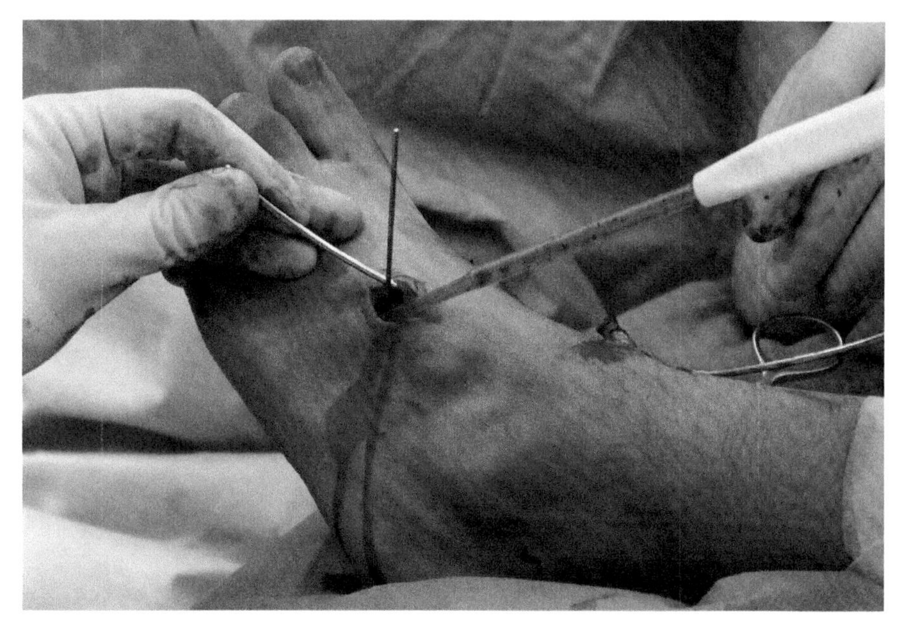

Fig. 11. The tendon passer is used and is guided carefully while rotating it, to stay under the retinaculum and within the tendon sheet.

pulled through separately. With the tendon mildly tensioned and the foot in neutral position the sutures are tied over the suture fixation button (**Fig. 12**).

The author prefers to add a bioresorbable interference screw (Arthrex Bio-Composite tenodesis screw; Arthrex) as an additional fixation of the tendon (**Fig. 13**). The interference screw is inserted with a gentle pull on the already securely tied plantar fixation to reduce the pressure of the suture button on the skin.

After irrigation and skin closure a soft dressing is applied in thin layers ensuring that there are no folds or wrinkles and fixed with a sterile cotton. A well-molded above-the-knee cast in maximum dorsiflexion and abduction is applied after surgery (**Fig. 14**).

If there is no swelling and pain the first cast change is performed only 4 weeks after surgery. At that time the plantar sutures, sponge, and suture button are removed, and a below-the-knee walking cast is applied for another 2 weeks. Walking is allowed and

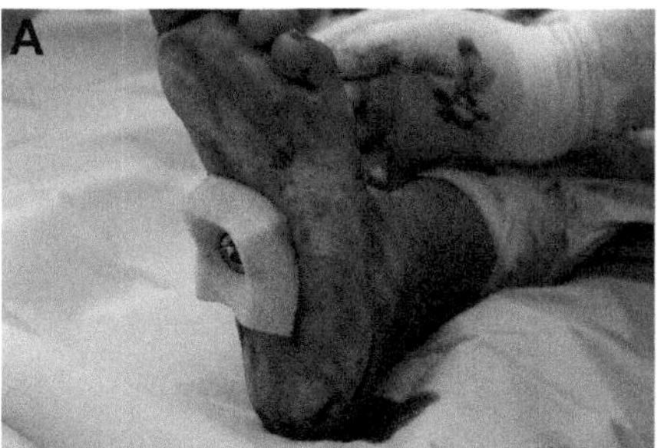

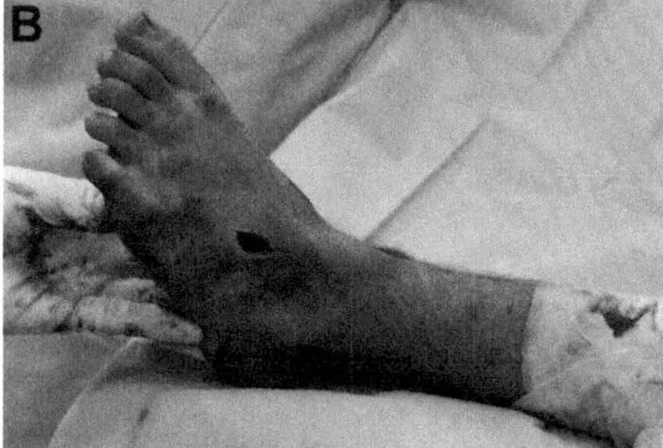

Fig. 12. (*A, B*): The sutures are tied with the foot in a corrected position. The foot should rest in neutral after the tendon is secured. Fixation in dorsiflexion limits plantarflexion after cast removal and should be avoided.

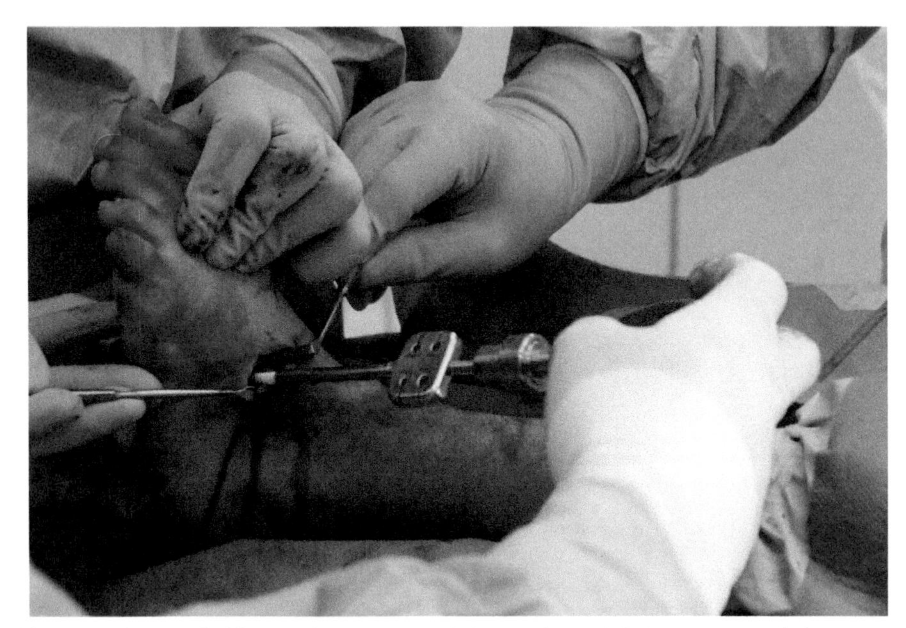

Fig. 13. A bioresorbable interference screw is inserted to minimize pressure of the suture button on the skin and to allow early removal of the plantar sutures.

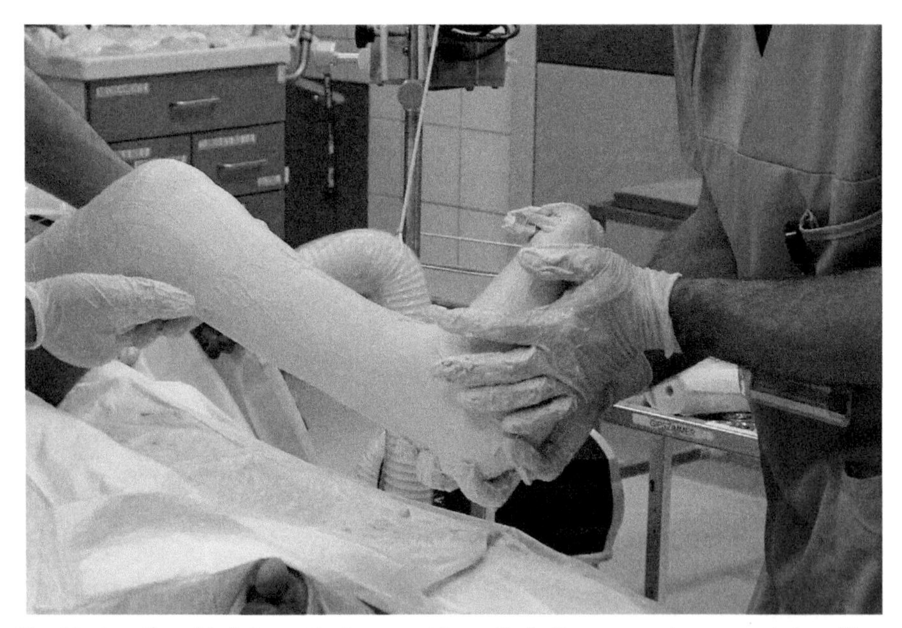

Fig. 14. A well-molded above-the-knee cast is applied after surgery in a corrected position.

encouraged in this cast. If a nighttime brace (ankle foot orthosis or nighttime single abduction dorsiflexion mechanism with abduction dorsiflexion mechanism sandal [MD Orthopedics, Inc, Wayland, IA]) is recommended brace measurements should be done during this cast change.

The described technique of tibialis anterior tendon transfer does deviate from the technique originally described by Ponseti.[16] The third cut above the extensor retinaculum was a tradition at my department and no need was felt to change it. The tendon might have a better angle when the rerouting starts more proximally and there might be less bow-stringing subcutaneously when the tendon runs within the extensor tendon sheet. Knutsen and coworkers[37] looked at three different techniques of routing the tendon in cadaveric specimen and found the three-incision whole transfer provided the most forefoot pronation. This might make the full transfer using three incisions the potentially most powerful, but also the most prone to overcorrection.

A split transfer might be indicated in rare cases in the previously mentioned scenarios to avoid overcorrection. In a biomechanical study the ideal insertion for split tibialis anterior tendon transfer was found at the fourth metatarsal axis,[38] which corresponds to the cuboid bone. If a split transfer is performed a similar technique can be used. Because the cuboid has an oblique bone surface the Kirschner-wire and drill hole can still be aimed at the middle of the foot.

The use of absorbable interference screws for tibialis anterior tendon transfer was first reported in 2004.[39] Herzenberg combined the traditional technique of fixation over a suture button with the fixation using an interference screw.[35] This has the advantage of minimizing plantar pressure of the suture button and thereby pressure sores, although still providing safe fixation without the risk of a pull out of the tendon. Interference screw fixation only would include the risk of loss of fixation especially in the age group 4 to 5 years where the ossific nucleus is still weak and/or in osteopenic bone after longer casting. In children age 2 to 3 years or if the ossific nucleus in the

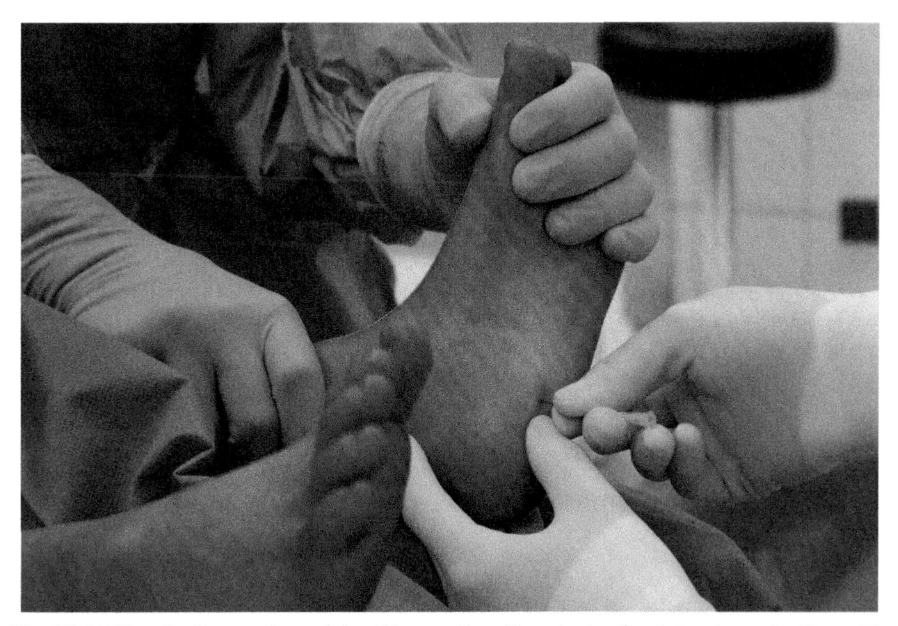

Fig. 15. With palpation and careful cutting motions the plantar fascia is released with an 18-gauge needle.

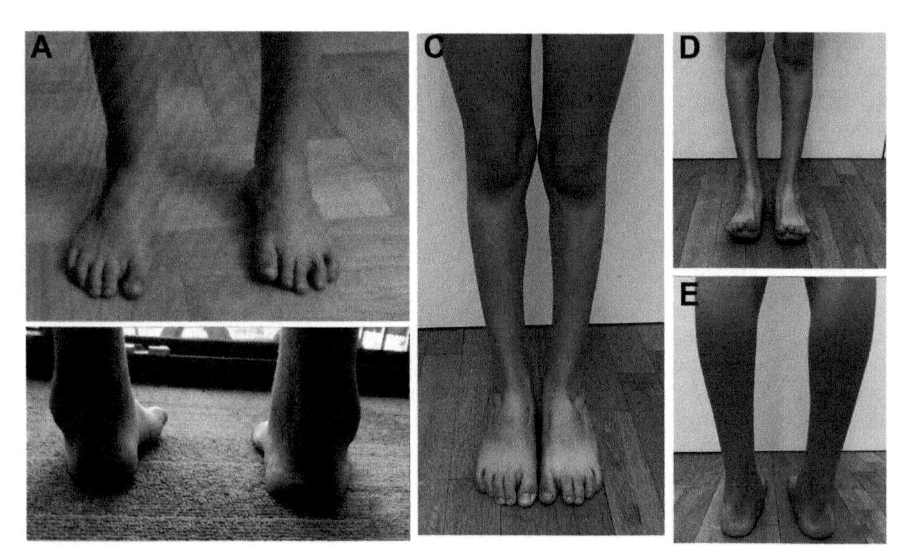

Fig. 16. This young girl was treated elsewhere with casting and a percutaneous tendo Achilles tenotomy and at the age of 3.5 years an open tendo Achilles lengthening and capsulotomy. However, another relapse developed (*A*) and she presented at the age of 5.5 years with heel varus and 0° of dorsiflexion on the left and 8° of dorsiflexion on the right (*B*). In walking there was severe adduction and supination on the left, no heel contact, and heel varus. The right side showed adduction and supination, heel varus during swing phase, but a neutral heel at initial contact. A percutaneous plantar fasciotomy, a three step-cut Hoke Achilles tendon lengthening, and a tibialis anterior tendon transfer were performed on both feet. (*C–E*) Follow-up 11 months after surgery showed a dorsiflexion of 23° on the left and 25° on the right side and a good muscle balance and heel position.

radiograph is too small interference screw fixation should be avoided. Whatever form of fixation is preferred, it should always include a drill hole and pull-out sutures to put the tendon in the right tension to bring the foot in neutral to mild plantar flexion after surgery.[40]

ADDITIONAL PROCEDURES

In case of additional cavus deformity a percutaneous planter fasciotomy is performed as the first step in the surgery using an 18-gauge needle (**Fig. 15**). Care must be taken not to go too deep because this might injure the medial planter nerve. In children older than the age of 6 to 7 years presenting with fixed midfoot adduction a cuboid closing wedge osteotomy might be added and is combined with a cuneiform medial opening wedge osteotomy if the adduction is more severe.[41] The piece of bone taken from the cuboid is inserted as a wedge at the medial cuneiform.

In patients showing adduction of the hallux during gait an abductor hallucis stripping might be added. Therefore, a 1-cm incision is performed just proximal to the prominence formed by the first metatarsal head. With a small mosquito clamp the abductor hallucis tendon is undermined, exposed, and cut.

SUMMARY

The described treatment regime covers about 95% of cases of recurrent congenital clubfoot in the authors experience (**Fig. 16**). Only cases with severe recurrent clubfoot after usually multiple previous surgeries and previously treated clubfoot in an adolescent age group might need more invasive procedures.[42] The conclusion of all papers or reviews on recurrence of clubfoot and its treatment must be the emphasis on preventing recurrence and residual deformity. This is achieved by strict adherence to the Ponseti method, ensuring and enforcing brace compliance, frequent follow-up, and early treatment of recurrence. Strict adherence to the Ponseti method does not stand in contrast to the knowledge gained, and the lessons learned in the last 15 to 20 years. We know now how to deal with the atypical/complex clubfoot and its iatrogenic relative, we know the prognostic value of the extensor function of the fourth and fifth toe after birth and the evertor muscle strength later on, we know that some feet do not recur even if the braces are stopped early and which feet and which families need closer attention, and we have been proven that recurrent and even neglected clubfoot is treated successfully using the Ponseti method. Finally, we have come to realize that the Ponseti method is not a casting technique for newborn clubfoot but a method to treat clubfoot and to prevent and treat relapse.

CLINICS CARE POINTS

- Prevent recurrence by regular follow-up and counseling.
- Check the brace at every visit and observe the parent applying it. There might be room for improvement.
- If you see recurrence, treat it. Loss of dorsiflexion and abduction after periods of bracing problems can easily be corrected with two to three casts and back to braces.
- Heel varus at initial contact in the gait cycle cries for attention. Casting or a tibialis anterior tendon transfer needs to be considered.
- Consider using the slow-motion video function of a phone device if you have no access to a gait laboratory.
- If the subtalar joint is not corrected (ie, not enough abduction of the calcaneus from underneath the talus) casting needs to be done before an Achilles tenotomy/lengthening or tendon transfer is performed.
- In tibialis anterior tendon transfer the tendon should be fixated under mild tension letting the foot rest near neutral, but not in dorsiflexion.
- Encourage starting a home stretching regime at the end of bracing.

DISCLOSURE

Consultant Smith and Nephew Europe. Consultant Nuvasive Inc.

REFERENCE

1. Zionts LE, Sangiorgio SN, Ebramzadeh E, et al. The current management of idiopathic clubfoot revisited: results of a survey of the POSNA membership. J Pediatr Orthop 2012;32(5):515–20.
2. Shabtai L, Specht SC, Herzenberg JE. Worldwide spread of the Ponseti method for clubfoot. World J Orthop 2014;5(5):585–90.
3. Sangiorgio SN, Ebramzadeh E, Morgan RD, et al. The timing and relevance of relapsed deformity in patients with idiopathic clubfoot. J Am Acad Orthop Surg 2017;25(7):536–45.
4. Siebert MJ, Karacz CM, Richards BS. Successful Ponseti-treated clubfeet at age 2 years: what is the rate of surgical intervention after this? J Pediatr Orthop 2020;40(10):597–603.

5. Hosseinzadeh P, Kiebzak GM, Dolan L, et al. Management of clubfoot relapses with the Ponseti method: results of a survey of the POSNA members. J Pediatr Orthop 2019;39(1):38–41.
6. Ponseti IV, Zhivkov M, Davis N, et al. Treatment of the complex idiopathic clubfoot. Clin Orthop Relat Res 2006;451:171–6.
7. Matar HE, Beirne P, Bruce CE, et al. Treatment of complex idiopathic clubfoot using the modified Ponseti method: up to 11 years follow-up. J Pediatr Orthop B 2017;26(2):137–42.
8. Dragoni M, Gabrielli A, Farsetti P, et al. Complex iatrogenic clubfoot: is it a real entity? J Pediatr Orthop B 2018;27(5):428–34.
9. Zionts LE, Dietz FR. Bracing following correction of idiopathic clubfoot using the Ponseti method. J Am Acad Orthop Surg 2010;18(8):486–93.
10. George HL, Unnikrishnan PN, Garg NK, et al. Unilateral foot abduction orthosis: is it a substitute for Denis Browne boots following Ponseti technique? J Pediatr Orthop B 2011;20(1):22–5.
11. Janicki JA, Wright JG, Weir S, et al. A comparison of ankle foot orthoses with foot abduction orthoses to prevent recurrence following correction of idiopathic clubfoot by the Ponseti method. J Bone Joint Surg Br 2011;93(5):700–4.
12. Mindler GT, Kranzl A, Lipkowski CA, et al. Results of gait analysis including the Oxford foot model in children with clubfoot treated with the Ponseti method. J Bone Joint Surg Am 2014;96(19):1593–9.
13. Feldbrin Z, Gilai AN, Ezra E, et al. Muscle imbalance in the aetiology of idiopathic club foot. An electromyographic study. J Bone Joint Surg Br 1995;77(4):596–601.
14. Gelfer Y, Dunkley M, Jackson D, et al. Evertor muscle activity as a predictor of the mid-term outcome following treatment of the idiopathic and non-idiopathic clubfoot. Bone Joint J 2014;96-B(9):1264–8.
15. Little Z, Yeo A, Gelfer Y. Poor evertor muscle activity is a predictor of recurrence in idiopathic clubfoot treated by the Ponseti method: a prospective longitudinal study with a 5-year follow-up. J Pediatr Orthop 2019;39(6):e467–71.
16. Ponseti IV. Congenital clubfoot: fundamentals of treatment. New York: Oxford University Press; 1996. p. p41, 84.
17. Radler C, Manner HM, Suda R, et al. Radiographic evaluation of idiopathic clubfeet undergoing Ponseti treatment. J Bone Joint Surg Am 2007;89(6):1177–83.
18. Staheli LT, Corbett M, Wyss C, et al. Lower-extremity rotational problems in children. Normal values to guide management. J Bone Joint Surg Am 1985;67(1): 39–47.
19. Farsetti P, De Maio F, Russolillo L, et al. CT study on the effect of different treatment protocols for clubfoot pathology. Clin Orthop Relat Res 2009;467(5):1243–9.
20. van Praag VM, Lysenko M, Harvey B, et al. Casting is effective for recurrence following Ponseti treatment of clubfoot. J Bone Joint Surg Am 2018;100(12): 1001–8.
21. Nogueira MP, Ey Batlle AM, Alves CG. Is it possible to treat recurrent clubfoot with the Ponseti technique after posteromedial release? A preliminary study. Clin Orthop Relat Res 2009;467(5):1298–305.
22. Hoke M. An operation for stabilizing paralytic feet. J Bone Jt Surg 1921;3: 494–507.
23. Chu A, Lehman WB. Persistent clubfoot deformity following treatment by the Ponseti method. J Pediatr Orthop B 2012;21:40–6.
24. Grigoriou E, Abol Oyoun N, Kushare I, et al. Comparative results of percutaneous Achilles tenotomy to combined open Achilles tenotomy with posterior

capsulotomy in the correction of equinus deformity in congenital talipes equinovarus. Int Orthop 2015;39:721–5.
25. Sætersdal C, Fevang JM, Engesæter LB. Inferior results with unilateral compared with bilateral brace in Ponseti-treated clubfeet. J Child Orthop 2017;11(3):216–22.
26. Jeans KA, Tulchin-Francis K, Crawford L, et al. Plantar pressures following anterior tibialis tendon transfers in children with clubfoot. J Pediatr Orthop 2014;34:552–8.
27. Ezra E, Hayek S, Gilai AN, et al. Tibialis anterior tendon transfer for residual dynamic supination deformity in treated club feet. J Pediatr Orthop B 2000;9:207–11.
28. Gray K, Burns J, Little D, et al. Is tibialis anterior tendon transfer effective for recurrent clubfoot? Clin Orthop Relat Res 2014;472:750–8.
29. Holt JB, Oji DE, Yack HJ, et al. Long-term results of tibialis anterior tendon transfer for relapsed idiopathic clubfoot treated with the Ponseti method: a follow-up of thirty-seven to fifty-five years. J Bone Joint Surg Am 2015;97:47–55.
30. Mindler GT, Kranzl A, Radler C. Normalization of forefoot supination after tibialis anterior tendon transfer for dynamic clubfoot recurrence. J Pediatr Orthop 2020;40(8):418–24.
31. Zionts LE, Jew MH, Bauer KL, et al. How many patients who have a clubfoot treated using the Ponseti method are likely to undergo a tendon transfer? J Pediatr Orthop 2018;38(7):382–7.
32. Luckett MR, Hosseinzadeh P, Ashley PA, et al. Factors predictive of second recurrence in clubfeet treated by Ponseti casting. J Pediatr Orthop 2015;35:303–6.
33. Masrouha KZ, Morcuende JA. Relapse after tibialis anterior tendon transfer in idiopathic clubfoot treated by the Ponseti method. J Pediatr Orthop 2012;32:81–4.
34. Cosma DI, Corbu A, Nistor DV, et al. Joint hyperlaxity prevents relapses in clubfeet treated by Ponseti method-preliminary results. Int Orthop 2018;42(10):2437–42.
35. Jindal G, Lamm BM, Herzenberg JE. Tibialis anterior tendon transfer for relapsed clubfoot after treatment with Ponseti method. In: Agrawal RA, editor. Pandey S: step by step Management of clubfoot by Ponseti technique. 5th edition. New Dehli (India): Jaypee Brothers Medical Publishers; 2007. p. 154–72.
36. Radler C, Gourdine-Shaw MC, Herzenberg JE. Nerve structures at risk in the plantar side of the foot during anterior tibial tendon transfer: a cadaver study. J Bone Joint Surg Am 2012;94(4):349–55.
37. Knutsen AR, Avoian T, Sangiorgio SN, et al. How do different anterior tibial tendon transfer techniques influence forefoot and hindfoot motion? Clin Orthop Relat Res 2015;473(5):1737–43.
38. Hui JH, Goh JC, Lee EH. Biomechanical study of tibialis anterior tendon transfer. Clin Orthop Relat Res 1998;349:249–55.
39. Fuller DA, McCarthy JJ, Keenan MA. The use of the absorbable interference screw for a split anterior tibial tendon (SPLATT) transfer procedure. Orthopedics 2004;27(4):372–4.
40. Mosca V. Anterior tibialis tendon transfer. In: Staheli L, editor. Clubfoot: Ponseti management. 3rd edition. Global Help Publications; 2009. p. 24–5.
41. McHale KA, Lenhart MK. Treatment of residual clubfoot deformity–the "bean-shaped" foot–by opening wedge medial cuneiform osteotomy and closing wedge cuboid osteotomy. Clinical review and cadaver correlations. J Pediatr Orthop 1991;11:374–81.
42. Radler C, Mindler GT. Treatment of severe recurrent clubfoot. Foot Ankle Clin 2015;20(4):563–86.

The Foot in Cerebral Palsy

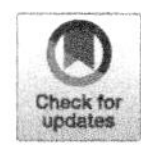

Julieanne P. Sees, DO[a], Freeman Miller, MD[b,*]

KEYWORDS

• Cerebral palsy • Planovalgus • Equinus • Equinovarus • Natural history

KEY POINTS

- The natural history for young children less than 5 years of age is for planovalgus to improve.
- Equinus contracture surgery should be conservative, carefully avoiding overlengthening.
- Flexible moderate-severity planovalgus correction surgery in adolescence provides good long-term correction when all concomitant deformities are also corrected.
- Planovalgus deformities that are severe, stiff, and in patients with low functional demand have excellent long-term outcome with fusions.
- Tendon transfer for equinovarus correction should be limited to children more than 8 years old in flexible deformities.

INTRODUCTION

Cerebral palsy (CP) is the result of a static insult or deformity to the immature brain where the child may have multiple system impairments. Motor function and musculoskeletal development are usually delayed, and there may be some permanent motor impairment.[1] Motor impairment severity is best described using the Gross Motor Function Classification System (GMFCS). GMFCS I is an individual who has almost normal gait and can navigate stairs without handrails; GMGCS II has limitation in walking on uneven surfaces and needs handrails for stairs; GMFCS III requires a walking aid such as crutches or a walker; GMFCS IV uses a wheelchair for most mobility, but can walk with assistance for transfers and exercise; and GMFCS V is an obligatory wheelchair user.[2] There are more detailed aged-related gradations, but the general gradation is most widely used in orthopedic communications. The pattern of motor impairment has traditionally used the term quadriplegia to describe involvement of all 4 limbs, diplegia for predominantly lower extremity involvement, hemiplegia for ipsilateral arm and leg involvement, and triplegia for 3-limb involvement. Because these definitions often blend together, the use of unilateral involvement

[a] Department of Orthopedics, Thomas Jefferson University, 111 South 11th Street, Philadelphia, PA 19107, USA; [b] Department of Orthopedics, Nemours/Alfred I. duPont Hospital for Children, BOX 269, Wilmington, DE 19899, USA
* Corresponding author.
E-mail address: fmiller@nemours.org

Foot Ankle Clin N Am 26 (2021) 639–653
https://doi.org/10.1016/j.fcl.2021.07.002
1083-7515/21/

and bilateral involvement has gained popularity[3]; however, the problem with the blending issue has not been eliminated but only reduced to 2 groups.

Because the insult to the brain in children with CP occurs, by definition, at an early age, neurologic maturation is significantly affected, with most children who gain the ability for independent ambulation being delayed 1 to 2 years in reaching this milestone. Motor control and the evolvement of the final pattern on the child's gait often are not apparent until the child is 3 to 5 years old, and major improvement in motor function may occur in some children up to age 7 to 9 years. Because of the variation in development, natural motor control, and skeletal maturation, treating musculoskeletal problems in children with CP requires an understanding of the typical direction of deformity patterns and possible change over time. This overview of treating foot deformities in children with CP also focuses on the known natural history of foot posture maturation, as well as the specific deformities encountered. Equinus, equinovarus, planovalgus, cavovalgus, and toe deformities are specifically addressed.

NATURAL HISTORY

Neurologic maturation and motor control progresses from proximal to distal, as shown by babies having better shoulder and hip muscle control than hand and foot control. Another aspect of this normal development is that infant and toddler feet do not have a developed medial arch and tend to have a foot pressure pattern with high variation and little anatomic definition. In children with CP, the development of mature foot posture typically is not completely apparent until the child is 7 to 8 years old.[4] The most common foot posture for children when initiating gait is ankle equinus, which is also a natural posture for some neurologically normal children. In children with CP, this equinus posture is also driven by increasing spasticity, commonly affecting the plantar flexors. This spasticity reaches its peak between 3 and 5 years of age and then slowly decreases through adolescence.[5,6] The equinus may be associated with a varus foot, which is most common in unilateral CP. The varus component tends to be very flexible and reduces when the equinus is reduced. It is important not to aggressively surgically treat this varus component before adolescence, especially in children with bilateral involvement, because the natural history is most commonly for the foot to fall into planovalgus during adolescence. When beginning to walk, some children have a severe collapse of the feet into planovalgus, but as spasticity increases up to age 5 years and better motor control develops, the planovalgus may completely resolve and, occasionally, the same child develops a varus foot deformity[4] (**Fig. 1**, case 1). A common associated malalignment in young children is internal tibial torsion, which may contribute to instability caused by equinus and foot varus. The natural history is for internal tibial torsion to correct with growth; however, the severity at times requires corrective surgery. After surgery, the tendency is for the tibia to continue to grow into external torsion, so it is important not to overcorrect the internal tibial torsion.[7] Some children do have external tibial torsion; however, just like internal tibial torsion, the tendency with growth in immature children is for the tibia to go into further external torsion. This deformity rarely self-corrects, even in young children.[8] To summarize the important natural history of feet in children with CP, equinus spasticity usually peaks at around age 5 years, often with significant contractures that are impairing function by age 5 to 8 years. The spasticity improves, but the contractures do not, and tend to get worse if untreated. Planovalgus foot deformities are common in young children less than age 5 years and these have a very unpredictable outcome, with most improving toward a normal foot posture up to age 5 to 7 years, then plateauing, and becoming more severe again during adolescent growth and weight gain.[9] Varus foot deformities

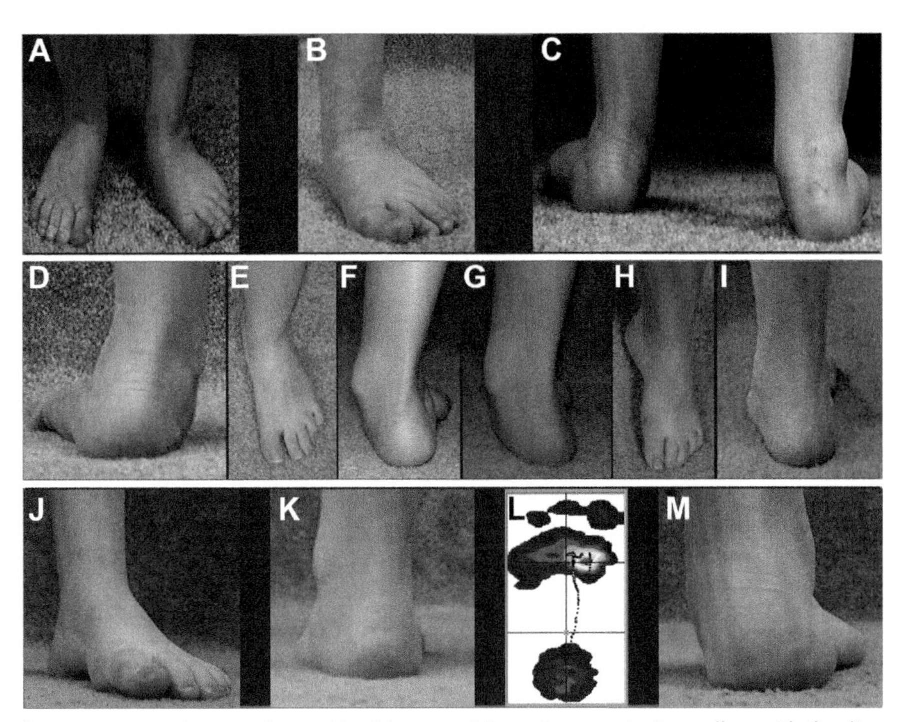

Fig. 1. Case 1. At 2 years of age, this girl was walking using a posterior walker with the diagnosis of an asymmetric spastic diplegic CP. The family was concerned about the severe planovalgus, especially of the left foot (*A, B, C*). The patient tolerated the use of an ankle-foot orthosis (AFO), and the family was also encouraged to allow her to walk barefoot part time to stimulate motor control. At 4 years of age, she continued to improve and was walking independently. The asymmetry was now more apparent, and the family was especially concerned about the severe hallux deformity (*B*). The hindfoot deformity appeared to be slightly improved and the family was reassured of the child's improved motor function and encouraged to continue AFO use (*D*). At age 5 years, there was increased toe walking for which she had bilateral hamstring and gastrocnemius lengthening, and, by age 6 years, the forefoot and hallux deformity had corrected (*E*); however, the hindfoot was now developing varus (*F*). By age 6 years, she was presenting with unilateral CP, with the right side having normal muscle tone and no contracture. By age 9 years, the hindfoot had developed increased varus, she was having trouble tolerating the AFO (*G*), and the forefoot developed supination (*H*). At age 10 years, she had a left split tibialis posterior tendon transfer to the peroneus brevis and repeat gastrocnemius recession. By age 13 years, she had a normal hindfoot (*I*), but mild residual cavus (*J*). At full maturity at age 18 years, the left foot has normal alignment (*K*), with a pedobarograph showing residual mild cavus and increased first ray pressure (*L*). At this time, the right side appears normal; however, the right foot has a mild planovalgus (*M*). This case shows the difficulty in defining the neurologic pattern in young children; however, at this age range, almost all children have natural improvement of planovalgus feet. This case also shows the increased likelihood of unilateral CP developing equinovarus; however, in bilateral CP, the feet are more likely to improve up to age 5 to 7 years, but will again collapse into more planovalgus during adolescence.

tend to persist in children with unilateral CP (see **Fig. 1**, case 1); however, in those with bilateral CP, they usually overcorrect into planovalgus without any intervention. In varus feet of children with bilateral CP, surgical intervention should be avoided before adolescence because of the high risk of overcorrection.[10]

EQUINUS

Toe walking, or equinus deformity, is the most common initially presenting functional symptom in children with CP. The initial management of equinus is with daytime plantar flexion–controlling orthotics, along with physical therapy instruction for caregivers on daily stretching.[11] Nighttime or rest time splinting or casting in dorsiflexion should not be used without inclusion of the knee splinted in full extension, or there will be progressive stretching of the soleus, encouraging gastrocnemius contracture, because these children always lie with full knee flexion. Children are able to tolerate this conservative, routine use of ankle-foot orthoses (AFOs) until age 6 to 8 years, when their tendency for toe walking has resolved or they are developing significant contractures of the gastrocnemius. In unilateral CP (hemiplegia), the soleus also tends to develop a contracture. Surgical lengthening is indicated when the foot can no longer tolerate plantigrade orthotics or develops midfoot break from the orthotics or therapy. Surgical procedures aim to restore neutral dorsiflexion; however, the muscle-tendon architectures are still dominated by short muscle fiber lengths, with the Achilles tendon being longer.[12] Surgical lengthening must focus on the specific contracted muscle. In bilateral CP (diplegia), typically only the gastrocnemius is contracted and thus requires a midcalf myofascial release; in unilateral CP, typically both gastrocnemius and soleus muscle contractures develop, thus a combined slightly more distal myofascial release in the conjoined tendon is preferred. The gastrocnemius recession should be performed when there is a difference of 10° or more with ankle dorsiflexion between the knee flexed and knee extended positions. In severe equinus, an open z-lengthening of the tendon Achilles is the optimal approach (**Fig. 2**). Long-term results suggest that, in spastic bilateral CP, intramuscular aponeurotic recession corrects the equinus while avoiding overlengthening, which is severely detrimental to gait.[13] In

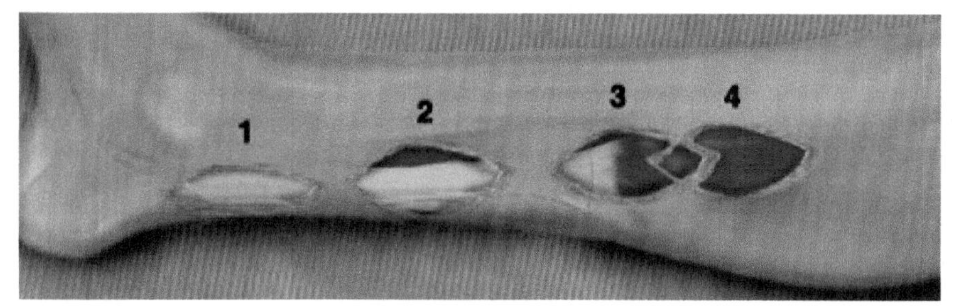

Fig. 2. The incision level for plantar flexor lengthening depends on the difference between dorsiflexion with the knee extended compared with the knee flexed. If there is a less than 10° difference and the equinus is more than −10° of dorsiflexion, open Z-plasty tendon Achilles lengthening is indicated (site 1). If there is more than 10° of difference, a distal fascial lengthening at level 2 is indicated, and, if there is zero dorsiflexion with the knee flexed and more than −10° dorsiflexion with the knee extended, a level 3 lengthening in which the gastrocnemius fascia is detached from the soleus and allowed to slide proximal. For patients whose gastrocnemius is spastic, but knee extended dorsiflexion comes to neutral or greater, the interval between the gastrocnemius and soleus is developed and only the fascia of the gastrocnemius is released at this level (level 4).

severe neglected cases, toe flexor lengthening and plantar fascia release may be needed. In adolescents with severe equinus contracture, concurrent shortening of the tibialis anterior tendon with Achilles tendon lengthening has been shown to improve ankle movement, and gait analysis indicates 93% of patients obtain active dorsiflexion with this combination, optimizing postoperative function.[14] Shortening of the tibialis anterior is performed between the extensor retinaculum and the insertion. Approximately 1.5 to 2 cm of shortening is usually required; the tendon should have some tension at neutral ankle dorsiflexion but allow some plantarflexion. The exact method of shortening is likely not important. The authors prefer to split the tendon and detach half distally then fold over the remaining half and suture it into place at the correct tension. The detached half is then used to reinforce the repair by weaving it into the distal segment. It is important not to make the tendon too tight or it will prevent plantarflexion and push-off during gait. It is extremely important to avoid overlengthening the plantar flexors (**Fig. 3**, case 3), and just as important is not neglecting severe equinus. The overall recurrence rate is 43%, with the highest rate among children with unilateral CP (62.5%), with a higher rate of recurrence in younger children treated before age 8 years compared with older children. Therefore, a second procedure performed by full skeletal maturity may be needed.[15]

EQUINOVARUS

Varus deformity of the feet with equinus is common in younger children, age 3 to 7 years; thus, at this age, treatment must follow the equinus protocol. The natural history of varus is for it to be stable or persist with hemiplegia, whereas, in children with diplegia, almost all overcorrect to valgus.[4] With equinovarus, the primary deformity is typically equinus, thus treatment of equinus should be of first consideration. Surgical lengthening of the plantar flexors is usually needed in addition to muscle balancing to address a more significant varus component. The age of the child is also an important factor to consider when trying to determine whether tendon transfers should be added to plantar flexor lengthening for supple varus feet. Children less than 8 years of age with equinovarus deformities have a very high risk of overcorrection into planovalgus

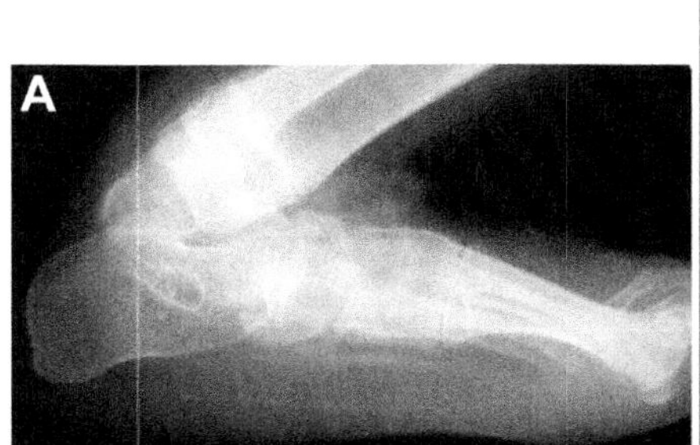

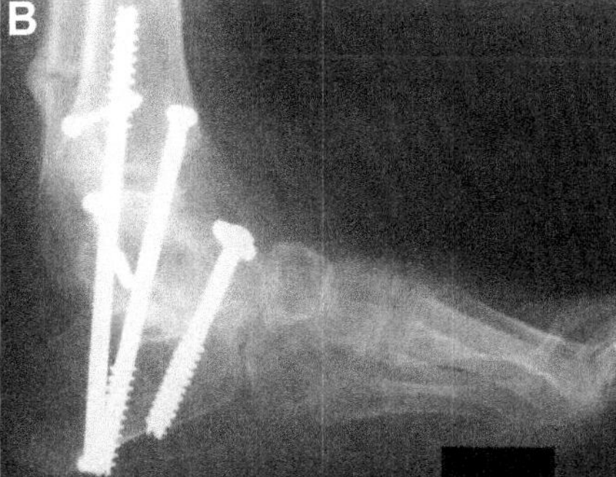

Fig. 3. Case 3. At 10 years of age, this boy was able to do some household ambulation with assistance and walk along furniture with a crouch gait and toe walking. He underwent bilateral percutaneous tendon Achilles lengthening, and, by age 12 years, he was no longer able to support his weight because of severe ankle plantarflexion (*A*). The treatment options for this overlengthening are limited to pantalar fusion (*B*). The risk of functional loss is very high if all aspects of the gait mechanics are not addressed, and are especially high with this type of uncontrolled plantar flexor lengthening.

when both release of the plantarflexion contracture and muscle transfers are combined to correct the varus position.[10] Before the age of 8 years, varus should only be addressed if there is a fixed deformity, in which the foot cannot be brought into a neutral position under anesthesia, after plantar flexor lengthening. The pattern of CP is also important, because the natural history of children with bilateral involvement, diplegia, or quadriplegia involves a very high risk of their feet going into planovalgus during the adolescent and teenage years; this can be magnified by early tendon transfers.[10] In children older than 8 years of age with unilateral CP, an attempt should be made to determine the cause of the varus position. If the varus deformity stems predominantly from the midfoot with forefoot supination, is most apparent during swing phase, and shows tibialis anterior electromyographic activity, which is always on or high and prolonged during swing phase, then a split-tendon transfer of the tibialis anterior tendon to the lateral side of the foot or peroneus longus tendon is preferred. A complete tibialis anterior tendon transfer to the midfoot, as is recommended for clubfoot in a spastic foot, may risk overcorrection. If the varus deformity is most apparent during stance phase and most severe in the hindfoot, with overactivity or out-of-phase electromyographic activity of the tibialis posterior, then a split transfer of the tibialis posterior routed around the posterior tibia and fibula to the antagonist peroneus brevis on the lateral side of the foot is recommended. In contrast with paralytic conditions and weak muscle conditions, performing tibialis posterior tendon transfers through the interosseous membrane in patients with spasticity is never recommended. In spastic feet, this may lead to severe overcorrections that are very hard to treat (**Fig. 4**, case 4).

The involvement pattern of CP, age at operation, foot flexibility, and preoperative status of ambulation are significant factors in the outcome of surgery. Split tibialis posterior tendon transfer is performed to balance a flexible spastic varus foot in unilateral CP in children older than 8 years of age.[10] Biomechanical studies have shown less sensitivity to correct tensioning of the transferred tendon compared with the moment

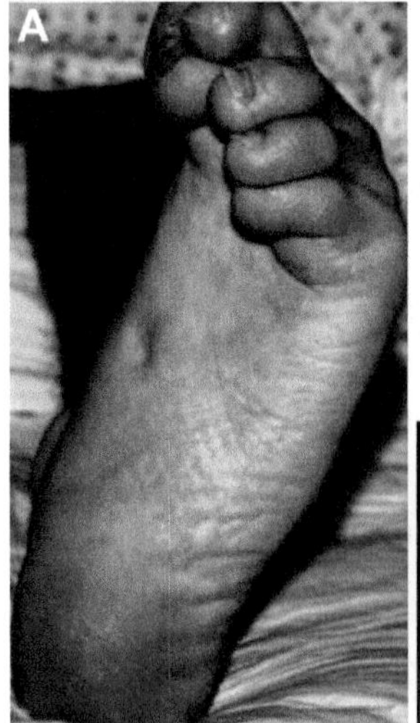

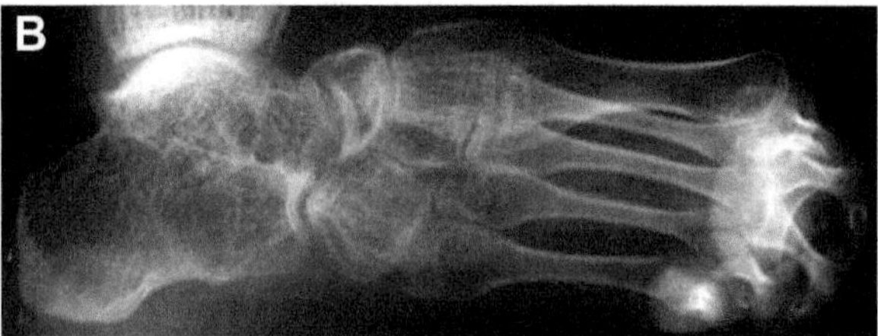

Fig. 4. Case 4. At age 12 years, this ambulatory boy with diplegia developed bilateral equinovarus and had a complete transfer of the tibialis posterior through the interosseus membrane as would be recommended for a peroneal nerve palsy. By age 16 years, his feet were so deformed that he had a hard time wearing shoes and walking (*A*, *B*).

arms of the transferred segment.[16] Failures following tendon transfers for flexible equinovarus result in planovalgus overcorrection, which occurs most commonly in patients younger than 8 years with bilateral involvement and split tibialis posterior transfer.[10] Undercorrection and residual deformity may occur when the transferred tendon ruptures or loses attachment. Tendon transfers for fixed deformities usually are not successful. Determining the cause of failure following tendon transfer is usually difficult because it tends to occur over several years rather than as an immediate failure. Fixed equinovarus foot deformities tend to occur in older, neglected feet, often in young adults. There are also rare nonambulatory children with GMFCS IV or V level function who develop severe equinovarus. Fixed equinovarus deformities in patients with ambulatory ability (GMFCS I–III) tend to cause significant disability with pain and limited walking endurance. These feet tend to require correction with osteotomy, either with joint preservation or triple arthrodesis. Each component of a fixed equinovarus deformity needs to be distinguished; should be identified; and a stepwise approach, including planter fasciotomy, equinus correction with plantar flexor lengthening, hindfoot varus with calcaneal osteotomy or subtalar fusion, midfoot supination correction with midfoot osteotomy, or a combination of cuboid closed wedge osteotomy or calcaneocuboid fusion, should be performed. A recent report shows good outcome with focusing on joint preservation osteotomies to correct these fixed equinovarus deformities.[17] Treatment of GMFCS IV and V patients should be focused on comfortable seating positions with wheelchair adaptations. Occasionally, a family is concerned about this deformity, in which case a triple arthrodesis is preferred. There are no reports comparing the outcome of arthrodesis versus extraarticular osteotomies for correction of severe, stiff equinovarus in CP.

PLANOVALGUS

Planovalgus foot deformity is common with many treatment options, each with substantiated benefits; however, the evidence for 1 rather than the other is not well documented. Planovalgus, known as a flatfoot, varies from mild to stiff and severe, whereby the foot cannot be placed in a shoe. Because of the variation in flexibility and severity, no 1 treatment fits all feet. Several disorders contribute to the deformity, beginning with the lateral displacement of the navicular on the talar head. This condition causes the talar head to become uncovered and prominent on the medial side of the midfoot. This relationship between radiographic and foot pressure measurements has been correlated using a simple linear regression model.[18] In our experience, pedobarography, also known as the foot pressure measurement, is the most objective method for assessing severity of the foot and change over time.[10]

Along with age and spectrum of severity, the natural history of planovalgus must be considered for every child being evaluated for treatment. The foot position in children with CP who are younger than 5 years of age is extremely variable and unpredictable.[4] As with young children with unilateral CP, planovalgus feet often resolve and even progress to a varus position later in childhood and adolescence (see **Fig. 1**, case 1). Often, the pattern of CP in 3-year-old children can be unclear. In some children, determining whether they are unilateral or bilateral may be difficult because of the high variation in foot position. This variability decreases by the time these children reach 5 to 7 years of age. Commonly, children with diplegia have planovalgus, which improves until age 5 or 6 years, then is stable into middle childhood before the planovalgus collapses into more severe deformity and may become progressively more painful during the growth period of adolescence.[4]

This collapse into planovalgus also causes lever arm dysfunction and may lead to progressive crouch gait in the teenage years.[19]

Based on our previous discussion of the natural history of planovalgus, it rarely requires surgical treatment before 9 or 10 years of age, and then only if the foot is painful or has progressive collapse causing decreased ambulatory function. In young children, the primary treatment of planovalgus feet is with the use of orthotics, usually an AFO. It is unclear whether the effect of orthotics on the natural history of the planovalgus foot is positive or negative. Protecting the planovalgus foot during the time when the joints are primarily in the cartilaginous stage from high pressures caused by abnormal posture during gait seems reasonable to avoid joint deformity. This rationale is common in orthotic management. However, in counterpoint, if the foot is constantly controlled with restrictive orthotics, the proprioceptive feedback, muscle strength, and motor control of the foot may not be stimulated to develop, thus leading to further weakness and more collapse ushering in a lifelong orthotics requirement for these individuals. At present, there is no objective evidence for either of these conflicting potential orthotic effects. It is in this light that the authors recommended using orthotics for one-half to three-quarters of the daytime hours while children are awake to take advantage of active walking. We usually start with full calf-height AFOs, then reduce to ankle height, supramalleolar, if there is adequate equinus control. The orthotics must be well fitted, and they are well tolerated by most children. The goal of the orthotic is to have the foot in a natural position, not overcorrected, and with a goal to provide stance stability during gait leading to better function. Nearly all children with a planovalgus deformity have contractures of the gastrocnemius, notable on a positive Silfverskiold test by passively correcting the planovalgus on examination. The treatment of this contracture, with regard to the impact on the natural history of planovalgus deformity, is unclear. However, some children have problems tolerating orthotics because of this equinus. In these cases, a gastrocnemius recession may improve comfort for orthotic use and sometimes leads to progressive improvement of the planovalgus deformity (see **Fig. 1**, case 1). However, treatment of the gastrocnemius contracture with surgical lengthening in isolation is not recommended if children are doing well with orthotics, with the goal of improving the planovalgus. There are no case studies reporting the impact of plantar flexor lengthening on planovalgus; however, it has been our experience that some feet, especially in older children, may develop increased planovalgus after plantar flexor lengthening, so the outcome is unpredictable. Almost all children who have surgical correction of planovalgus need gastrocnemius lengthening as part of the combined procedures to correct hindfoot position. Every foot needs careful examination to make certain it can come to plantigrade position after surgical correction of the planovalgus, and, if not, the appropriate muscle lengthening should be performed.

Planovalgus feet that are painful during ambulation, unable to tolerate adequate orthotic management, or lack mechanical stability leading to lever arm dysfunction, which in turn affects the ability to achieve optimal gait, have indications for surgical correction. Planovalgus deformity has varying degrees of hindfoot varus, forefoot abduction, and supination with apparent shortening of the lateral column caused by posterior subluxation of the calcaneus on the talus and collapse of the medial arch. Other frequently associated deformities include external tibial torsion, ankle joint valgus, and hallux valgus. All aspects of the deformity should be considered when surgically planning a correction. Another important factor to be considered is the child's functional level, because higher-functioning ambulatory children (GMFCS I, II, and III) are the best candidates for joint-preserving corrections. Children who have more limited ambulation and weight-bearing ability (GMFCS IV and V) are better candidates for fusion procedures. Also, deformities that are flexible and not severe, usually in younger patients 10 to 16 years of age, are better candidates for joint-preserving procedures. Surgical correction of planovalgus is uncommon in children less than 10 years of age, because most younger children tolerate the orthotics, and correction at younger ages has a higher recurrence rate in our experience.

Our preferred joint-preserving procedure is a lateral calcaneal lengthening. The calcaneal lengthening usually requires 1 to 1.5 cm of distraction and blocking with bone graft. The osteotomy can be fixated with an intraosseous screw, or Kirschner wire, or a plate (**Fig. 5**, case 5). Lengthening of the peroneus brevis tendon often allows easier distraction of the osteotomy; however, care should be taken to avoid any damage to the peroneus longus because this will lead to increased forefoot supination. After fixing the lateral column lengthening, many feet have a prominent medial navicular tuberosity and first-ray elevation with forefoot supination or medial column instability. If any of these are present, the navicular tuberosity should be resected and the tibialis posterior tendon advanced to provide medial arch support. If there is forefoot supination with elevation of the first ray, a medial column plantar-based wedge resection is performed, which can be completed at the medial cuneiform or at the naviculocuneiform joint as desired (see **Fig. 5**, case 5). Next, if the foot is unable to come to plantigrade because of plantarflexion contracture of the gastrocnemius, a gastrocnemius recession should be performed with caution not to overlengthen or cause excessive dorsiflexion, which is more detrimental than mild plantarflexion tightness. In addition, careful examination of the tibial torsion is required, and, if needed, a tibial derotation is added. If desired, bunion correction can also be added. Postoperative management includes using a short-leg cast for 6 to 8 weeks, allowing weight bearing as tolerated.

The outcome of the lateral calcaneal lengthening procedure as described has good long-term outcome, with the primary complication being recurrent deformity.[9] Ambulatory children have significantly better clinical and radiographic outcomes with calcaneal lengthening for correction of mild to moderately flexible planovalgus deformities than nonambulating children.[9,20] Surgical correction of planovalgus by calcaneal lengthening with peroneus brevis lengthening is an effective procedure for milder deformities, as reported previously. In this report, feet with a 23° anteroposterior talus-first metatarsal angle, 36° lateral talus-first metatarsal angle, and 72% naviculocuboid overlap did better with additional procedures.[21] Another study noted that a talonavicular lateral abduction of more than 24° and calcaneal pitch of less than −5° were independent predictors that could be used to identify planovalgus deformities that were indicators of poor ability to restore normal alignment by lateral lengthening.[22] The goal of planovalgus correction is to improve foot contact, which is best measured by pedobarography; the radiologic measure that best correlates with reduced medial midfoot pressure is the talonavicular uncoverage index, which can be used as an intraoperative measurement of adequate correction.[18]

For children with lower levels of motor function, who mostly do weight-bearing transfers or exercise ambulation (GMFCS IV or V levels) and have painful feet or severe deformities with limited standing ability, a subtalar fusion is indicated, followed by medial column correction with fusions as needed (**Fig. 6**, case 6). For very severe planovalgus foot deformities, a medial column fusion may encompass the first metatarsal to the talus, and, for moderate feet, the talus to the medial cuneiform may be completed. With more severe deformities, there must also be an evaluation for

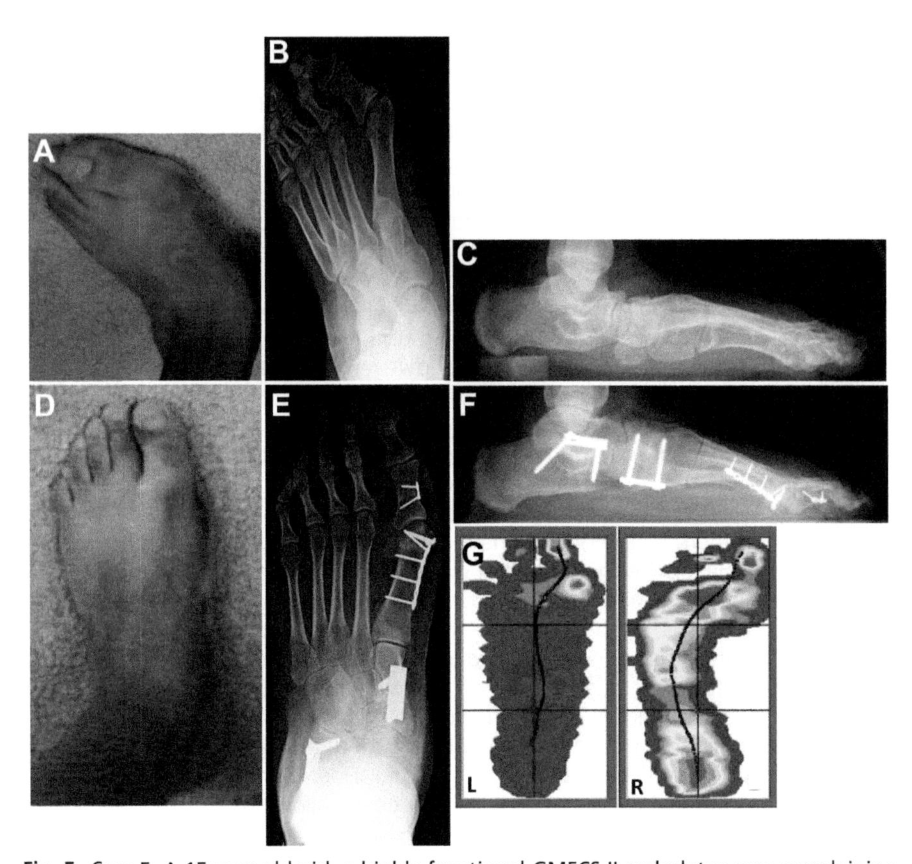

Fig. 5. Case 5. A 15-year-old girl, a highly functional GMFCS II ambulator, was complaining of pain in her feet with intense activity. Her feet were both similar with severe planovalgus and severe bunions (*A, B*). She also had a midfoot break (*C*). Both feet were corrected concurrently by starting with hindfoot correction with calcaneal lengthening, which brings the forefoot over and corrects the talonavicular joint. However, the medial column still had a break at the naviculocuneiform joint. This joint was resected with a plantar medial closing wedge fixed with a plantar medial plate. By bringing the forefoot down in line with the hindfoot, she now had limited dorsiflexion with the knee extended, which required gastrocnemius release at midcalf. The next step in the reconstruction was to correct the severe bunion, but, because of her high function, we elected to do realignment osteotomies instead of a fusion. She had a distal closing medial displacement osteotomy fixed with a plate and proximal phalangeal (Akin type) osteotomy. At 1-year follow-up, she had no pain with ambulation with good medial arch presentation and a mild residual hallux valgus (*D–F*). She is happy with the outcome and her plantar pressures have almost normalized (*G*) compared with the severe planovalgus pattern preoperatively (*L*, preoperative; *R*, postoperative). Another important element of this case was that correcting the bunion was not possible without correcting the hindfoot and midfoot deformities. Although the pain from activity may be mainly in the midfoot, failing to correct the hallux valgus often leads to an unhappy patient because this is the deformity the patient sees even when it is not painful. A good outcome should include a patient who is happy with the outcome; therefore, it is important to pay attention to the forefoot.

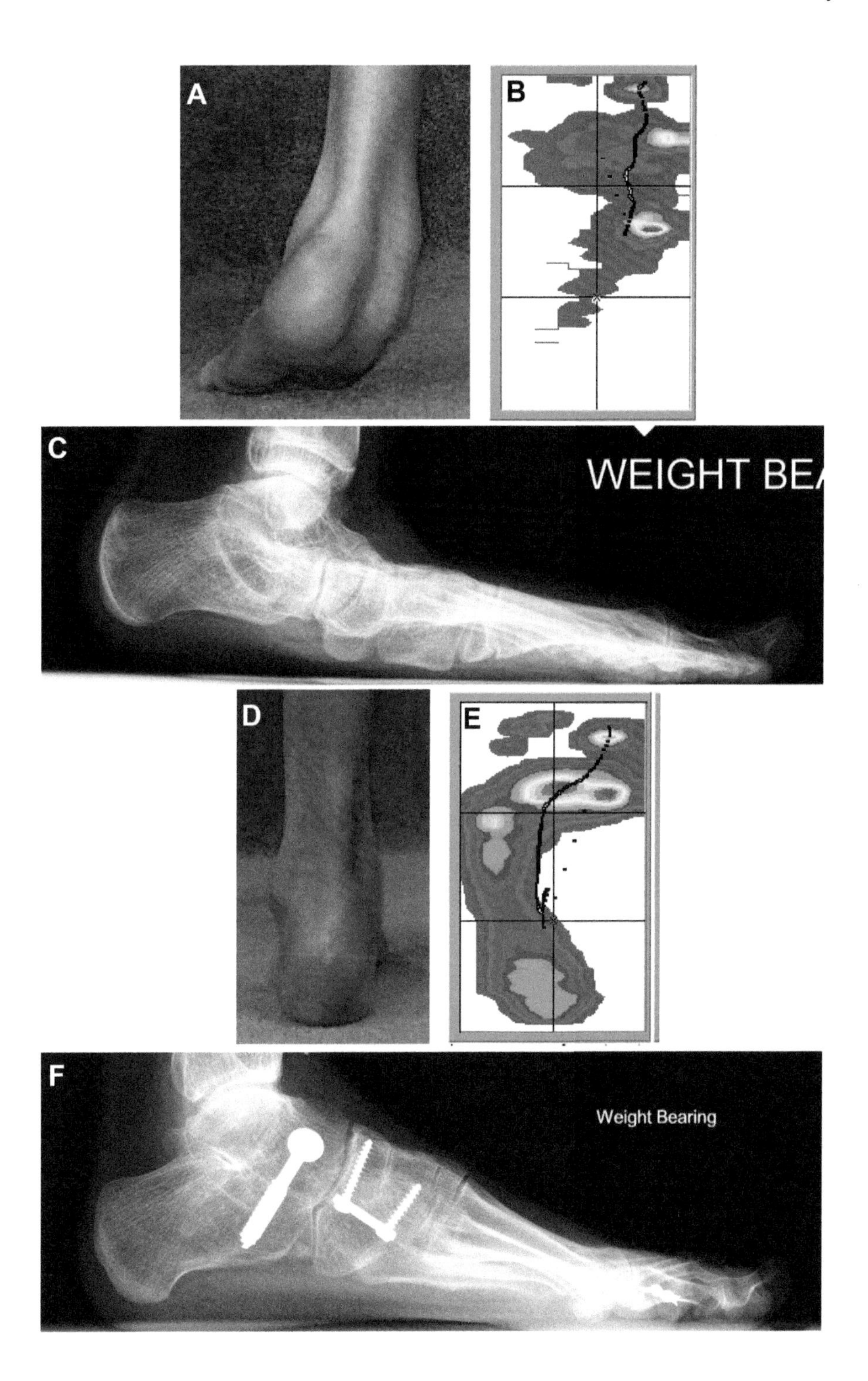
A
B
C
WEIGHT BE
D
E
F
Weight Bearing

correction of plantarflexion contractures or tibial torsion, which should not be left uncorrected. Major problems occur after surgical corrections in a few cases. The postoperative management is similar, with a short-leg cast for 6 to 8 weeks allowing weight bearing as tolerated. The outcome of the fusion procedure shows less recurrence and few complications.[9] However, this procedure likely places more stress on the ankle joint with a possible high risk of arthritis in very active individuals, which is the reason the authors prefer joint sparing in more functional ambulators. There are a few individuals (GMFCS V) with very severe feet that are painful with all shoe wear who desire correction. The authors think these are best managed with arthrodesis, usually more than a triple because the forefoot supination often also requires resection and fusion. There is a group of children with weakness and hypotonia who develop a cavovalgus deformity with collapse through the subtalar joint, but with no forefoot deformity except mild increased cavus. These feet respond well to subtalar fusion (**Fig. 7**, case 7).

The overall goal for planovalgus correction is to improve the function of the patient. In a few children with severe crouch, the lever arm dysfunction may be the primary cause and good stable correction of the foot may lead to correction of the crouch without other procedures. These patients tend to have severe planovalgus but no knee flexion contractures or significant hamstring contractures.[19] Recurrence of the deformity is most common with calcaneal lengthening,[9] and our preferred treatment is a subtalar fusion. Another recurrent issue is failure to correct associated deformities such as tibial torsion, medial column collapse, and plantarflexion contractures.

Other options for treatment of planovalgus include consideration of the use of subtalar arthroereisis. Some reports on short-term follow-up have found outcomes similar to subtalar fusion[23] or similar to arthroereisis for normal pediatric flatfeet.[24] One report with average 4-year follow-up found 96% good outcome; however, some of the children were as young as 2 years old.[25] Another report found 40% poor outcome in children with spastic CP.[26] The authors have no experience with performing implants for arthroereisis; however, we have seen several children in whom these were painful and required removal. Based on this experience, we have noted that the subtalar joint is usually stiff and the foot does remain corrected. Another option is the calcaneocuboid-cuneiform (triple-C) osteotomy, in which compensatory osteotomies are made for the subluxated joints. Good functional and radiologic results have been reported.[27] We have not used this technique and cannot comment further because there are also few publications.

Fig. 6. Case 6. A 16-year-old boy, GMFCS II, with left-side unilateral CP type IV, who is having increased pain with ambulation. He has a severe equinoplanovalgus foot (*A*), with all the pressure on the medial forefoot (*B*) and collapse of the midfoot (*C*). Based on a full gait analysis, he had a left femoral derotation, hamstring lengthening, tibial derotation, tendon Achilles Z-plasty lengthening, subtalar fusion, naviculocuneiform fusion, and bunion correction. The fusion was chosen rather than calcaneal lengthening because of the severe and stiff nature of the deformity. At 1-year postoperative follow-up, he had a neutral plantigrade foot (*D*) with near-normal foot pressure (*E*) and a reconstituted midfoot arch. (*F*) He is walking pain free. This case shows the frequent need for full limb correction rather than only focusing on the foot. Good correction of the planovalgus requires correction of the equinus, lateral column, and medial column. For good patient satisfaction, attention should also be paid to toe deformities.

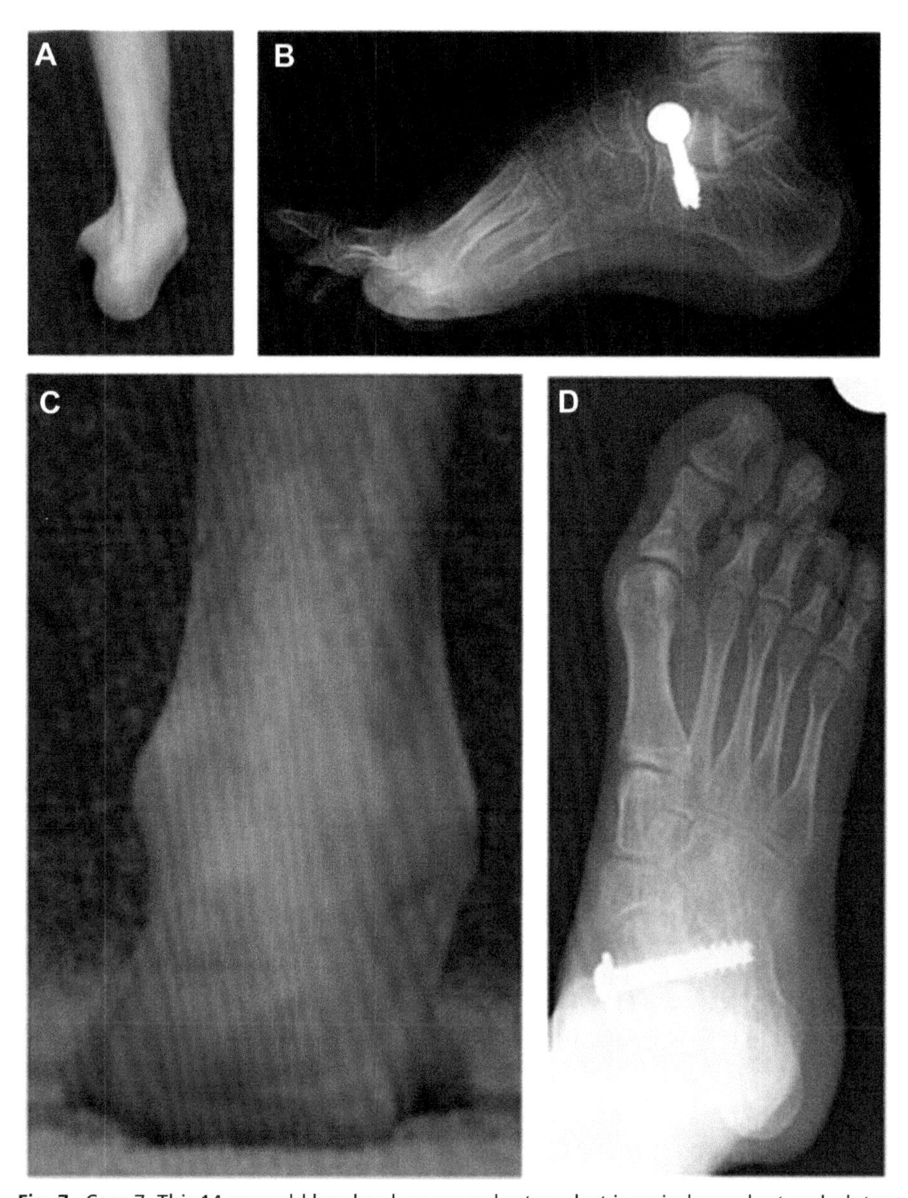

Fig. 7. Case 7. This 14-year-old boy has low muscular tone but is an independent ambulator. He has become unwilling to walk with his AFO and his mother feels it is causing him pain. Because of his cognitive limitations, it is not possible for him to express his level of pain or whether he has pain. As he has grown and gained weight, his feet have collapsed into cavovalgus posture (*A*). He has no contractures and no spasticity. This collapse is entirely through the subtalar joint and responded extremely well to reduction and fusion (*B*). Following subtalar fusion, he was back to normal ambulation without the need for orthotics (*C*). Note that the fixation screw crosses the foot transversely through the anterior facet (*D*). This position provides maximum prevention of recurring deformity because it is farthest away from the center of rotation of the deformity. Screws placed longitudinally may allow recurring deformity because they are along the axis of the deformity.

SUMMARY

Deformities of the feet are the most common musculoskeletal problem in children with CP, and it is important to have an understanding of the natural history of the deformity. With this review, the management concepts require a combination of observation, orthotics, and surgical interventions depending on the child and the foot.

CLINICS CARE POINTS

- Avoid overlengthening plantar flexors, especially in bilateral CP, because this may lead to severe crouch gait. It is far better for the gait function to have undercorrection and need a second lengthening than overcorrection.
- In young children less than 6 years old, foot surgery for planovalgus or varus should rarely be performed because many of these children are still developing motor control and may improve the deformity as part of the natural evolution.
- Tendon transfers for equinovarus feet have a high overcorrection rate in bilateral CP and in children less than 8 years of age, and the transfers should generally be split-tendon transfers, not whole-tendon transfers to avoid overcorrection.
- Correction of planovalgus feet usually requires lengthening of the plantarflexors, and lateral and medial column correction. Abnormal tibial torsion is a common concurrent problem that should be evaluated after foot correction. Careful assessment and correction of all deformities in the limb should occur at the time of surgical correction of the planovalgus.

DISCLOSURE

The authors have nothing to disclose.

REFERENCES

1. Bax M, Goldstein M, Rosenbaum P, et al. Executive Committee for the Definition of Cerebral Palsy. Proposed definition and classification of cerebral palsy, April 2005. Dev Med Child Neurol 2005;47:571–6.
2. Wood E, Rosenbaum P. The gross motor function classification system for cerebral palsy: a study of reliability and stability over time. Dev Med Child Neurol 2000;42:292–6.
3. Beckung E, White-Koning M, Marcelli M, et al. Health status of children with cerebral palsy living in Europe: a multi-centre study. Child Care Health Dev 2008;34: 806–14.
4. Church C, Lennon N, Alton R, et al. Longitudinal change in foot posture in children with cerebral palsy. J Child Orthop 2017;11:229–36.
5. Linden O, Hagglund G, Rodby-Bousquet E, et al. The development of spasticity with age in 4,162 children with cerebral palsy: a register-based prospective cohort study. Acta Orthop 2019;90:286–91.
6. Hagglund G, Wagner P. Spasticity of the gastrosoleus muscle is related to the development of reduced passive dorsiflexion of the ankle in children with cerebral palsy: a registry analysis of 2,796 examinations in 355 children. Acta Orthop 2011;82:744–8.
7. Er MS, Abousamra O, Rogers KJ, et al. Long-term outcome of internal tibial derotation osteotomies in children with cerebral palsy. J Pediatr Orthop 2017;37: 454–9.
8. Er MS, Bayhan IA, Rogers KJ, et al. Long-term outcome of external tibial derotation osteotomies in children with cerebral palsy. J Pediatr Orthop 2017;37:460–5.

9. Kadhim M, Holmes L Jr, Miller F. Long-term outcome of planovalgus foot surgical correction in children with cerebral palsy. J Foot Ankle Surg 2013;52:697–703.
10. Chang CH, Albarracin JP, Lipton GE, et al. Long-term follow-up of surgery for equinovarus foot deformity in children with cerebral palsy. J Pediatr Orthop 2002;22:792–9.
11. Sees JP, Miller F. Overview of foot deformity management in children with cerebral palsy. J Child Orthop 2013;7:373–7.
12. Wren TAL, Cheatwood AP, Rethlefsen SA, et al. Kay RM Achilles tendon length and medial gastrocnemius architecture in children with cerebral palsy and equinus gait. J Pediatr Orthop 2010;30:479–84.
13. Dreher T, Buccoliero T, Wolf SI, et al. Long-term results after gastrocnemius-soleus intramuscular aponeurotic recession as a part of multilevel surgery in spastic diplegic cerebral palsy. J Bone Joint Surg Am 2012;94:627–37.
14. Rutz E, Baker R, Tirosh O, et al. Tibialis anterior tendon shortening in combination with Achilles tendon lengthening in spastic equinus in cerebral palsy. Gait Posture 2011;33:152–7.
15. Joo SY, Knowtharapu DN, Rogers KJ, et al. Recurrence after surgery for equinus foot deformity in children with cerebral palsy: assessment of predisposing factors for recurrence in a long-term follow-up study. J Child Orthop 2011;5:289–96.
16. Piazza SJ, Adamson RL, Moran MF, et al. Effects of tensioning errors in split transfers of anterior and posterior tendons. J Bone Joint Surg Am 2003;85:858–65.
17. Thamkunano V, Kamisan N. Approach to bone procedure in fixed equinovarus deformity in cerebral palsy. J Orthop 2018;15:1008–12.
18. Kadhim M, Holmes L Jr, Miller F. Correlation of radiographic and pedobarograph measurements in planovalgus foot deformity. Gait Posture 2012;36:177–81.
19. Kadhim M, Miller F. Pes planovalgus deformity in children with cerebral palsy: review article. J Pediatr Orthop B 2014;23:400–5.
20. Ettl V, Wollmerstedt N, Kirschner S, et al. Calcaneal lengthening for planovalgus deformity in children with cerebral palsy. Foot Ankle Int 2009;30:398–404.
21. Sung KH, Chung CY, Lee KM, et al. Calcaneal lengthening for planovalgus foot deformity in patients with cerebral palsy. Clin Orthop Relat Res 2013;471:1682–90.
22. Luo CA, Kao HK, Lee WC, et al. Limits to calcaneal lengthening for treating planovalgus foot deformity in children with cerebral palsy. Foot Ankle Int 2017;38:863–9.
23. Wen J, Liu H, Xiao S, et al. Comparison of mid-term efficacy of spastic flatfoot in ambulant children with cerebral palsy by 2 different methods. Medicine (Baltimore) 2017;96:e7044.
24. Kubo H, Krauspe R, Hufeland M, et al. Radiological outcome after treatment of juvenile flatfeet with subtalar arthroereisis: a matched pair analysis of 38 cases comparing neurogenic and non-neurogenic patients. J Clin Orthop 2019;13:346–52.
25. Vedantam R, Capelli AM, Schoenecker PL. Subtalar arthrodesis for the correction of planovalgus foot in children with neuromuscular disorders. J Pediatr Orthop 1998;18:294–8.
26. Molayem I, Persiani P, Lior Marcovici L, et al. Complications following correction of the planovalgus foot in cerebral palsy by arthrodesis. Acta Orthop Belg 2009;75:374–9.
27. El-Hilaly R, El-Sherbini MH, Abd-Ella MM, et al. Radiological outcome of calcaneo-cuboid-cuneiform osteotomies for planovalgus feet in cerebral palsy children: relationship with pedobarography. Foot Ankle Surg 2019;25:462–8.

The Pediatric Foot in Neurologic Disorders

Leonard Doederlein, MD

KEYWORDS

- Neurologic foot deformities • Spastic foot deformities • Flaccid foot deformities
- Tendon transfers • Central and peripheral neurologic disorders
- Pediatric neuromuscular conditions • Muscle imbalance • Surgical management

KEY POINTS

- The first steps are a clinical and technical evaluation of a neurologically involved foot.
- A working diagnosis must be followed by a concise treatment plan.
- Treatment consists of planning and executing definite surgical steps.
- After-treatment mostly includes orthotic protection. Regular follow ups are mandatory.
- Pitfalls and problems should be recognized early followed by adequate solutions.

INTRODUCTION

Neurogenic and neuromuscular disorders may produce numerous different foot abnormalities that often mimic primary foot deformities, although their causes, the pathomechanisms, and treatment principles are fundamentally different.[1–5]

A thorough knowledge of the possible underlying disorders regarding their differential diagnostics as well as their indication and management principles seems essential for any foot specialist. In contrast to primary foot problems, the underlying neuromuscular deficits often affect not only the foot but also concomitantly the proximal joints and even the whole musculoskeletal system.[6–9] In addition, nonmotor functions, such as the sensory-vegetative, the gastrointestinal, the cardiopulmonary, and other systems, may be disturbed. Therefore, additional medical professional advice and often also long-term care for these patients will be necessary.[9,10] Therefore, the pediatric foot is frequently only 1 important aspect of a more generalized disorder.

CAUSE AND CLASSIFICATION OF NEUROLOGIC AND NEUROMUSCULAR DISORDERS

Although the term "neuromuscular" is commonly used for all neurogenic and neuromuscular deficits, a distinction between both is of interest for a clear communication among the members of the treatment team.

Orthopaedic Hospital Aukammklinik, Leibnizstrasse 21, Wiesbaden D-65191, Germany
E-mail address: doederlein@orthopaedie-aukamm.de

Foot Ankle Clin N Am 26 (2021) 655–683
https://doi.org/10.1016/j.fcl.2021.08.003
1083-7515/21/

Neurogenic problems arise from deficits within the central nervous system, including the brain, the brainstem, and the long spinal tracts.[6,11]

Neuromuscular disorders, on the other hand, may affect any lower level from the spinal anterior horn cell down to the striated skeletal muscles.[8,9,12]

Both disorders can occur in isolation or (rarely) combined and may have a progressive or a nonprogressive course. It is important to note that growth mechanisms, such as weight and height gains, often mimic an underlying progressive disorder.

The causes are multifactorial, and sometimes combinations among different disorders occur (eg, cerebral palsy plus sensorimotor neuropathy).

The etiologic spectrum varies from traumatic, congenital, vascular, malformative, infective, toxic-metabolic, and iatrogenic, which all may give rise to neurogenic or neuromuscular problems. Therefore, differential diagnostics, if possible, with the help of the multidisciplinary team are often among the first steps.[4,13,14]

It should be noticed that these disorders may not only affect the neuromuscular system but also impact the sensorimotor and autonomous areas. Therefore, the author suggests classifying each individual according to the underlying deficits[7] (**Tables 1** and **2**).

ASPECTS OF NEUROLOGIC FOOT INVOLVEMENT, PATHOMECHANICS, AND FUNCTIONAL CONSEQUENCES

Foot involvement and neurogenic or neuromuscular disorders can occur in isolation or combined with proximal and contralateral problems.[6,11,13,16] This must always be exactly ruled out, because it has a critical impact on the functional goals of treatment. Any combinations of foot together with proximal joint problems must be treated concurrently and not isolated.

The leading motto must always be the following: a foot can only function correctly if the joints above are correctly aligned in 3 planes ("There is a whole child above the foot". [17]

> Therefore, in almost every case, the creation of a straight leg should precede or accompany every effort to reconstruct a deformed foot.

The characteristics of foot involvement in neurologic disorders of children can be grouped according to joint, muscle, and sensation status as follows[17,18]:

Joint Conditions

- Joint stiffness (eg, in arthrogrypotic or myelodysplastic feet)[19,20]
- Normal joint mobility
- Excessive joint mobility (hyperlaxity)
- Joint instability/joint disintegration (eg, in Charcot joints)

Muscle Power

- Absent muscles (eg, in amyoplasia)
- Muscular atrophy with flaccid paralysis
- Reduced muscle power (weakness; Medical Research Council [MRC] grading from 0 to 5)
- Normal muscle power
- Normal motor control
- Impaired motor control

Muscle Tone

- No muscle tone (flaccidity-flail joint)

Table 1
Classification of neurogenic and neuromuscular problems according to localization of neurologic defects and causes[15]

Defect Localization ▶ Causes ▼	Brain/ Central Nervous System	Extrapyramidal System	Long Tracts	Anterior Horn Cell	Peripheral Nerve	Neuromuscular Junction	Skeletal Muscle
Congenital							
Traumatic							
Vascular							
Infectious							
Toxic/metabolic							
Iatrogenic							
Tumorous							
Stationary							
Progressive							
Other							
Unclear							

Table 2
Classification of neurogenic and neuromuscular problems according to localization of neurologic defects and peripheral functional deficits

Definition Localization ▶ Deficits ▼	Brain/ Central Nervous System	Extrapyramidal System	Long Tracts	Anterior Horn Cell	Peripheral Nerve	Neuromuscular Junction	Skeletal Muscle
Muscle tone							
Voluntary control							
Patterned movements							
Muscle power							
Muscle balance							
Sensation							
Vegetative functions							
Vision							
Hearing							
Epilepsy							
Balance							
Other							

- Reduced muscle tone (hypotonia)
- Normal muscle tone
- Increased muscle tone (spasticity)
- Rigid muscle tone (lead pipe type; muscle rigor/rigidity)

Sensation and Autonomous System

- Absent sensation (anesthesia)
- Reduced sensation (hypoesthesia)
- Normal sensation
- Increased sensation (hyperesthesia; dysesthesia)
- Reduced pain sensation
- Absent pain sensation
- Sweating absent (eg, in autonomous dysfunction; hereditary sensoric-autonomous-neuropathy - congenital insensitivity to pain with anhidrosis = congenital insensitivity to pain with anhidrosis)[7,8]

Neurologic foot deformities mostly develop gradually in initially normal-shaped feet. Exceptions are congenital stiff feet in amyoplasia (arthrogryposis) or in myelomeningocele (spina bifida), whereby the children are born with extremely deformed feet.[21,22]

The mechanisms that lead to a gradual deterioration of a deformity can be categorized into the following 5 groups[2,6]:

- Congenital factors
- Neurogenic/neuromuscular factors
- Biomechanical factors[16]
- Growth
- Iatrogenic factors

Although most of the time several of these components act together, it is useful to separate them in every individual case (examples in **Figs. 1–3**).

Most often a combination of muscle weakness or muscle imbalance and biomechanical consequences of weight, shear forces, and gravity on an already deformed foot acts self-perpetuating, like a vicious circle, which terminates in an end position of the joints (= position of joint stop). Here, the agonist muscles are maximally shortened, and their antagonists are correspondingly elongated, which makes both muscle components completely nonfunctioning and therefore extremely weak[4,23] (**Figs. 4** and **5**).

DIAGNOSIS AND CLASSIFICATION OF FOOT DEFORMITIES

Diagnostic steps in neurogenic and neuromuscular pediatric foot deformities consist of clinical and instrumented techniques.[24,25] The clinical workup includes a neurologic overview (see box) and a clear description of the deformity under non-weight-bearing and weight-bearing conditions, a detailed examination of joint range of motion (ROM) and stability, and an estimation of muscle power (MRC scale 0–5). Sensation and reflex status must be considered as well. The status of the proximal joints and a general motor function survey are also necessary.[4,13]

Some basic neurologic examination steps in neuromuscular deformities[3,4,7,13,15] include the following (sensorimotor functions, spine, upper extremities, cranial nerves, behavioral abnormalities):

- Muscle tone (normal, increased, hypotonic, flaccid)
- Tendon and cutaneous reflexes (patella and Achilles tendon, Babinski, withdrawal response)

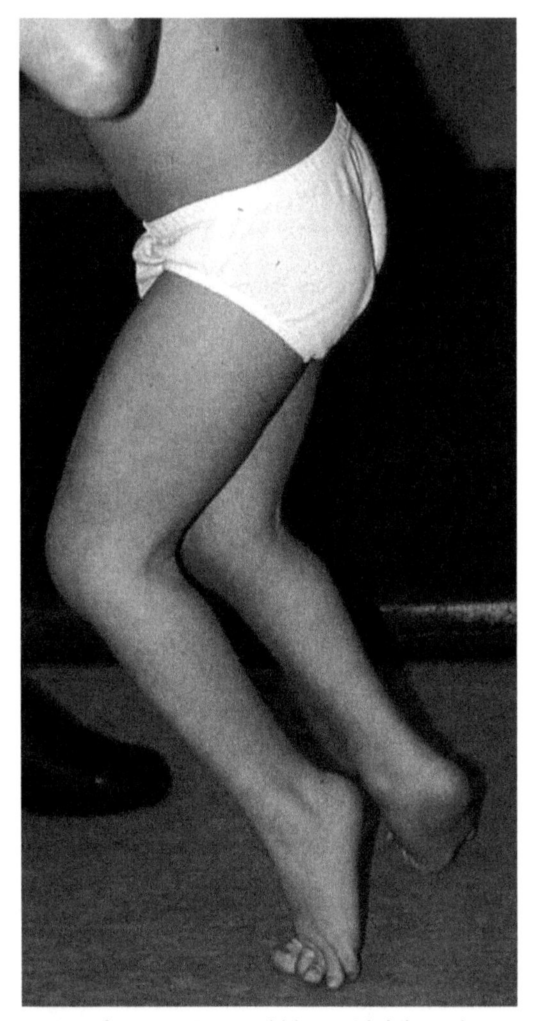

Fig. 1. Neurogenic equinus feet in a 6-year-old boy with bilateral spastic cerebral palsy.

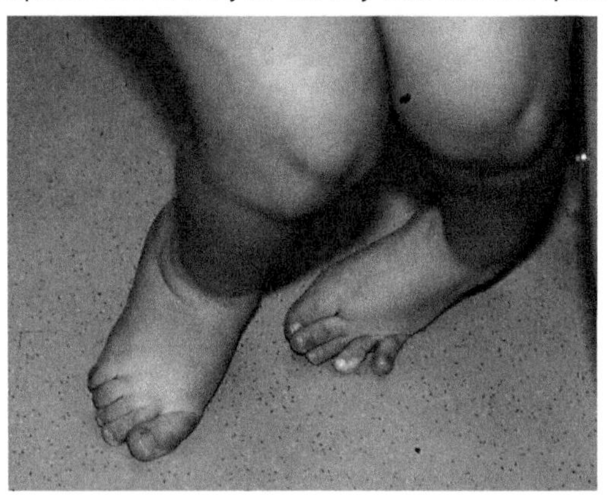

Fig. 2. Opposite foot deformities through vertical forces acting biomechanically upon already deformed feet with a muscle imbalance (8-year-old girl with bilateral spastic cerebral palsy).

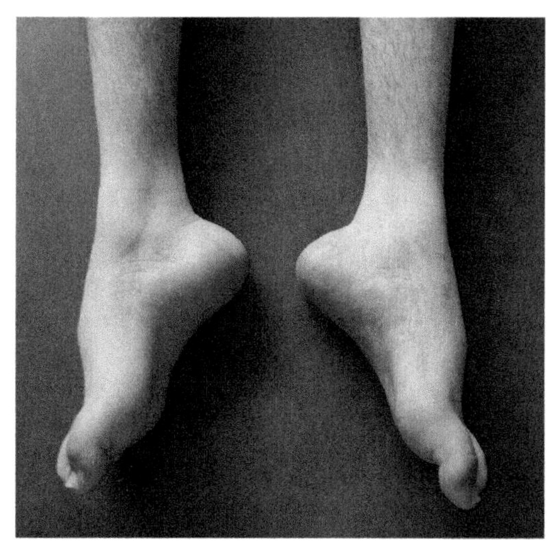

Fig. 3. Neuromuscular muscle imbalances and their pathologic effects on growth in a boy with hereditary sensorimotor neuropathy.

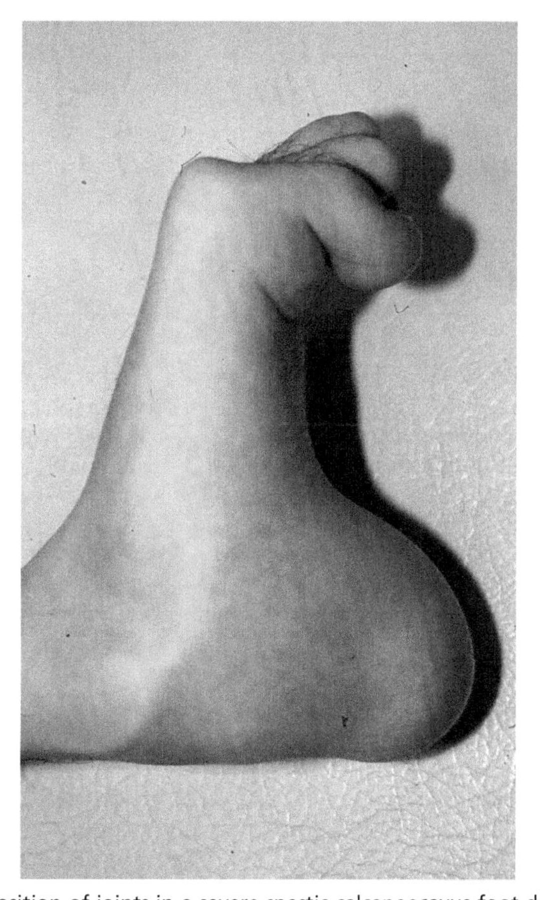

Fig. 4. The end position of joints in a severe spastic calcaneocavus foot deformity.

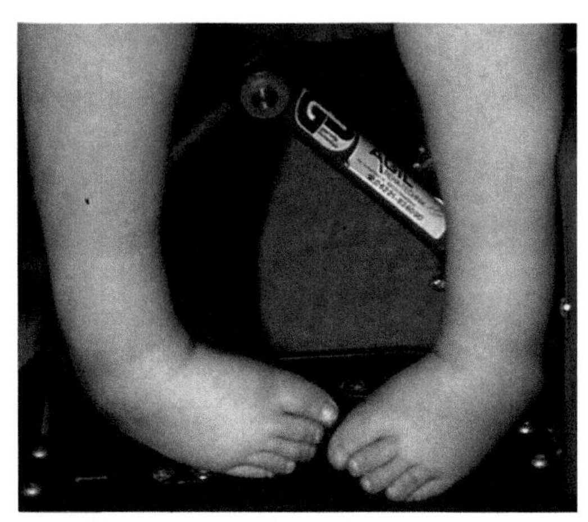

Fig. 5. The end position of joints in flaccid clubfeet in muscular dystrophy.

- Muscle activity (selective, patterned, not to be determined)
- Sensation (normal, hypersensitive, reduced, loss of sensation/proprioception)
- Signs of spinal dysraphism at lower lumbar spine
- Bladder and bowel functions
- Hands and fingers (shape, active function, weakness, fingernails, scars)
- Spinal deformities (scoliosis; kyphosis; lordosis)
- Basic locomotor functions
- Additional neurologic deficits (epilepsy; deafness, vision; cognition)
- Psychiatric abnormalities

Instrumented diagnostics include standard weight-bearing radiographs in 2 planes, in special cases accompanied by MRI and computed tomographic scans. In selected cases, especially for preoperative diagnostics, 3-dimensional (3D) dynamic movement analysis may be useful, but this is always complementary and does not replace a detailed clinical workup. Every extensive diagnostic method must begin with a specific question the method is intended to answer.

A straightforward classification of any deformity facilitates further goal setting, therapy, and evaluation (see **Tables 1** and **2**).

Different classifications[11,15–17] must be distinguished (**Table 3**) as follows:

- Classifications of the shape and severity of the presenting deformity (slight, moderate, severe)
- Etiologic classification (central or peripheral motor disorder, sensory and/or motor disorder, and so forth)
- Classification of passive reducibility (over-correctable, completely correctable, partly-correctable,stiff/rigid[22])
- Classification according to age of patient (infantile, juvenile, adolescent)

In terms of treatment planning, the author also advises a detailed description of all affected parts of the foot in all 3 planes.[1,16]

Table 3
Regional and clinical classification of neurogenic/neuromuscular foot deformities

Joint▶ Deformity▼	Ankle Joint	TaloCalcaneal Joint	Talonavicular and Calcaneo-Cuboid Joints	Naviculo-Cuneiform Joints	Tarsometatarsal Joints	Metatarsophalangeal Joints	Proximal and Sistal Interphalangeal Joints
Sagittal							
Frontal							
Transverse							
Stable							
Mobile							
Restricted							
Stiff/rigid							
Hypermobile							
Unstable							
Deformed							
Other							

INDICATION AND SELECTION OF TREATMENT

Defining a treatment indication must be based on a realistic expectation on the side of the surgeon, the patient, and his or her parents. Today, any result of a surgical procedure is rarely evaluated only locally, but mostly, it is accompanied by an estimation of its effects on the functional activities and participation levels (international classification of functioning - children and youth grading = classification of the results according to the international classification of function in children and adolescents).[17,26,27]

The fact that the causative disorder mostly cannot be cured by any surgical management makes it necessary to define realistic short- and long-term goals.

The indication for the correction of a pediatric neuromuscular foot deformity must be based on one of the following situations (**Figs. 6–8**):

- Preventive indication (with a high risk for deterioration of deformity and/or functional loss)
- Therapeutic-corrective indication (in an established deformity with a corresponding functional deficit)
- Palliative indication (if the situation makes any "complete correction" or "restoration" impossible and necessitates a palliative measure; see **Fig. 8**).

Treatment selection must then be founded on the presenting features of the problem and on the knowledge of the surgeon but also on the feasibility of the treatment methods.

Mostly a combination of surgery and conservative measures will be necessary, although in the lower degrees of a deformity combined conservative management may be very effective (for example, Botulinum injections plus plaster casts followed by orthotics).[28–30]

Appropriate selection of treatment should consider local and functional aspects, including the amount of passive correctability and any muscle imbalances and sensation deficits. Functional aspects should concentrate on muscular weakness, restricted passive joint ROM, and proximal joint problems. In muscle disorders, an equinus deformity is often functionally important to compensate for the weakness of proximal muscle groups. **Fig. 9** shows equinus deformities in a boy with Duchenne muscular dystrophy.

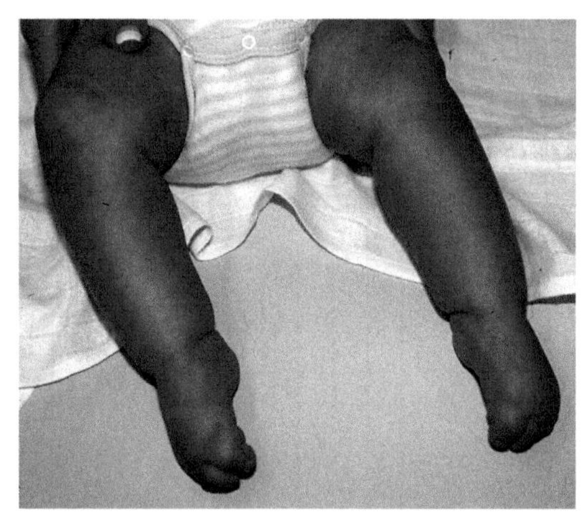

Fig. 6. Preventive indication of bilateral passively correctable equinus feet in a 3-year-old girl with myotonic dystrophy.

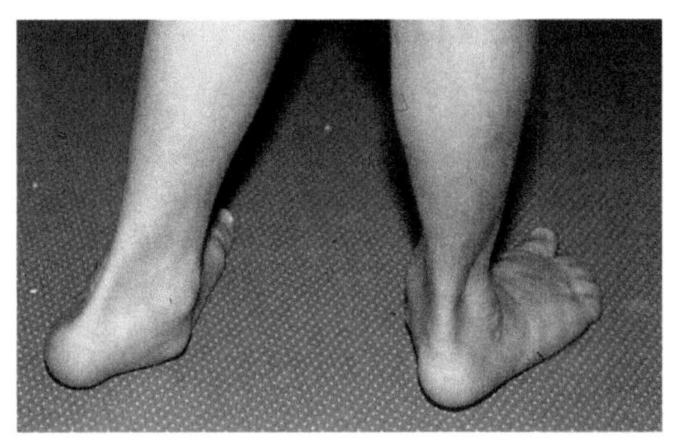

Fig. 7. Therapeutic-corrective indication of a severe equinovalgus deformity in an 8-year-old boy with unilateral spasticity.

The most important step toward proper treatment selection is the decision between observation, conservative, and surgical treatments. The following guidelines may help in this respect:

- Observation: Slight deformity, no progression, little or almost no functional impairment
- Conservative: Moderate deformity, passively complete or almost complete correction, no tendency toward deterioration, slight to moderate impairment of standing/walking function

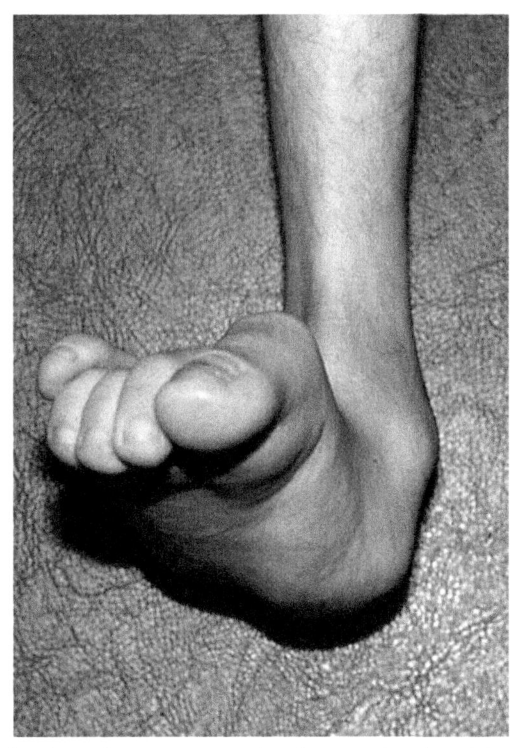

Fig. 8. Palliative indication of an extreme rocker bottom foot in a 15-year-old boy with severe spastic cerebral palsy.

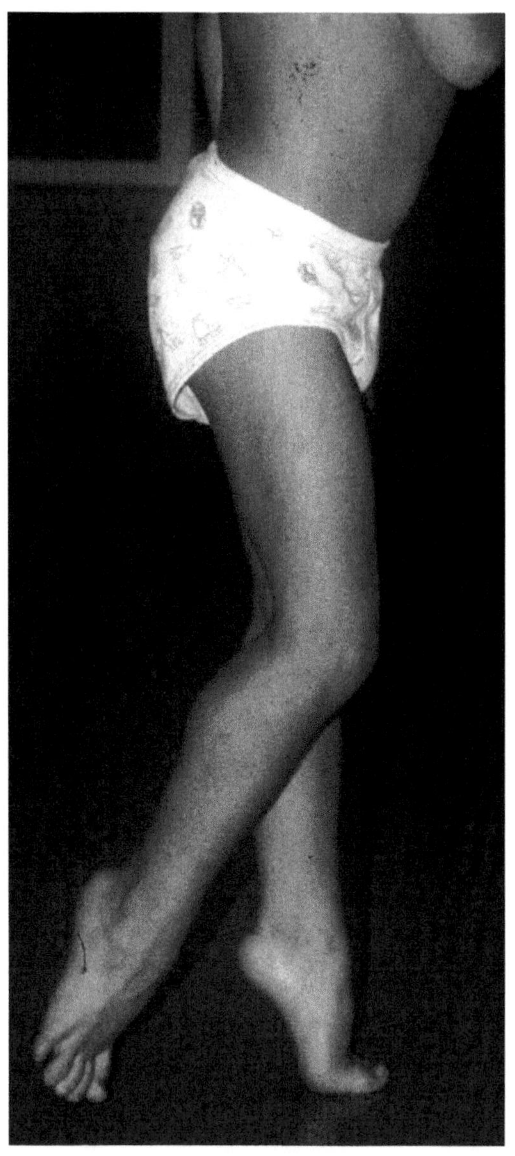

Fig. 9. Every indication must respect local and functional aspects: a 7-year-old boy with Duchenne muscular dystrophy and typical bilateral equinus deformities together with weak knee extensors.

- Surgical: Any significant or severe deformity with marked functional loss, any progressive deformity, always if conservative treatment fails

MANAGEMENT: PRINCIPLES AND TECHNIQUES

As in most orthopedic conditions, management principles are far more important than methods.[1,4,16,17,29] The particular characteristics of pediatric neurogenic/

neuromuscular foot deformities do not justify standard treatment protocols, which are appropriate for idiopathic deformities (eg, congenital clubfoot; idiopathic planovalgus foot). An often striking similarity to idiopathic forms must not mislead the surgeon.[1,17,31,32] An example may be the use of the universal Ponseti technique, which is successful in more than 90% of idiopathic clubfeet but fails in a high percentage of neurologic clubfeet.[19,33,34]

Another example is the structural equinus deformity, which is commonly treated by Achilles tendon lengthening. However, this technique fails with a high risk of overcorrections in neurologic and especially spastic equinus feet.[35–37] The author therefore urgently advises any surgeon to study the treatment principles before rushing into surgical adventures.

The treatment principles of pediatric neuromuscular foot deformities may be summarized as follows[5,11,16,17,20]:

- Correction of any existing and functionally restricting deformity
- Eliminating or reducing pain and pressure sores
- Balancing of any muscle imbalance
- Stabilizing joints that are deformed and/or cannot be stabilized voluntarily
- Improving or at least preserving muscle power
- Reestablishing and retaining important joint mobility for walking (eg, ankle joint; metatarso-phalangeal [MTP] joints)

(NOTE: Muscular weakness is a peculiar feature of nearly all neurogenic and neuromuscular disorders. This must always be kept in mind especially when muscle weakening procedures are contemplated.)

Management plans of neurologic pediatric foot deformities can be subdivided divided into the following:

- Conservative treatments
- Conservative plus surgery
- Surgery alone
- Soft tissue surgery
- Bony surgery
- Combinations of surgical techniques

All these methods and their combinations have their indications and contraindications.[4] They are only rarely interchangeable. The author summarizes the methods and their advantages and disadvantages as follows[15,17,38]:

Conservative Treatments

Physiotherapy, manual mobilizations, neurodevelopmental techniques, massage, applications of hot and cold packs, orthotics, special shoe wear, and medications. **Fig. 10** provides an example.

All these methods can be used either in isolation or in combination. The indications are passively correctable deformities with no or little tendency to deteriorate, good acceptance of these techniques, and knowledgeable experience to administer. The imminent risk for deterioration makes compliance and regular follow-ups quite important.[24,29,39]

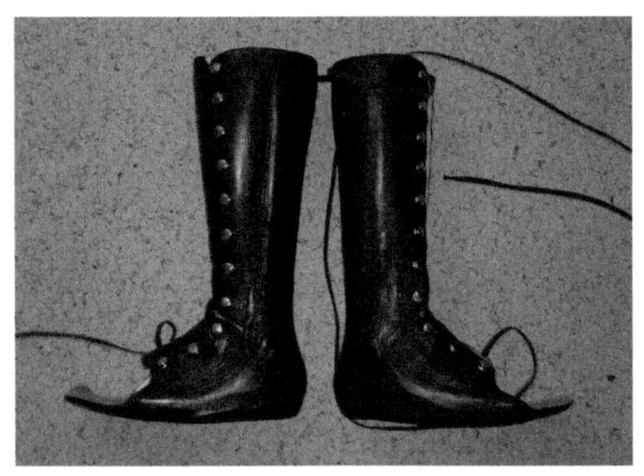

Fig. 10. Conservative measures include orthotics. Stiff orthoses are only indicated in advanced deformities because they further promote weakness. Therefore, articulated designs should be preferred if feasible.

Conservative Plus Surgery

This combination is the most often used procedure in pediatric neurologic deformities. **Fig. 11** shows an example of a combined surgical-orthotic solution. Any successful surgical result may fade because of a progressive underlying disorder or because of growth effects. The author therefore recommends protecting every surgical result by adequate orthotics during the growth period.[17,37,40]

Surgery Alone

This option is justified if the patient is toward the end of his growth, if the underlying disorder is controllable, and if adequate bony surgery has produced a stable plantigrade foot.[41,42] **Figs. 12** and **13** show an indication for bony reconstructive surgery.

Soft Tissue Surgery

Soft tissue surgery is either performed in isolation or more often combined with bony procedures. Any joint deformity that is caused by a muscle imbalance will recur if the muscular problem is not respected.[17,32] Isolated soft tissue surgery is only appropriate if the deformity is flexible or muscular balance surgery enables full correction. Protective orthotics are advisable following most soft tissue surgeries.[25,37]

Bony Surgery

The main question in osseous procedures is always: to fuse and correct or only to correct[17]? Although this question cannot be answered in a generalized manner, the following tips should be observed:

- Osteotomy only if adequate and strong enough voluntary motor function is present.[1,27,40]
- Fusion if complexity of the deformity exceeds your patient's capabilities (simplify motion; J.R. Gage, personal communication, 2004) or if there are not adequate muscle functions or severe structural joint deformities or instabilities.[43–45]

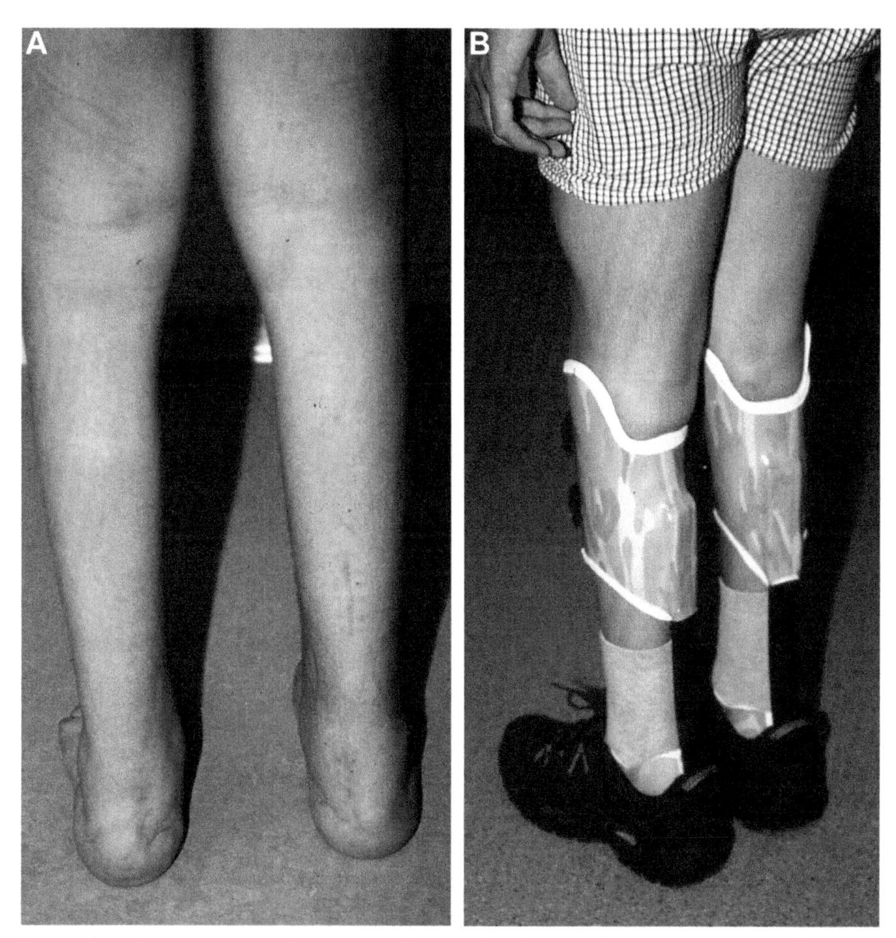

Fig. 11. (*A*, *B*) An example of a combined surgical-orthotic solution: a 12-year-old boy with spina bifida level L5 after bony correction of calcaneovalgus feet; dynamic AFOs are required postoperatively.

Remember J.E. Omer's advice: "Simplicity is the key to success: complexity invites failure."[46]

The author would rather tend to fuse, even at a younger age, but never the ankle or the MTP joint line, if this is in question.

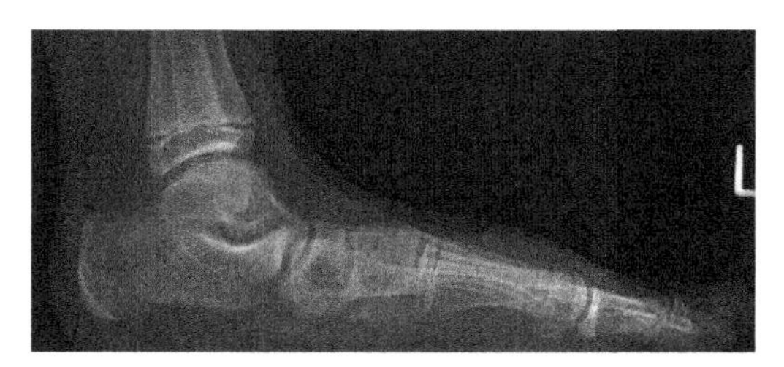

Fig. 12. Indication for bony surgery in unstable flatfeet in a girl with a psychomotor deficit.

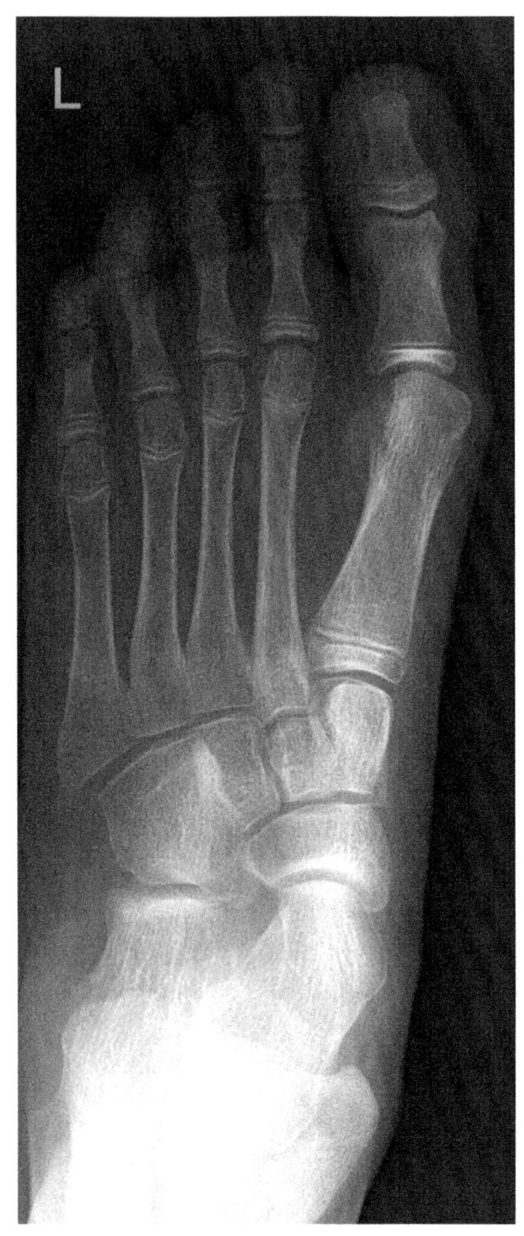

Fig. 13. Indication for bony surgery in unstable flatfeet in a girl with a psychomotor deficit.

Remember: Fusion does not need to remove large bone wedges. Any fusion technique should disintegrate the involved bones and put them together in an anatomically correct fashion.

But: No matter whether fusions or osteotomies are undertaken, any muscular imbalances must always be corrected as well.[17,47]

Some Technical Aspects

Orthotics and pediatric foot deformities

An AFO is the foremost orthotic. In every sagittal deformity (equinus or calcaneus), orthotic ankle joints with adequate joint stops are recommended[15,36]:

- Calcaneus deformity → ankle dorsiflexion stop
- Equinus deformity → ankle plantarflexion stop
- Drop foot deformity → ankle dorsiflexion spring assist

The author recommends the subtalar joint and the forefoot be placed in a custom-molded circular embracing fashion with the forefoot-hindfoot twist = hindfoot inverted and forefoot pronated.

Surgical Technical Pearls in Pediatric Foot Conditions

- Delicate soft tissue handling is recommended, especially of the skin (skin stitches instead of retracting hooks).[16,17]
- Avoid tension on the skin edges at all costs.
- atraumatic technique, including frequent irrigation.
- A tourniquet is not always recommended, especially in delicate paralytic tissues.[1,40]
- Bony surgery should be length preserving without larger bone resections.
- Larger bone wedge resections can be replaced by generously mobilizing the affected joints and rearranging them an anatomically correct position.
- Bony fixation needs rarely more than just a few K-wires.[32,40,48]
- Plates and screws may only be necessary in flatfoot reconstructions.[49,50]
- Children relearn tendon transfers much easier than adolescents or adults do.
- Immobilization should never exceed 6 weeks maximum.[40,41,48]
- Orthotic protection after surgery is mandatory (regularly for 6–9 months in feet at risk until the end of growth).[11,16,32]
- Neuromuscular foot procedures are not rarely associated with proximal surgeries (soft tissue and bone).[6,13,17,37]

Frequently Performed Surgical Procedures in this Patient Group Include the Following:

Soft tissues (**Figs. 14** and **15**)

Soft tissue surgeries comprise muscle, tendon, and musculotendinous lengthenings.

- Elongations of the triceps surae and Achilles tendon complex[51–53]
- Balancing procedures of dorsiflexing and plantarflexing inverting and everting muscles (split or complete tib ant and tib post transfers[54–56])
- Augmentation of weak triceps surae (tendo Achilles shortening and augmentation by tib post, FHL, FDL, PL, or/and PB[36,57])
- Drop foot reconstructions: TP plus FHL transfer, PL and PB transfer, Hibbs and Jones procedures[58]
- Flexor tendon transfers in flexible claw toes D I-V[40,59]

Figs. 16 and **17** provide examples of bony surgery K-wires that are mostly sufficient for intraoperative stabilization.

- Supramalleolar osteotomies (frontal or transverse planes)[11,17]
- Calcaneal shift osteotomies (medially or laterally)[60]
- Subtalar reposition and stabilization (eg, Grice procedure)[45,50]

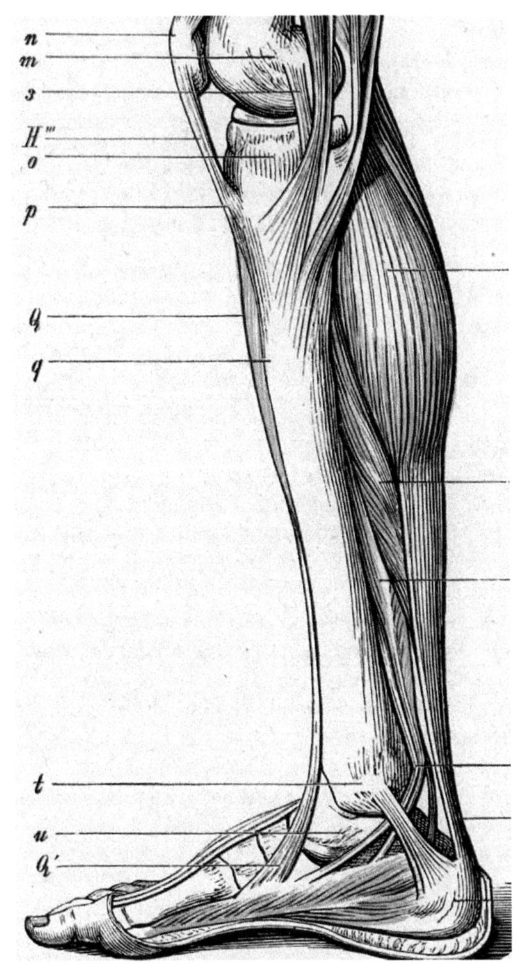

Fig. 14. Soft tissue surgeries comprise muscle lengthenings. In the triceps surae, the proximal intramuscular techniques create less weakness (after Froriep, 1905).

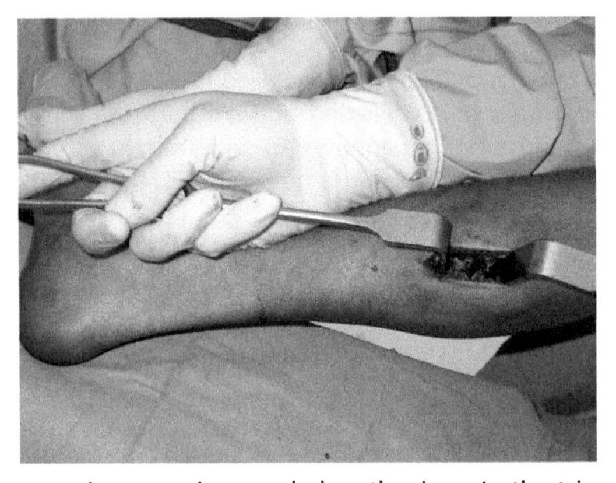

Fig. 15. Soft tissue surgeries comprise muscle lengthenings. In the triceps surae, the proximal intramuscular techniques create less weakness (after Froriep, 1905). Intramuscular aponeurotic tenotomy of gastroc-soleus muscle.

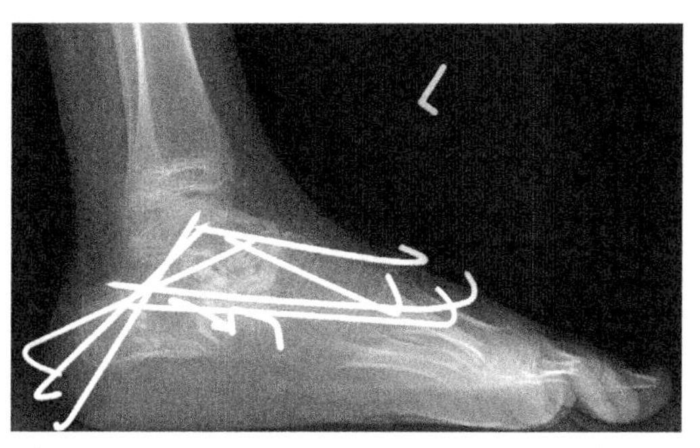

Fig. 16. Examples of bony surgery; K-wires are mostly sufficient for intraoperative stabilization.

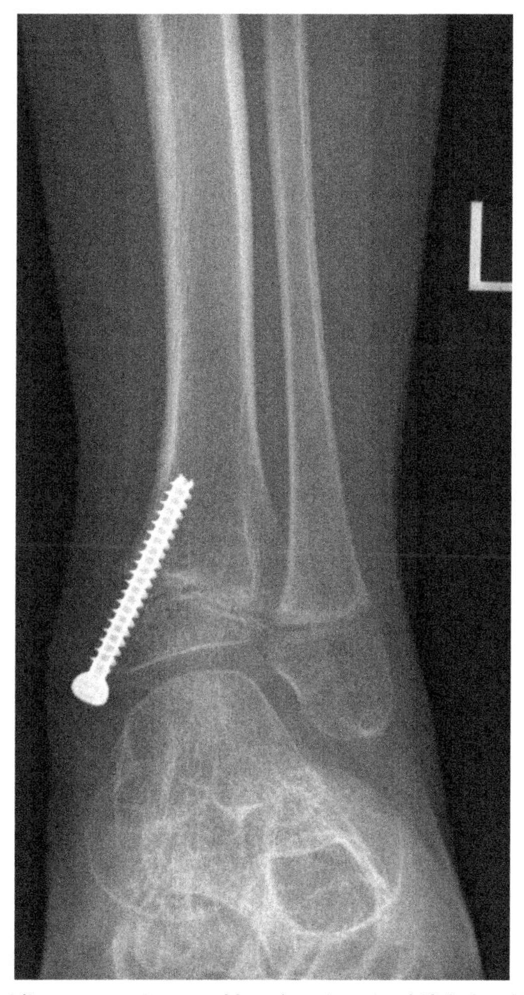

Fig. 17. Growth guiding surgery in an ankle valgus in spina bifida level L5.

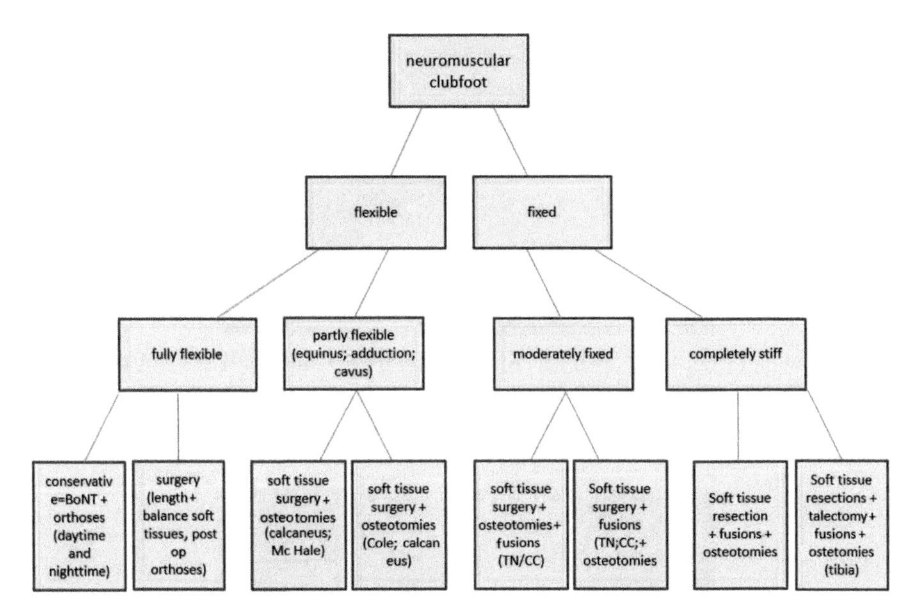

Fig. 18. Management algorithm for a neuromuscular clubfoot deformity. CC, calcaneocuboid; Cole, midtarsal 3D wedge osteotomy; ot, osteotomy; McHale, combined opening wedge med. cuneiform and closing wedge cuboid osteotomy; soft tissue surgery, tendo Achilles/Gastroc/Soleus lengthening; tib post and tib ant elongation or split transfers; Steindler, plantar fasciotomy; posterior capsulotomy of ankle joint; TN, talonavicular.

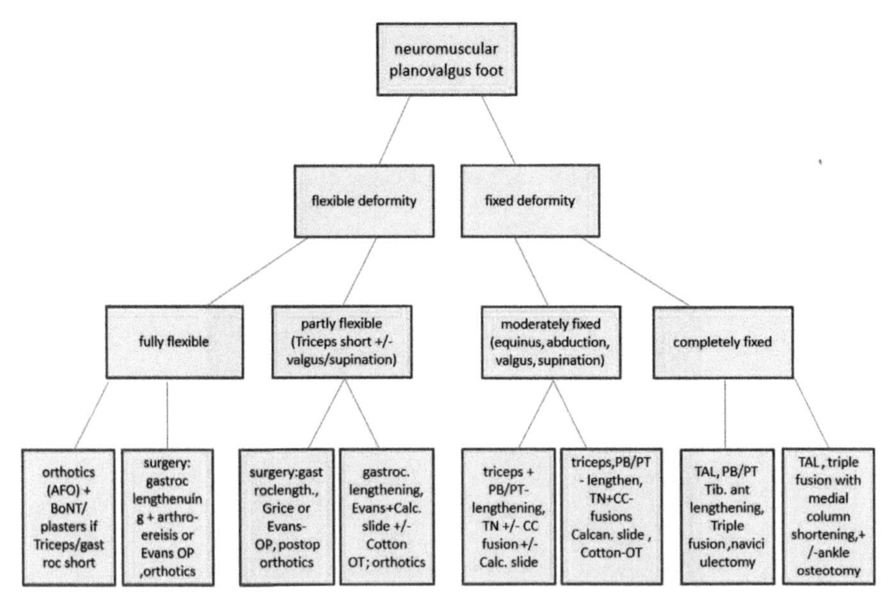

Fig. 19. Management algorithm for neuromuscular planovalgus deformity. Ant., anterior; BoNT, ; calcaneal slide, medial + plantar slide of posterior calcaneus; Cotton, open wedge plantarflexing osteotomy of medial cuneiform; Evans, calcaneal lengthening osteotomy; Grice, extraarticular subtalar fusion; OP, ; PB/PT, peroneus brevis and peroneus tertius; TAL, tendo Achilles lengthening.

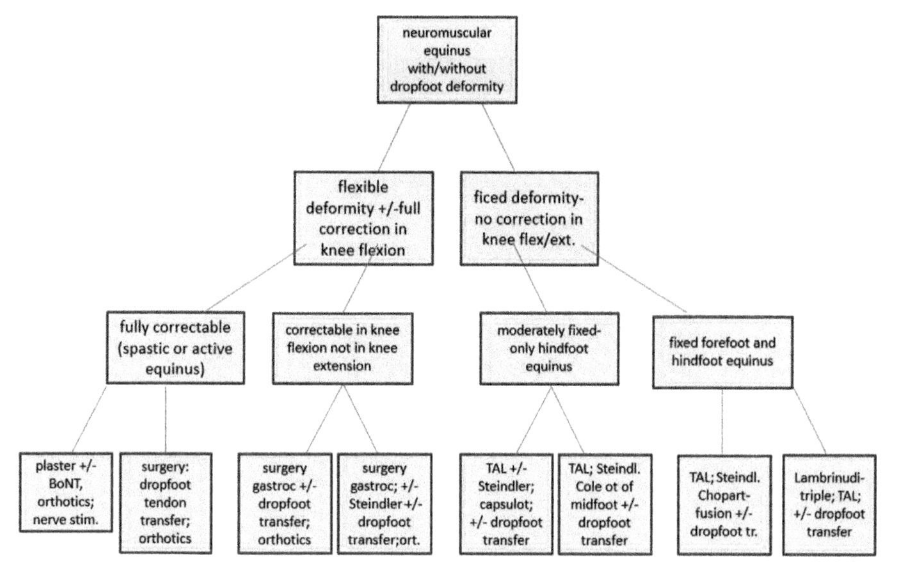

Fig. 20. Management algorithm for neuromuscular equinus/drop foot deformity. Chopart-fusion, talonavicular and calcaneocuboid 3D midtarsal fusion; drop foot transfer; flexor/extensor; TP + FDL transfer or PL transfer to dorsiflexors; nerve stim, peroneal nerve stimulating orthosis; orthotics; Steindler (plantar fascia release); tr., transfer .

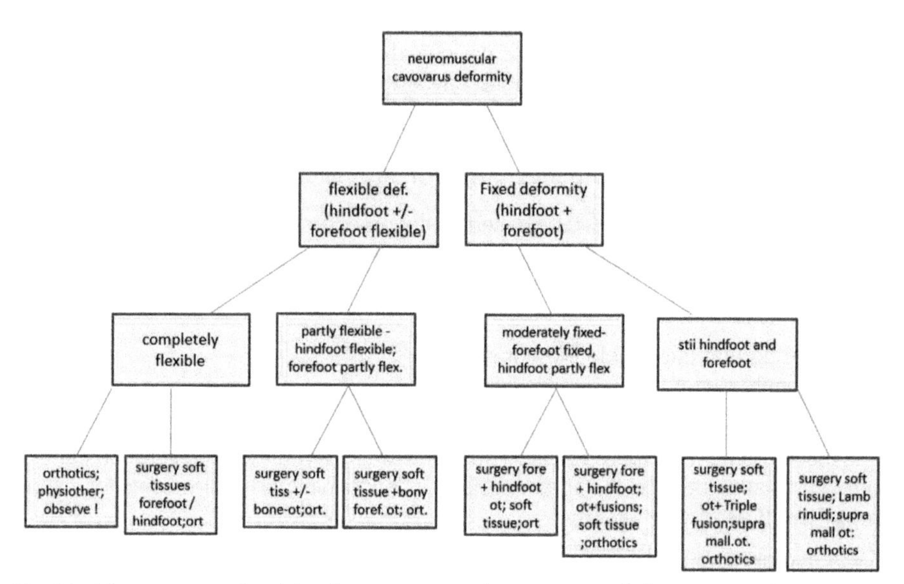

Fig. 21. Management algorithm for neuromuscular cavovarus deformity. Forefoot surgery: Hibbs transfer of extensor digitorum longus tendons to dorsum of the foot; Jones transfer of EHL to MT I; Flexor transfer, transfer of long flexor tendons to base of first phalanx or dorsal extensor hood; forefoot ot, elevating osteotomy of first MT or dorsiflexing ot of med. cuneiform; hindfoot soft tissue procedures = tib. post tendon transfer to dorsiflexors; Steindler plantar fasciotomy; Peroneus longus to brevis tendon transfer; Hindfoot bony procedures: Chopart (TN + CC corrective fusion; calcaneal lateral slide procedure, always together with tarsal tunnel release medially); Lambrinudi triple fusion for equinus component; supramalleolar osteotomy to internally rotate foot complex in external rotation.

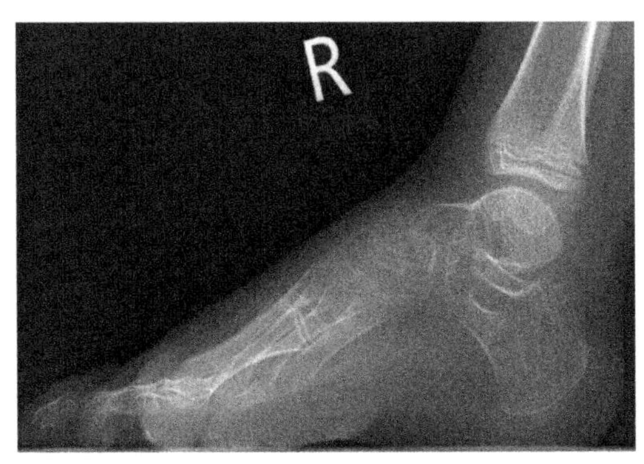

Fig. 22. A severe overcorrection of a paralytic clubfoot in myotonic dystrophy; generous tendo Achilles lengthening led to a calcaneocavus deformity, which needs another extensive surgery.

- Evans calcaneal lengthening[48,61]
- Chopart/midfoot-joint triplane fusion[40,62]
- Midtarsal wedge osteotomy (Cole)[27,40]
- Naviculo-cuneiform corrective fusion (Lichtblau operation [OP])[17]
- Temporary epiphyeodesis at ankle, medially or ventrally[63]
- Talectomy and calcaneo-cuboid (CC) fusion in severe neurogenic clubfeet[64,65]

In the algorithms (**Figs. 18–21**), the author gives a few therapeutic algorithms for the most common neurogenic/neuromuscular pediatric foot deformities, which are clubfoot, planovalgus foot, equinus foot, and cavus foot.

TREATMENT EVALUATION, EVIDENCE, AND CONTROVERSIES

Any treatment evaluation should be based on the preoperative findings and on the previously defined realistic treatment goals.[66,67] A clear description of the basic prerequisites for an acceptable surgical result for a paralytic foot deformity has been given by Joseph[4]:

- A plantigrade and stable foot for stance
- Adequate foot and toe dorsiflexion during swing
- Facilitating a strong pushoff

As these points refer more to (near) normal feet and even the best surgeon cannot correct persisting deficits, the author prefers to define minimal requirements for a successful result as follows:

- A straight and plantigrade foot with adequate stability
- Which is oriented with a correct line of progression
- No plantar pressure points
- No pain
- Adequate shape to wear normal or adjusted shoes or (sometimes) orthoses
- Adequate mobility of major joints (especially ankle and MTP line)
- Patient and parents satisfied with the result

In recent years, there has been a shift from simply estimating the local result of the surgery toward evaluating the outcome with its impact on activity and participation.

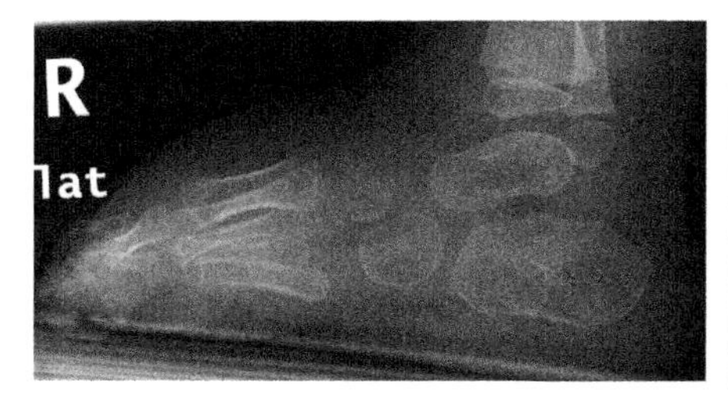

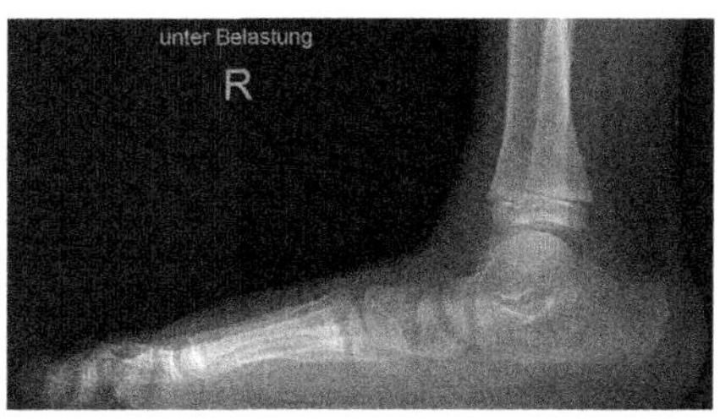

Fig. 23. Spontaneous improvement of a severe paralytic clubfoot. Through the use of orthotics and the impact of body weight on the foot, the deformity spontaneously overcorrected into valgus after 3 years. Regular follow ups are necessary in most neuromuscular conditions.

Simply creating a plantigrade foot is of course only one of the treatment goals, but incorporating the surgical result into the patient's individual life makes the difference.[26]

Considering the treatment results, the author should always incorporate the local result into everyday life.[26,67]

In growing patients, short- and midterm results do not give the complete information. Only if growth is completed can the result be regarded as definitive.[17,47]

> Of course, a plantigrade foot can only be achieved if the leg upon it is straight and correctly aligned. If this is not the case, the appropriate joint alignment must be achieved before or together with any foot surgery. This basic principle should never be violated.[4,17]

RECOGNIZING PROBLEMS AND TROUBLESHOOTING

Problems that occur after surgical management of neurologic pediatric foot deformities are by no means rare.[54,68] **Fig. 22** shows a severe overcorrection of a paralytic clubfoot into a calcaneocavus foot. According to the nature of the problems, they may be divided into the following:

- Initial undercorrection = the foot has never been corrected adequately
- Initial overcorrection = the foot has been overcorrected during the time of surgery
- Recurrent deformity after an adequate initial correction
- Secondary overcorrection = gradual worsening after adequate initial correction
- Initial malcorrections ("hell of a foot")
- Combination of undercorrection and overcorrection in the same foot may occur (eg, at forefoot and hindfoot regions)

> Only surgeons who follow their patients will recognize successful cases and failures.

Troubleshooting in Surgical Problems and Failures

- Recurrence: mild = observe; moderate to severe = reoperate
- Initial undercorrection = reoperate
- Initial overcorrection = if significant reoperate
- Secondary overcorrections = observe if progressive reoperate
- Initial malcorrections = reoperate or better refer to a specialist

> When encompassing problems, a wait-and-see and hope-for-the-best attitude is the best way to increase trouble.

Any problem should be identified in time. Here, the author draws attention to the post-operative compartment syndrome after extensive surgical corrections, especially in recurrent clubfoot deformities. Excessive pain, swelling, and skin blisters are signs of suspicion.[68] To detect further problems, the treating surgeon must be able to follow his or her patients at certain (ie, not more than yearly) intervals.

Obvious problems may be visible spontaneously, whereas hidden problems may be found only after standardized questioning and evaluation.

Recognizing a problem merits that the surgeon must be honest to the patient and to himself or herself as well.

In most instances, nothing will be gained from waiting and hoping for spontaneous improvement. Most cases deserve a new surgical concept, which is unfortunately often more extensive than the initial procedure and has less probability for a complete success. This is called "the more and less principle," which means more deformity needs more surgery but with less prospect for success.[11]

In the case of a complex new deformity, it is wise to seek the advice of an expert.[47]

How to proceed with problems and failures after surgery[16,17]:

- Detailed interview of patient and parents concerning the impact of the new problem
- Detailed clinical examination to identify the causative factors
- Standardized radiographic documentation
- Definition of a working diagnosis
- Formulating a treatment plan and considering alternatives
- Carrying out the necessary procedures and aftertreatment
- Evaluation of the result and adjustment of treatment if necessary

SUMMARY AND OUTLOOK

Pediatric neurogenic/neuromuscular foot deformities may occur at any age and with any possible picture and severity. The basic disorder and any remaining growth may constantly change the evolution of the foot. In most instances, the deformity tends to worsen and to stiffen. Therefore, an early workup of the presenting problems is advocated, including consideration of accompanying disorders of the proximal joints and nonorthopedic signs and symptoms. This necessitates a team approach because an isolated management of the foot problem is rarely sufficient. The treatment of the foot deformity must therefore be embedded in a concise treatment plan.

The principles of management of pediatric neurologic foot deformities rest on 5 factors:

- Full correction of the existing deformity
- Stabilization of unstable, severely deformed, or actively not controllable joints
- Balance of every deforming muscle imbalance
- Improvement of weakness and preservation of muscle power
- Retention of functionally important joint mobility

Indications for treatment may have preventive, therapeutic, or palliative goals. Orthotic protection will often remain necessary despite successful surgery. Consideration of any accompanying involvement of the proximal or contralateral joints is as important as regular follow-ups at least until the end of growth because new problems may always occur. **Fig. 23** show spontaneous improvement of a severe paralytic club-foot through the use of orthoses.

Management of unexpected postoperative problems will mostly necessitate new surgery, which often is more challenging than the initial one. Advice of an expert is recommended in doubtful cases.

There might be an optimistic view toward artificial intelligence because estimating a multitude of signs and symptoms and integrating them in a diagnostic and targeted therapeutic plan might be greatly improved.

Collecting patient data among different centers, especially for rare disorders, will enhance the care of patients. For further development of diagnostic and treatment algorithms, expert panels may be helpful.

MANAGEMENT ALGORITHMS

The following management algorithms are supplemental to the sections above. They should be used to facilitate decision making; however, each case must be viewed individually. Consider the following common neurologic foot deformities that frequently occur in childhood.

CLINICS CARE POINTS

Pearls

- Make sure that the foot deformity has a neurologic cause by successfully testing motor functions, sensibility, and reflexes.
- Always look for associated deficits at the proximal and contralateral joints.
- Treatment should be performed in the following order:
- Correction of any limiting deformity
- Stabilization of any deformed or unstable or voluntarily not controllable joint
- Balance of muscular imbalances
- Preservation of joint mobility and muscle power
- Treatment is mostly a combination of surgery plus conservative measures, including orthoses.

Pitfalls

- Correction without respecting muscular imbalance will lead to recurrence.
- Deformity correction precedes any muscle balancing procedure.
- Always correct accompanying proximal deformities simultaneously, or in advance orthotics are necessary postoperatively.
- Regular follow-ups until the end of growth will help to avoid failures.

DISCLOSURE

The author states that there are no conflicts of interest.

REFERENCES

1. Dimeglio A, Florensa G. Concepts de base dans le traitement du pied paralytique de l'enfant. In: Claustre J, Sinmon L (eds). Pied neurologique, trophique et vasculaire. Masson: Paris; 1984. pp. 21–34.
2. Döderlein L. Prinzipien der Behandlung schlaffer Lähmungen. Orthopäde 2014; 43:611–24.

3. Georgopoulos G. Myelomeningocele. In: Mc Carthy JJ, Drennan JC, editors. Drennan's the child's foot and ankle. Philadelphia: Wolters Kluwer; 2010. p. 219–29.
4. Joseph B. General principles of management of lower motor neuron paralysis. In: Joseph B, Nayagam S, Loder RT, et al, editors. Paediatric orthopaedics-a system of decision making. London: Hodder-Arnold; 2009. p. 363–77.
5. Joseph B. The paralysed foot and ankle. In: Joseph B, Nayagam S, Loder RT, et al, editors. Paediatric orthopaedics-a system of decision making. London: Hodder-Arnold; 2009. p. 378–85.
6. Graham HK. Mechanisms of deformity. In: Crutton D, Damiano D, Mayston M, editors. Management of the motor disorders of children with cerebral palsy; Clinics in developmental medicine no 161. 2nd edition. London: Mc Keith press; 2004. p. 105–29.
7. Pourmand R. Neuromuscular diseases-expert clinicians'views. Boston: Butterworth-Heinemann; 2001. p. 1–50.
8. Shapiro F, Bresnan MJ. Orthopaedic management of childhood neuromuscular disease-part 2—peripheral neuropathies, Friedreich's ataxia and arthrogryposis. J Bone Joint Surg 1982;64-A(6):949–53.
9. Shapiro F, Bresnan MJ. Orthopaedic management of childhood neuromuscular disease—part 3—diseases of muscle. J Bone Joint Surg 1982;64-A(7):1102–7.
10. Schafer MF, Dias LS. Myelomeningocele-orthopaedic treatment. Baltimore: Williams &Wilkins; 1983. p. 160–213.
11. Döderlein L. Der Fuß bei der Zerebralparese in Döderlein L.: Infantile Zerebralparese. Heidelberg: Springer; 2015. p. 257–79.
12. Shapiro FBresnan MJ. Orthopaedic management of childhood neuromuscular disease—part 1—spinal muscular atrophy. J Bone Joint Surg 1982;64-A(3): 785–9.
13. Joseph B. General principles of management of upper motor neuron paralyses. In: Joseph B, Nayagam S, Loder RT, et al, editors. Paediatric orthopaedics-a system of decision making. London: Hodder-Arnold; 2009. p. 407–23.
14. Mortier W. Muskel- und Nervenerkrankungen im Kindesalter. Stuttgart: Thieme; 1994. p. 15–47.
15. Lusardi MM, Bowers DM. Orthotics in the management of neuromuscular impairment. In: Lusardi MM, Nielsen CC, editors. Orthotics and prosthetics in rehabilitation. St. Louis: Saunders-Elsevier; 2007. p. 263–331.
16. Davids JR. Biomechanically based clinical decision making in pediatric foot and ankle surgery. In: Sabharwal S, editor. Pediatric lower limb deformities. Heidelberg: Springer; 2016. p. 153.
17. Mosca VS. Principles and management of pediatric foot and ankle deformities and malformations. Philadelphia: Wolters Kluwer; 2014.
18. Staheli LT, Hall JG, Jaffe KM, et al. Arthrogryposis. Cambridge: Cambridge University Press; 1998. p. 67–73.
19. Moroney PJ, Fogarty EE, Kelly PM. A single center prospective evaluation of the Ponseti method in non idiopathic congenital talipes equinovarus. J Pediatr Orthop 2012;32:636.
20. Joseph B. The spastic foot and ankle. In: Joseph B, Nayagam S, Loder RT, et al, editors. Paediatric orthopaedics-a system of decision making. London: Hodder-Arnold; 2009. p. 412–23.
21. Schrantz WF. Arthrogryposis. In: Mc Carthy JJ, Drennan JC, editors. Drennan's the child's foot and ankle. Philadelphia: Wolters Kluwer; 2010. p. 247–60.

22. Van Bosse HJ. Syndromic feet: arthrogryposis and myelomeningocele. Foot Ankle Clin 2015;20:619–44.
23. Dimeglio A, Florensa G. Le pied du dysraphisme. In: Claustre J, Sinmon L, editors. Pied neurologique, trophique et vasculaire. Paris: Masson; 1984. p. 102–7.
24. Ries AN, Novachek TF, Schwartz MH. The efficacy of ankle foot orthoseson improving the gait of children with diplegic cerebral palsy; a multiple outcome analysis. PM R 2015;7:922–9.
25. Dreher T, Buccoliero T, Wolf SJ, et al. Long-term results after gastrocnemius-soleus intramuscular aponeurotic recession as a part of multilevel surgery in spastic diplegic cerebral palsy. J.Bone Joint Surg 2012;94-A:627–37.
26. Hollenweger J, Kraus de Camargo O. ICF-CY-Internationale Klassifikation der Funktionsfähigkeit,Behindeung und Gesundheit bei Kindern und Jugendlichen. Bern: Hans Huber; 2011.
27. Wicart P. Cavus foot: from neonates to adolescence. Orthop Traumatol Surg Res 2012;98:813–28.
28. Lin RS. Ankle-foot orthoses. In: Lusardi MM, Nielsen CC, editors. Orthotics and prosthetics in rehabilitation. St. Louis: Saunders-EElsevier; 2007. p. 219–36.
29. Milne N, Miao M, Beattie E. The effects of serial casting on lower limb function for children with cerebral palsy: a systematic review with meta-analysis. BMC Pediatr 2020;20:324–47.
30. Bjornson K,, Hays R, Graubert C,, et al. Botulinum neurotoxin for spasticity with cerebral palsy: a comprehensive evaluation. Pediatrics 2007;120:49–58.
31. Bosse HJP, Marangoz S, Lehmann WB, et al. Correction of arthrogrypotic clubfoot with a modified Ponseti technique. Clin Orthop Rel Res 2009;467:1283–93.
32. Döderlein L, Wenz W, Schneider U. Der Klumpfuss. Heidelberg: Springer; 1999.
33. Gerlach DJ, Gurnett CA, Limpaphayom N, et al. Early results of the Ponseti method for the treatment of clubfoot associated with myelomeningocele. Bone Joint Surg 2009;91-A:350–9.
34. Gurnett CA, Boehm S, Connolly A, et al. Impact of congenital talipes equinovarus etiology on treatment outcomes. Dev Med Child Neurol 2008;50:498–502.
35. Borton DC, Walker K, Pirpiris M, et al. Isolated calf lengthening in cerebral palsy-outcome analysis of risk factors. J Bone Joint Surg 2001;83-B(3):364–70.
36. Döderlein L, Wenz W, Schneider U. Der Spitzfuß, der Hackenfuß. Heidelberg: Springer; 2004.
37. Rutz E, McCarthy J, Shore BJ, et al. Indications for gastrocsoleus lengthening in ambulatory children with cerebral palsy; a Delphi consensus study. J Child Orthop 2020;14(5):405–14.
38. Morakis E, Foster A. Evidence-based treatment for feet deformities in children with neuromuscular conditions. In: Alshryda S, Huntley JS, Banaszkiewicz PA, editors. Pediatric orthopaedics; an evidence based approach for clinical questions. Switzerland: Springer; 2017. p. 375–92.
39. Figueiredo EM, Ferreira GB, Maia Moreira RC, et al. Efficacy of ankle foot orthoses on gait of children with cerebral palsy: a systematic review of literature. J Pediatr Phys Ther 2008;20:207–23.
40. Döderlein L, Wenz W, Schneider U. Der Hohlfuss. Heidelberg: Springer; 2001.
41. Dussa C, Doederlein L, Forst R, et al. Management of severe equinovalgus in patients with cerebral palsy by naviculectomy in combination with midfoot arthrodesis. Foot Ankle Int 2017;38(9):1011–9.
42. Hall JE, Calvert PT. Lambrinudi triple arthrodesis:a review with particular reference to the technique of operation. J Pediatr Orthop 1987;7:19–25.

43. Tenuta J, Shelton YA, Miller F. Long term follow up of triple arthrodesis in patients with cerebral palsy. J Pediatr Orthop 1992;13:713–6.
44. Seitz DG, Carpenter EB. Triple artrhrodesis in children-a ten year review. South Med J 1974;67:1420–5.
45. Senaran H, Yilmaz G, Nagai MK, et al. Subtalar fusion in cerebral palsy patients: results of a new technique using corticocancellous allograft. J Pediatr Orthop 2011;31(2):205–10.
46. Omer GE. The palsied hand in C McCollister Evarts: surgery of the musculoskeletal system, vol. 2. New York: Chrurchill Livingstone; 1983. p. 411.
47. Rang M, Silver R, de la Garza J. Cerebral palsy. In: Lovell WW, Winter RB, editors. Pediatric orthopedics, 2.Aufl. Philadelphia: Lippincott; 1986. p. 345–96.
48. Zeifang F, Breusch SJ, Döderlein L, et al. Evans calcaneal lengthening procedure for spastic flexible flatfoot in 32 patients (46 feet). Foot Ankle Int 2006;27(7): 500–7.
49. Döderlein L, Wenz W, Schneider U. Der Knickplattfuß. Heidelberg: Springer; 2002.
50. Kadhim M, Miller F. Pes planovalgus deformity in children with cerebral palsy: review article. J Pediatr Orthop 2014;23 B:400–5.
51. Baumann JU, Koch H. Gventrale aponeurotische Verlängerung des M.Gastrocnemius. Oper Orthop Traumatol 1989;1(4):254–8.
52. Dussa CU, Boehm H, Doederlein L, et al. Is shortening of tibialis anterior in addition to calf muscle lengthening required to improve the active dorsal extension of the ankle joint in patients with cerebral palsy? Gait Posture 2021;83:210–6.
53. Firth GB, Mc Mullan M, Chin T, et al. Lengthening of the gastrocnemius-soleus complex: an anatomical and biomechanical study in human cadavers. J Bone Joint Surg Am 2013;95(16):489–96.
54. Chang CH, Albarracin JP, Lipton GE, et al. Long term follow up of surgery for equinovarus foot deformity in children with cerebral palsy. J Ped Orthop 2002; 22:792–9.
55. Scott AC, Scarborough N. The use of dynamic EMG in predicting the outcome of split posterior tibial tendon transfers in spastic hemiplegia. J Pediatr Orthop 2006;26:777–80.
56. Vlachou M, Beris A, Dimitriadis D. Split tibialis posterior tendon transfer for correction of spastic equinovarus hindfoot deformity. Acta Orthop Belg 2010; 76:651–7.
57. Park KB, Park HW, Joo SY, et al. Surgical treatment of calcaneal deformity in a select group of patients with myelomeningocele. J.Bone Joint Surg 2008;90A: 2149–59.
58. Birch R. The dropfoot from common peroneal nerve palsy. In: Birch R, editor. Surgical disorders of the peripheral nerves. London: Springer; 2011. p. 598–605.
59. Hossain M, Huntley JS. Evidence based treatment for pes cavus. In: Alshryda S, Huntley JS, Banaszkiewicz PA, editors. Paediatric orthopaecdics-An evidence based approach to clinical questions. New York: Springer; 2017. p. 183–92.
60. Torosian CM, Dias LS. Surgical treatment of severe hindfoot valgus by medial displacement osteotomy of the os calcis in children with myelomeningocele. J Pediatr Orthop 2000;20:226–9.
61. Yoo WJ, Chung CY, Choi IH, et al. Calcaneal lengthening for the planovalgus foot deformity in children with cerebral palsy. J Pediatr Orthop 2005;25(6):781–5.
62. Steinhäuser J. Die Arthrodesen der Chopart'schen Gelenklinie;Bücherei des Orthopäden Band 20. Stuttgart: Thieme; 1978.

63. Ebert N, Ballhause M, Babin K, et al. Correction of recurrent equinus deformity in surgically treated clubfeet by anterior distal tibial hemiepiphysiodesis. J Ped Orthop 2020;40(9):520–5.
64. Cassis N, Capdesvila R. Talectomy for clubfoot in arthrogryposis. J Pediatr Orthop 2000;20:652–5.
65. Trumble T, Banta JV, Raycroft JF, et al. Talectomy for equinovarus deformity in myelodysplasia. J Bone Joint Surg 1985;67-A:21–9.
66. Morris C, Doll H, Davies N, et al. The Oxford ankle-foot questionnaire for children: responsiveness and longitudinal validity. Qual Life Res 2009;18:1367–76.
67. Novachek TF, Stout JL, Tervo R, et al. Reliability and validity of the Gillette Functional Assessment Questionnaire as an outcome measure in children with walking disabilities. J Pediatr Orthop 2000;20:75–81.
68. Livingstone K, Glotzbecker M, Miller PE, et al. Pediatric non-fracture acute compartment syndrome, a review of 39 cases. J Pediatr Orthop 2016;36(7):685–90.

The Surgical Treatment of Brachymetatarsia

Hubert O. Klauser, MD

KEYWORDS

- Brachymetatarsia • Callus distraction • Internal fixator • External fixator
- One-stage lengthening

KEY POINTS

- There are 3 operative procedures for the correction of brachymetatarsia.
- The correction of short longitudinal bone defects of a metatarsal bone up to 10 mm can be performed by lengthening osteotomy or interposition of autologous or allogenic bone graft with various surgical techniques.
- The correction of longitudinal bone defects more than 10 mm is ideally performed through distraction osteogenesis using an external fixator or internal titanium minifixator.
- Callus distraction with an internal fixator facilitates length compensation more than 20 mm and results in far fewer complications within 1 year. Postoperative treatment is way more comfortable with early full weight-bearing.
- The internal fixator is suitable for callus distraction of all metatarsal bones and, if necessary, for simultaneous correction of up to 3 metatarsal bones.

INTRODUCTION

Brachymetatarsia is a deformity with a longitudinal defect of one or multiple metatarsal bones.[1,2] It is characterized by short metatarsal bones, clinically resulting in an apparent ray truncation, which usually is not visible in newborns and becomes visible between the age of 3 and 5 years (**Fig. 1**).[3,4] This pathology is either congenital or acquired. The congenital or idiopathic form is caused by a premature fusion of the epiphyseal plate (**Fig. 2**).[5,6] The acquired one is either post-traumatic or associated with systemic diseases that have an impact on bone metabolism. Association with syndromes such as Turner syndrome, Down's syndrome, pseudohypoparathyroidism, poliomyelitis, multiple epiphyseal dysplasia, Larsen syndrome, and Albright osteodystrophy has to be mentioned as well.[4,5,7] Brachymetatarsia is present if the distance between the affected metatarsal bone and the metatarsal parabola is more than 5 mm

HAND- UND FUSSZENTRUM BERLIN, Schlüterstr. 38, Berlin 10629, Germany
E-mail addresses: sekretariat@hfz-berlin.de; klauser@hfz-berlin.de

Foot Ankle Clin N Am 26 (2021) 685–704
https://doi.org/10.1016/j.fcl.2021.07.003

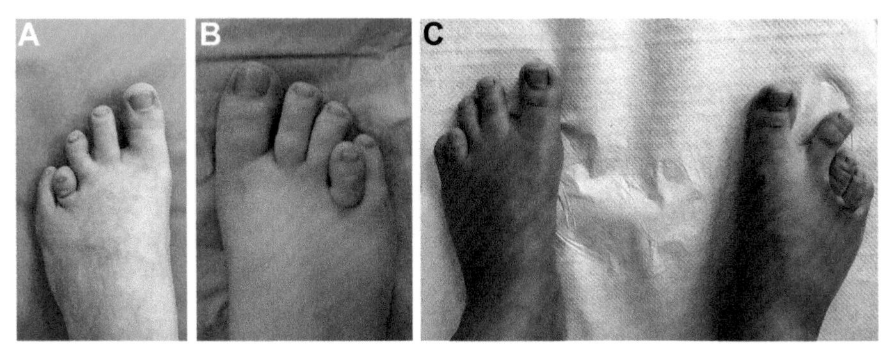

Fig. 1. Brachymetatarsia of the fourth metatarsal bone on an 8-year-old girl left (*A*), on a 10-year-old girl right (*B*), brachymetatarsia of the fourth metatarsal bone left, of the third and fourth metatarsal bone right on a 14-year-old girl (*C*).

(**Fig. 3**). It often occurs bilaterally, can coexist with brachydactyly and short metacarpal bones (brachymetacarpia; see **Fig. 2** and **Fig. 4**).[2,8] The fourth metatarsal bone is most commonly affected as it lies on the phylogenetic and embryogenetic axis, along which the preaxial and postaxial foot structures differentiate in the course of rotation and torsion development of the lower extremity (see **Figs. 1**, **2**, and **4**).[9] At a ratio of 1:25, girls are far more likely to have brachymetatarsia than boys. It can affect all metatarsal bones, whereas multiple metatarsals can be involved either adjacent or nonadjacent (**Figs. 5–7**). The incidence of brachymetatarsia is between 0.02% and 0.05%.[2,4,5,10,11]

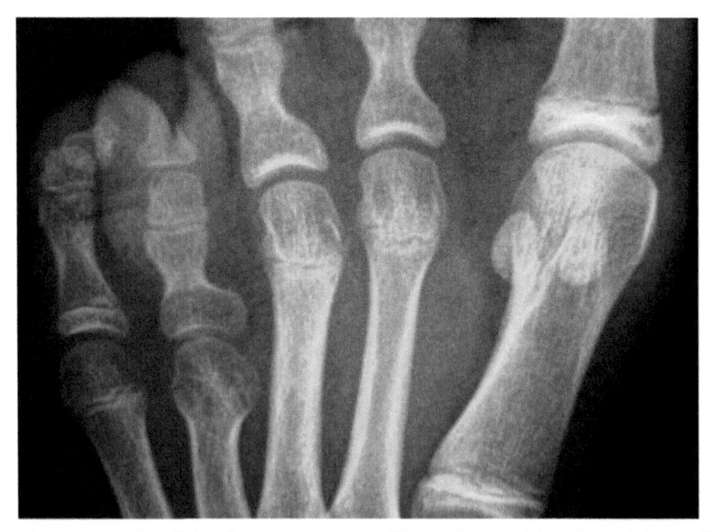

Fig. 2. Brachymetatarsia of the fourth metatarsal bone in combination with brachydaktyly (brachybasophalangy) of the fourth toe (8-year-old female). The growth plate of the fourth metatarsal bone is closed in contrast to the other bones.

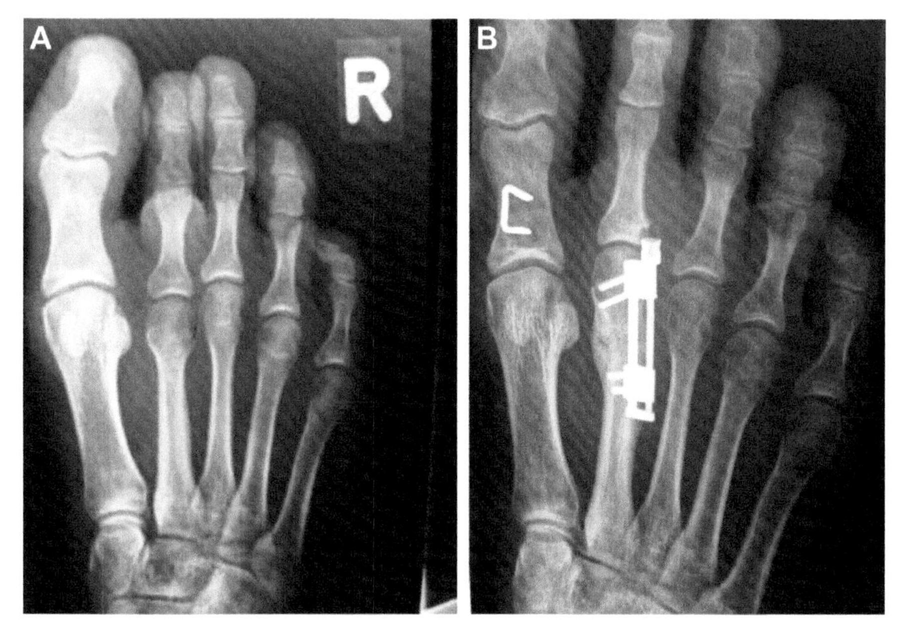

Fig. 3. A short metatarsal bone or borderline brachymetatarsia of the second metatarsal bone (*A*) and the reconstruction using an internal fixator on an 11-year-old female patient (*B*).

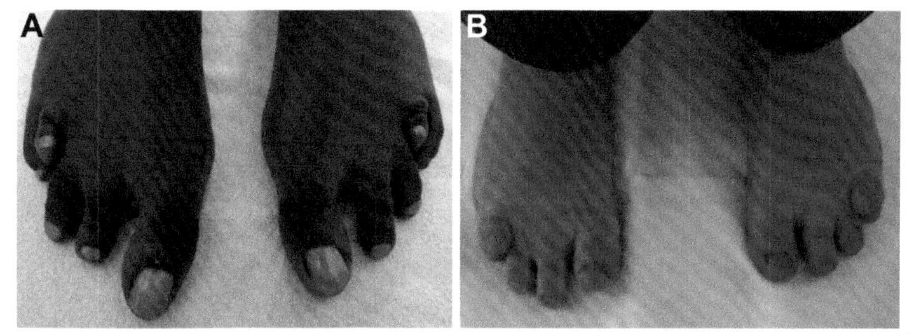

Fig. 4. Bilateral brachymetatarsia of the fourth metatarsal bone on a 15-year-old (*A*) and 9-year-old (*B*) girls.

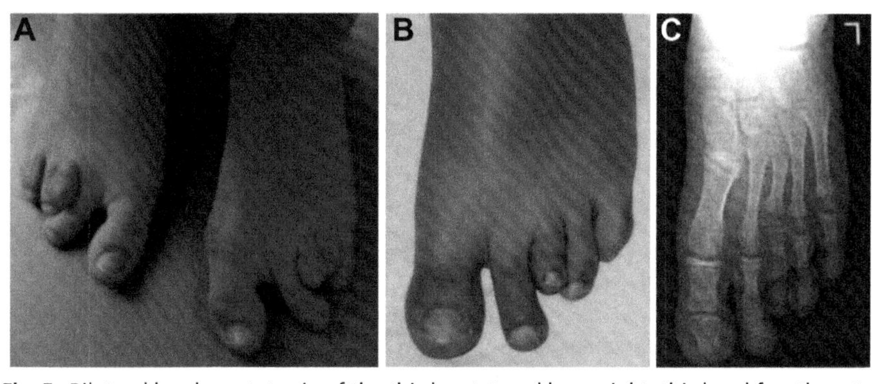

Fig. 5. Bilateral brachymetatarsia of the third metatarsal bone right, third and fourth metatarsal bone left on a 12-year-old girl (*A*), a unilateral brachymetatarsia of the third metatarsal bone on an 8-year-old girl (*B, C*).

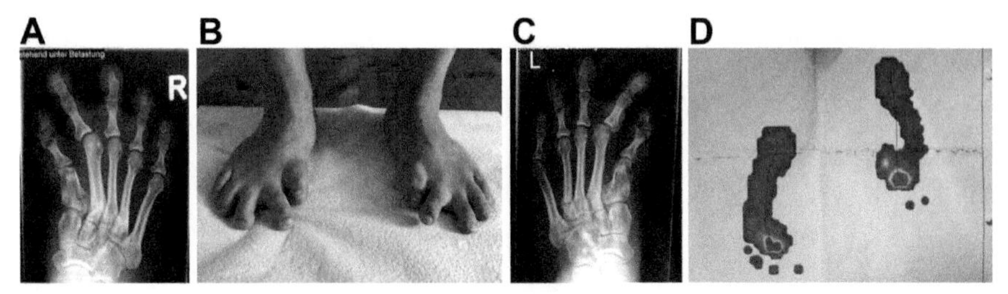

Fig. 6. Bilateral brachymetatarsia of the first metatarsal bones in combination with a macrometatarsia of the second metatarsal bones and brachydactyly of the first toes on a 19-year-old girl (*A–C*), gait analysis of the same patient (*D*).

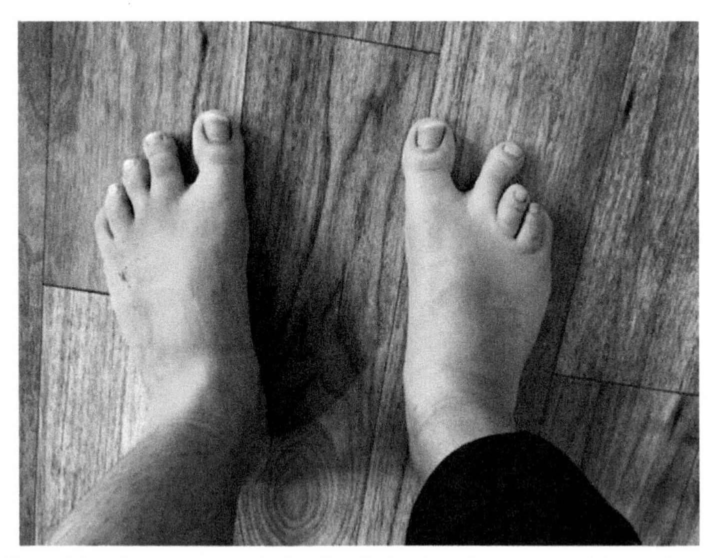

Fig. 7. Bilateral brachymetatarsia, left side of the fourth metatarsal bone (correction by callus distraction with an internal minifixator still in situ), right side of the third and fourth metatarsal bones on a 14-year-old girl.

CLINICAL AND RADIOLOGICAL PRESENTATION

The clinical presentation of brachymetatarsia involves the length of the affected foot ray, which is shortened and often exhibits in a typical elevated position, with a rotation deformity of the toe, as well as brachydactyly, which makes the toe appear misshapen with increased dorsal soft tissue wrinkling.[2,8,10,11] If the third or fourth metatarsal bones are affected, the adjacent medial toe is usually showing axis deviation to lateral and the adjacent lateral one a misalignment to medial, the fifth toe is indicating a rotation deformity. The affected toe as a typical sign of brachymetatarsia cannot be seen when observing from a plantar view.[2] In addition, it is not uncommon to see plantar callosity, especially at the level of 2nd and 3rd metatarsal bones as a sign of overload in the case of brachymetatarsia of the fourth metatarsal (**Figs. 8–10**).[2,10,11] This problem can be clearly presented by a pedobarography (see **Figs. 6**, **9**, and **10**).[2] The severity of the clinical presentation and secondary changes of the foot varies widely and depends on the age of the child or adolescent as well as on the extent of the deformity. For example, the involvement of the first metatarsal bone is very adverse not only for the foot itself but also for the entire affected lower extremity. Overload or even insufficiency of the medial column lead to hallux valgus deformities and transfer metatarsalgia from the second through fourth metatarsals as well as to hindfoot and genu valgum deformity as a result of the significant disorder in proprioception (see **Figs. 9** and **10**).[2,10–12]

In the radiological presentation, the metatarsal bone results were too short showing a bright area throughout the entire head of the metatarsal compared with the other metatarsals as a sign of reduced mineral content. This radiological phenomenon of the altered trabecular structure and lower density is considered as a result of low stress on the affected ray and pathologic alignment of the metatarsals to each other.[2] In accordance with the etiology of the diseases, the epiphyseal plate compared to the other metatarsal bones is not visible, as it stops growing prematurely (see **Fig. 2**, **Fig. 11**).[2,3,8,10,11] Consequently, this primary, congenital, longitudinal defect becomes clinically visible from about 4 years of age.[4,6,8,11] Hypoplasia—micrometatarsia—of the entire affected metatarsal bone may additionally be present.[2]

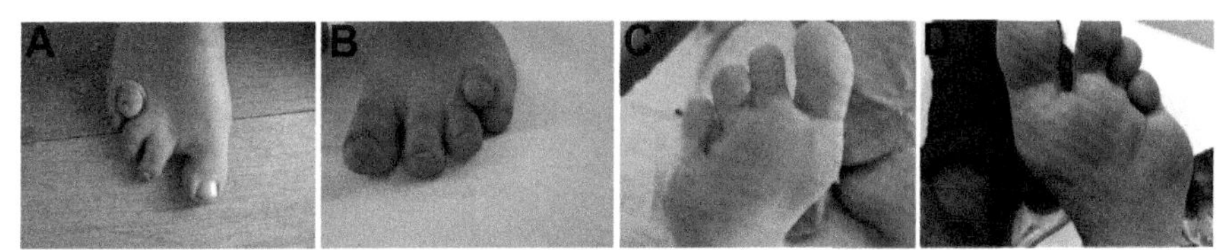

Fig. 8. Brachymetatarsia of the fourth metatarsal bone with typical characters of shortening, dorsal extension, rotation and wrinkling of the affected toe, axis deviation, and malrotation of the adjacent toes medial and lateral side (*A*, *B*), plantar callosity (*C*, *D*).

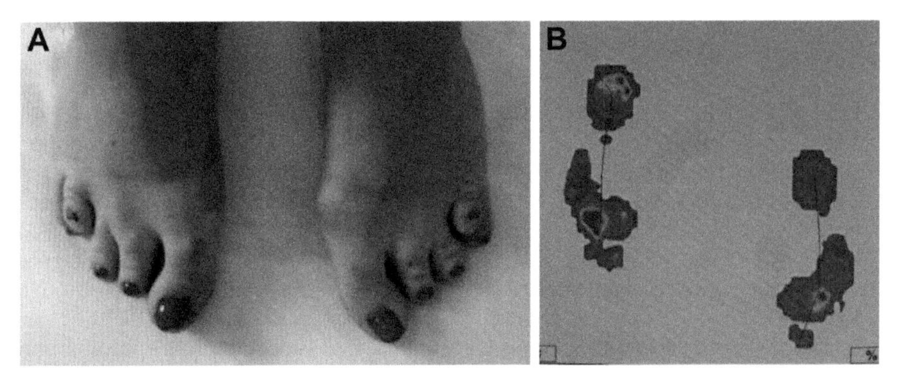

Fig. 9. Bilateral brachymetatarsia of the fourth metatarsal bones with secondary hallux valgus deformity left more than right (*A*) and in the gait analysis an overload of the second and third metatarsal head right more than left on a 21-year-old girl (*B*).

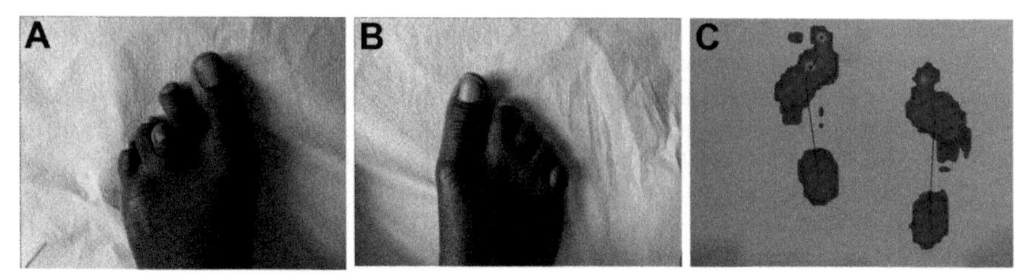

Fig. 10. Brachymetatarsia of the third metatarsal bone left side (*A*) with a secondary hallux valgus deformity compared to the right side (*A, B*) and an overload of the second metatarsal head in the gait analysis (*C*).

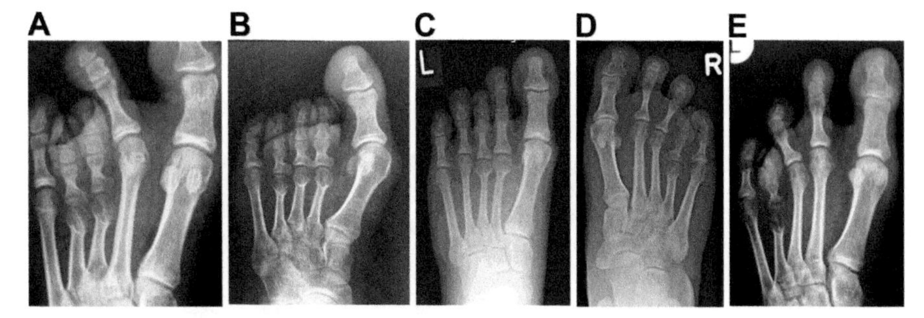

Fig. 11. Typical radiological characters of brachymetatarsia of the third and fourth metatarsal bone on a 12-year-old female patient (*A*), brachymetatarsia of the second, third, and fourth metatarsal bones on a 17-year-old female patient (*B*), brachymetatarsia of the second and third metatarsal bones on a 15-year-old female patient (*C*), brachymetatarsia of the fourth metatarsal bone on a 16-year-old girl (*D*), brachymetatarsia of the fourth metatarsal bone on a 14-year-old girl (*E*).

TREATMENT

Early operative intervention of this congenital defect is desirable. This allows to prevent local secondary changes of the affected foot, but also to avoid proprioception disorders through ascending muscle chains and fascias with secondary changes of the entire locomotor system, especially regarding body posture and physical development of the child and adolescent.[2] Clinical symptoms like metatarsalgia, painful callus formation in the plantar forefoot area, and a conflict of the elevated toes in the shoe are rare. When they occur, causal treatment with the correction of the disrupted anatomic structures is necessary in addition to symptomatic treatment (see **Fig. 8**, **Fig. 12**).[2,4,8,10–13] Conservative treatment options only reduce local symptoms and cannot prevent long-term damages. With regard to the prevention of these problems, an early reconstruction of the metatarsal parabola around the age of 10 years is appropriate.[2,6]

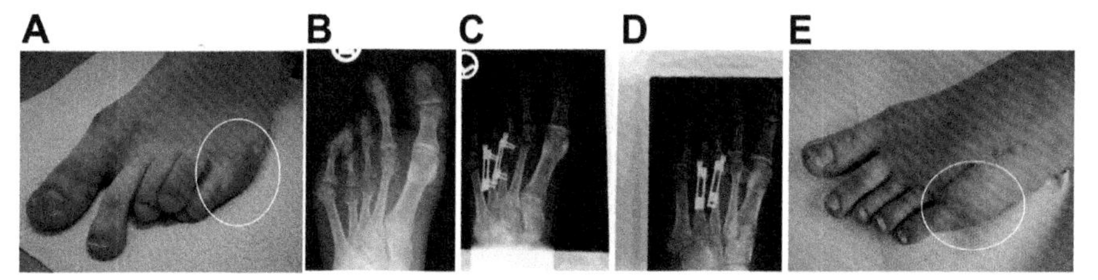

Fig. 12. Painful callosity of the fifth metatarsophalangeal joint lateral with a secondary malrotation of the fifth toe on a 14-year-old boy (*A, B*) and the result after callus distraction of the third and fourth metatarsal bones using 2 internal fixators for callus distraction (*C–E*).

SURGICAL TREATMENT

There are 3 main operative techniques for the surgical correction of brachymetatarsia: lengthening osteotomy, lengthening with interposition of bone graft, and callus distraction.[14] Lengthening osteotomy and lengthening by bone graft interposition are suitable for defects up to 10 mm (**Fig. 13**).[8,10–15] Both procedures are referred to as one-stage lengthening or single-step lengthening. The benefit of these 2 operative techniques is the immediate length compensation resulting in an instant reconstruction of the metatarsal parabola in one step.[14–17] The disadvantage, when using an autologous bone graft, may be related to the donor site morbidity. In this case, the problem can be avoided by performing surgery with an allogenic bone graft.[14,16,18] The high tension force of the bones and soft tissues, especially in adolescent patients, makes the choice of the target length of the interposition bone graft as well as the intraoperative lengthening of the bone itself a further challenge. Consequently, a complete intraoperative correction of the length of the metatarsal bone is not always achievable. Fixation of the bone graft by a plate osteosynthesis or intramedullary K-wire is performed during surgery but there are other surgery-related risks. Pseudoarthrosis and dorsal, plantar, medial, or lateral deviation of the toe can occur because of the very high and immediate compression on the metatarsophalangeal

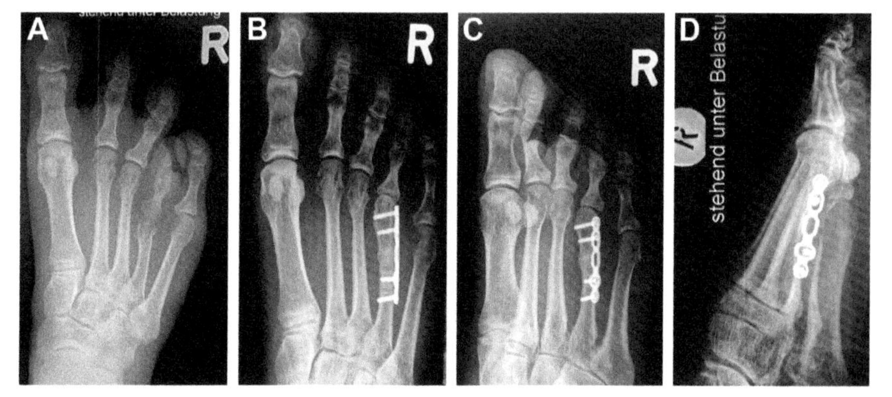

Fig. 13. Interposition of tricortical crest graft and fixation by one-stage lengthening with a locking plate for reconstruction of the metatarsal parabola arch and correction of brachymetatarsia of the fourth metatarsal bone on a 17-year-old girl (*A–D*).

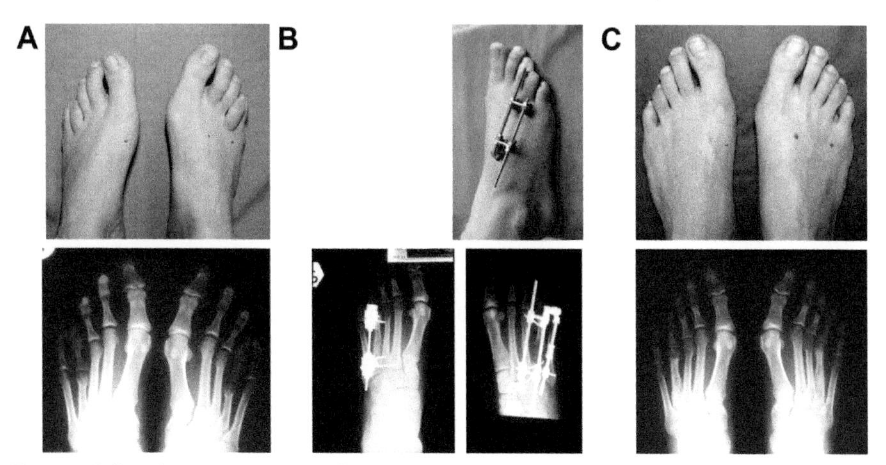

Fig. 14. Callus distraction using different external fixator for correction of bilateral brachymetatarsia of the fourth metatarsal bone on a 17-year-old female. Clinical and radiological course. Preoperative situation (*A*), during the callus distraction (*B*) and the result (*C*). Case from A. Kirienko, Milan, Italy.

joint.[19,20] Pseudoarthrosis is mostly caused by an osteotomy of the short metatarsal bone in the diaphyseal area, and due to the occurrence of osseous circulatory disorders on bone fragments caused by inserting of the graft.[21] Additional soft tissue corrections, especially the extensor tendon lengthening and the arthrolysis of the metatarsophalangeal joint, are regularly necessary during the bone graft interposition to avoid axis deviation of the toe.[10,11,17] To a lesser extent, this also applies to a lengthening osteotomy.[14,16,20] If the brachymetatarsia is accompanied by rare hypoplasia of the affected metatarsal bone, additional bone graft apposition is required for this correction process.[14]

The benefit of the callus distraction as per the principles of Ilizarov is the gentle and gradual lengthening of the metatarsal bone as well as of the soft tissue structures like

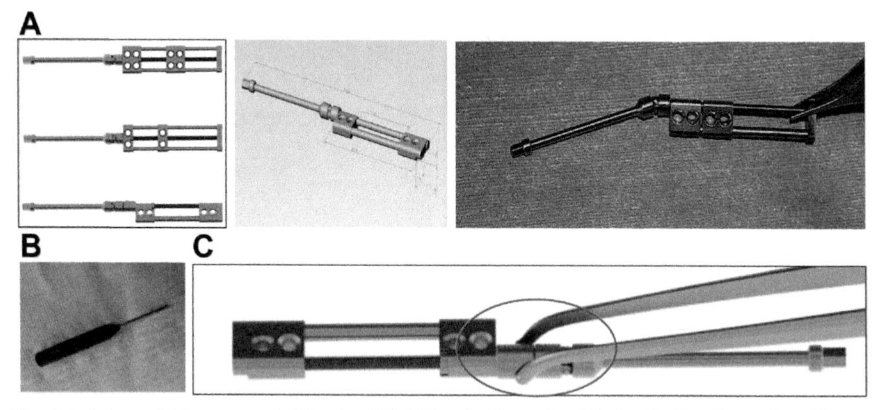

Fig. 15. Internal titanium minifixator (KLS Martin Group) with 2 spindles for callus distraction of the second to the fifth metatarsal bones and 3 spindles for metatarsal 1 (*A*), activator driver (*B*), special forceps for removing the activator rod (*C*).

tendons, vessels, and nerves.[22] This procedure can also be referred to as distraction osteogenesis or callotasis and is suitable for bone defects from 10 mm to over 20 mm of all metatarsal bones, especially in children (**Fig. 14**).[2,10,11,23,24] The risk of vessel and nerve damage as well as skin and soft tissue problems with secondary wound healing and circulatory disorders is minimized considerably by gradual lengthening. Another benefit is the exact reconstruction of the metatarsal parabola by target length compensation of the shortened metatarsal bone. However, additional soft tissue corrections are often necessary to avoid axis deviation of the metatarsal and the toes. This is caused by the compression of soft tissue structures and especially of the metatarsophalangeal joint which can result in joint stiffness.[24,25] The disadvantages of the procedure related are the prolonged postoperative process over several months to reach full bone healing, as well as the uncomfortable handling for the patient, especially if the Ilizarov ring fixator or other external fixator systems are used; in fact, they involve a lot of risks and complications during the distraction and remodeling phase until full bone consolidation.[26–30] However, in the last 15 years, with the development of an internal minifixator for callus distraction of metatarsal and metacarpal bones, the complications of external fixator systems have been minimized significantly (**Fig. 15**).[6] The major advantage is the postoperative comfort for children and adolescents during the distraction, neutralization, and remodeling phase, with a total of 3 operations. The significantly improved stability of the callus distraction using a locked angle stable internal minifixator allows postoperatively an early full weight-bearing of the affected lower extremity in a cast or special shoe. Owing to these major innovations and advantages, callus distraction with an internal fixator has been established as an excellent option for the surgical treatment of brachymetatarsia.[2,11] All metatarsal bones and up to 3 metatarsals simultaneously can successfully be reconstructed with the gradual lengthening surgery using an internal fixator (**see Fig. 12, Fig. 16**).[2]

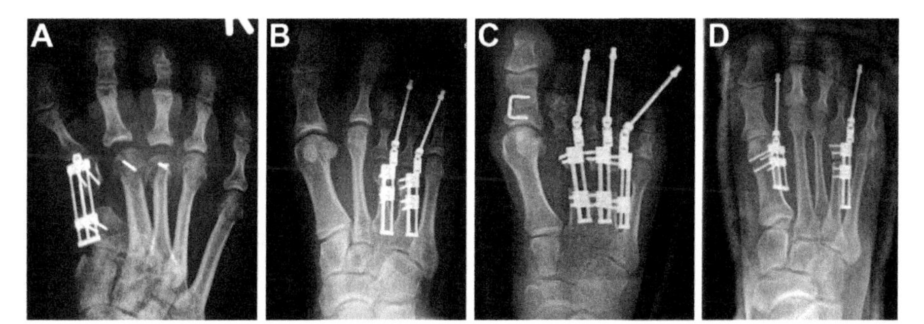

Fig. 16. Correction of brachymetatarsia of the first metatarsal bone (*A*), third and fourth metatarsal bones (*B*), second, third, and fourth metatarsal bones (*C*), first and fourth metatarsal bones (*D*) by gradual lengthening with an internal fixator.

LENGTHENING OSTEOTOMY—ONE-STAGE LENGTHENING

A dorsal approach is used to perform a modified scarf or oblique sliding osteotomy of the affected diaphyseal metatarsal bone. A distraction of the metatarsal bone up to nearly 10 mm is possible with gradual manual traction of the ray, which should be continuously performed not less than 10 minutes and using a bone spreader. Arthrolysis of the metatarsophalangeal joint of the affected ray should be accompanied by a lengthening Z-plasty of the extensor tendon. Tendon lengthening will be stitched following a successful lengthening osteotomy and fixation under correspondingly reduced tension. The apposition of bone graft or cancellous bone graft cubes is recommended to increase the stability of the lengthening osteotomy and minimize the risk of pseudoarthrosis.[14] The osteosynthesis can be fixed with screws or, to make it considerably more stable, with a laterally applied locking plate. Alternatively to autologous bone grafts acquired from the tibial head or the iliac crest, allogenic material can be used to reduce donor-site morbidity.[16] The postoperative aftercare is uncomplicated with an immobilization over 6 weeks, first in a plaster splint for 2 weeks followed by 4 weeks in a postoperative shoe gradually increasing partial weight-bearing. Physiotherapy should start immediately after surgery with traction of the metatarsophalangeal joint and the toe.

LENGTHENING OSTEOTOMY WITH INTERPOSITION OF BONE GRAFT—ONE-STAGE LENGTHENING

After acquiring a tricortical iliac crest graft having the length of the longitudinal bone defect, but not longer than 10 mm, a longitudinal dorsal approach just above the shortened metatarsal is used for the osteotomy in the metadiaphyseal area lateral to the short and long extensor tendon. The previously acquired tricortical iliac crest graft is pressed into the osteotomy gap under continuous traction and simultaneous distraction of the osteotomy with a bone spreader. This process should be carried out during a period of up to 30 minutes as the elasticity of the soft tissue depends on the age of the child or adolescent.[31–33] Different autologous bone grafts from sites such as the calcaneus, fibula, tibia, the proximal phalanx of the adjacent toe or adjacent metatarsal bone are described but the primary donor site is the iliac crest.[34–39] The one-stage lengthening osteotomy can be combined with the truncation of adjacent metatarsals using extracted bone grafts for interposition into the metatarsal bone, which is being distracted for reconstruction of the metatarsal parabola. Removal of bone graft from other locations is not necessary with this procedure.[32] The extensor tendon should be incised in a Z-plasty and then, after inserting the bone graft combined with an arthrolysis of the metatarsophalangeal joint, stitched in the lengthened position to simplify the interposition of the bone graft and to prevent axis deviation of the toe.[10–12,17,33] The graft should be fixed temporarily with an intramedullary K-wire before the final osteosynthesis with a locking plate on the lateral side to make this procedure easier.[4,33] (see **Fig. 13**). Truncation of the interposition bone graft is often necessary, as the desired length cannot always be used due to excessive bone and soft tissue tension. It is described to use an allogenic interposition bone graft or to combine this lengthening technique with a shortening of the adjacent metatarsals because of the donor-side morbidity.[4,17,26] A plaster splint should be modeled postoperatively, followed by a cast after 14 days. Alternatively, in the event of stable osteosynthesis, the patient can be mobilized in a special shoe. Increasing full weight-bearing is allowed after 2 weeks if using a locking plate, intensive physiotherapy should immediately be provided for the affected metatarsophalangeal joint.

CALLUS DISTRACTION WITH AN EXTERNAL FIXATOR—GRADUAL LENGTHENING

This surgical technique starts with a dorsal approach directly above the affected metatarsal bone. The fixator screws are positioned proximally and distally to the planned osteotomy. It is not recommended to apply the fixator screws directly dorsal, as

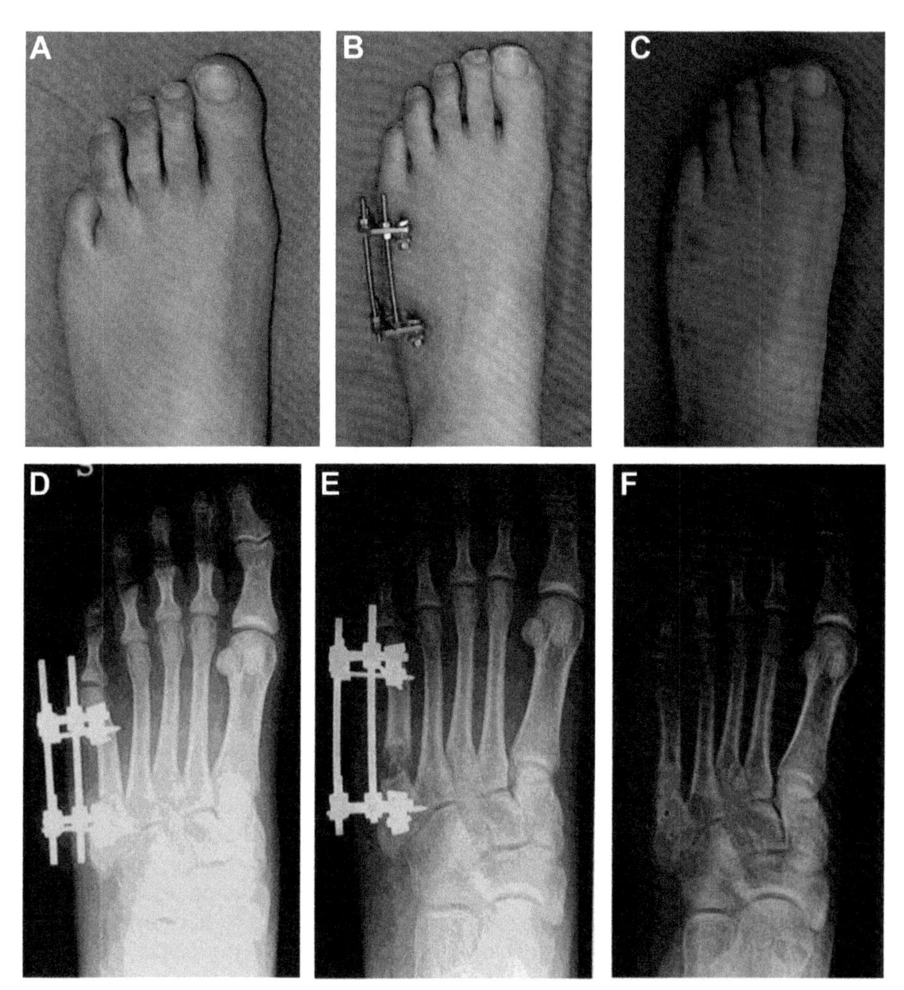

Fig. 17. Callus distraction using an external fixator for correction of brachymetatarsia of the fifth metatarsal bone (19-year-old female). Clinical (*A–C*) and radiological (*D–F*) course. Case from A. Kirienko, Milan, Italy.

you have to consider the oval anatomy of the metatarsal bones. The screws are applied with a slight dorsolateral inclination, which corresponds to the arch of the foot and the metatarsal parabola (see **Fig. 14**, **Fig. 17**).[11,25] Using a monolateral external minifixator entails the application of 2 screws each distally and proximally to the planned osteotomy of the affected metatarsal bone. Therefore, the osteotomy on the shortened metatarsal can only be performed diaphyseal and not metaphyseal, as it would be ideal to prevent pseudoarthrosis.[40] Intraoperative x-ray should be used to check the correct position of the external fixator. The osteotomy is conducted with an oscillating saw and cooling, or with a Gigli saw,[40,41] which is followed by callus distraction (**Fig. 18**).[22] A Z-plasty lengthening of the extensor digitorum tendon and arthrolysis of the metatarsophalangeal joint of the affected ray must be performed after estimating the target length by the push-up and traction test of the affected toe. Callus distraction with an external fixator allows a lengthening of the shortened

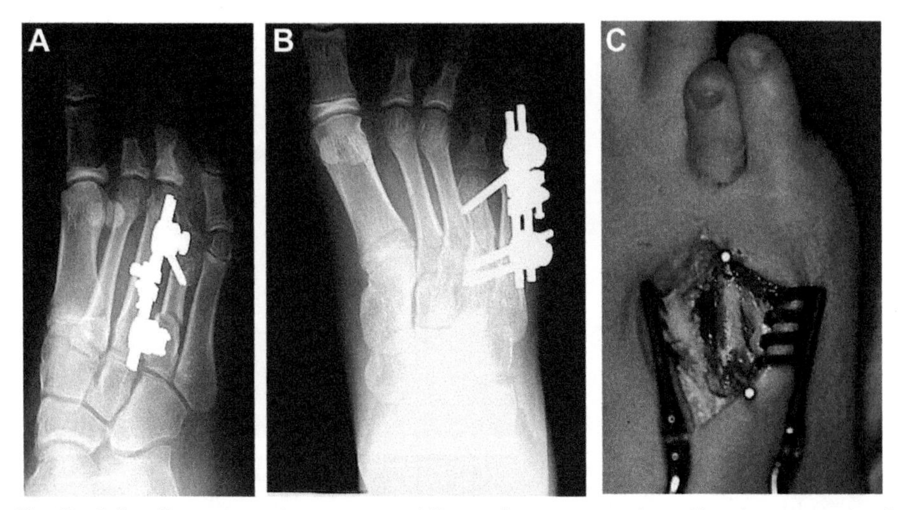

Fig. 18. Callus distraction using an external fixator for reconstruction of brachymetatarsia of the fourth metatarsal bone on a 12-year-old girl. Osteotomy metaphyseal (*A, B*), position of the pins (*C*).

metatarsal bone over 20 mm. It is not uncommon to observe lateral or medial axis deviations of the metatarsal during callus distraction with an external fixator. In literature, the possibility of an additional intramedullary splinting and axis guidance with a 1.5 mm K-wire percutaneously from the tip of the toe to the base of the metatarsal before application of an external fixator is described.[11,20,41,42] A dorsal lower leg plaster splint is applied postoperatively. Wound care and skin incisions along the fixator screws during callus distraction is necessary. After a resting period of 5 days in which the regenerate develops, the distraction osteogenesis begins. The metatarsal is distracted by 0.5 mm or 0.75 mm every day until the metatarsal parabola, and thus the length of the metatarsal bone is reconstructed.[11,41,43] The fixator remains in situ throughout the entire length compensation process, even if the callus distraction has been completed, until full bone consolidation, which may take several months, is reached. Young patients are mobile during the callus distraction and until bone consolidation, after 6 to 8 weeks full weight-bearing is allowed while wearing a cast or special shoe, although the limitations for an implanted external fixator and any additional K-wire throughout this period are significant.[11,25,41] This also concerns the risk of pin infections, soft tissue and skin irritation, and postoperative stiffness of the metatarsophalangeal joint.[19,23–27,42,43] There are various external fixator systems for gradual lengthening, such as the Ilizarov external minifixator, the monolateral external fixator, and the external ring fixator, each having its benefits and disadvantages, whereby the unilateral external minifixator has become more established because of its postoperative comfort (see **Figs. 14**, **17** and **18**).[30,40,41,44–46]

CALLUS DISTRACTION WITH AN INTERNAL FIXATOR—GRADUAL LENGTHENING

To minimize the complications of callus distraction with an external fixator and maximize the comfort of postoperative aftercare, a new innovative internal fixator has been established 15 years ago and reported first time in 2009 by Klauser and Mellerowicz.[2] Dorsal skin incision is made along the lateral side of the affected metatarsal bone in direction of the respective interdigital space. In addition, a 1 cm long skin incision in

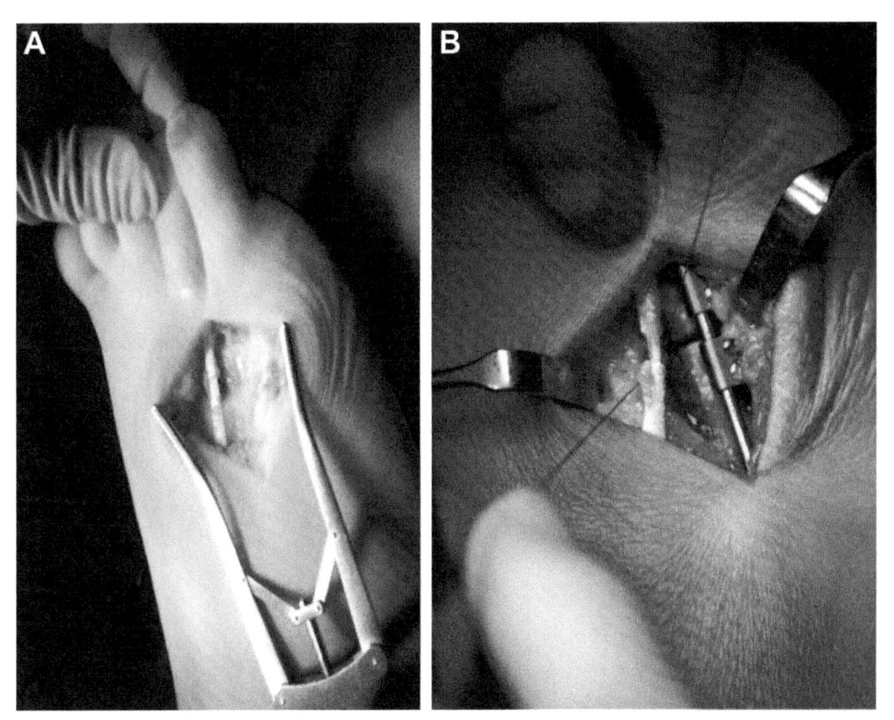

Fig. 19. Dorsal approach to the metatarsal 4, preparation of the extensor tendon 4, traction test (*A*), extensor tendon lengthening by Z-plasty (*B*).

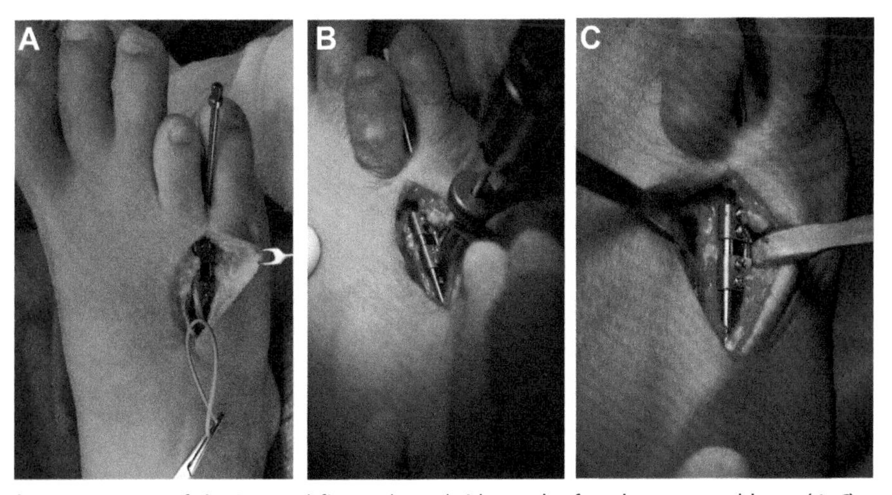

Fig. 20. Fixation of the internal fixator lateral side on the fourth metatarsal bone (*A–C*).

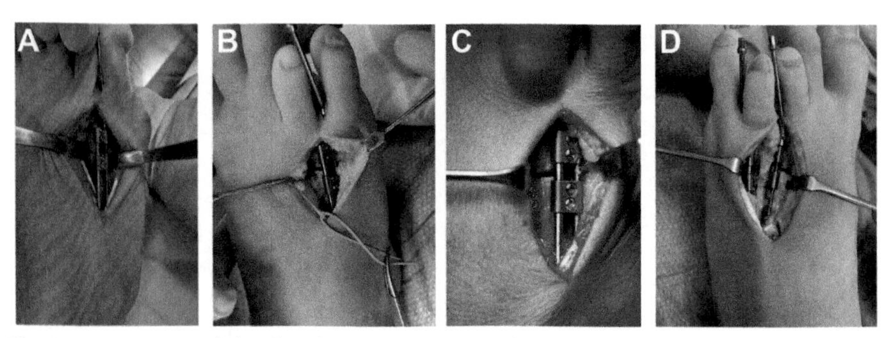

Fig. 21. Osteotomy of the fourth metatarsal bone (*A–C*), simultaneously of the third and fourth metatarsal bones (*D*), between the guide jaws from dorsal and adjusting the regenerate preliminary stage up to 2 mm (*B–D*).

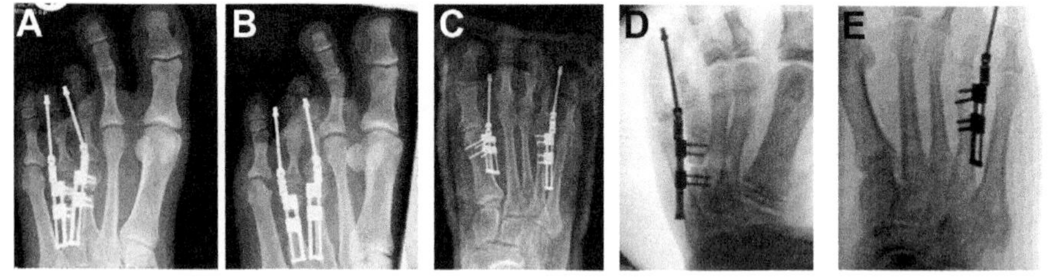

Fig. 22. Intraoperative x-ray pictures, which demonstrate the regenerate preliminary stage and the correct position of the internal minifixator (*A–E*).

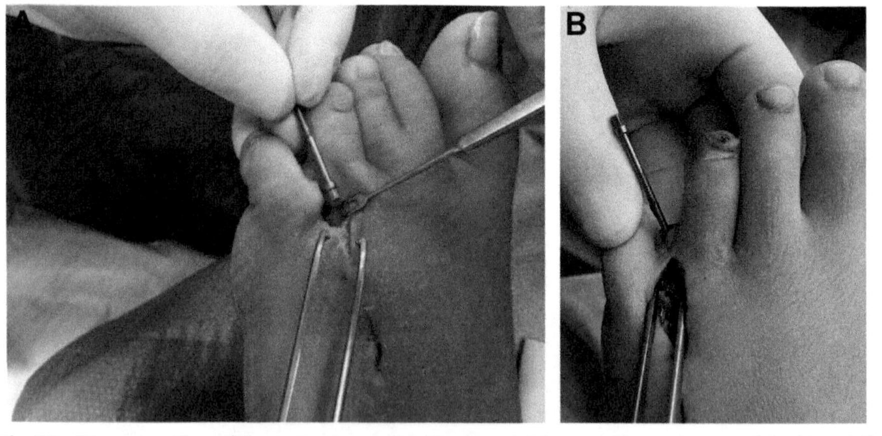

Fig. 23. Disconnection of the activator rod with a special forceps through a small incision (*A*) or big incision (*B*) if an arthrolysis of the metatarsophalangeal joint is necessary.

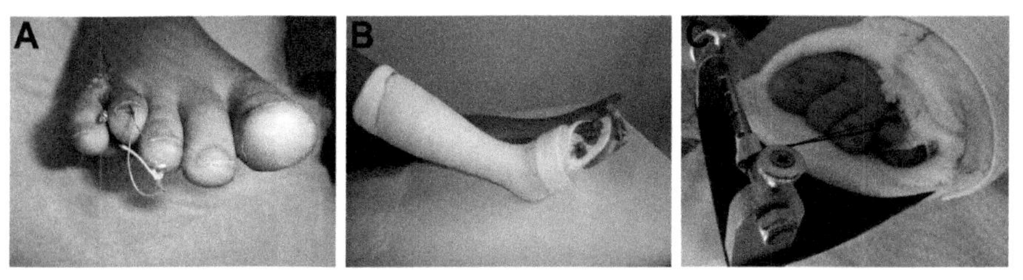

Fig. 24. Special cast postoperative with traction of the affected short fourth toe by thread extension through the toenail (*A–C*).

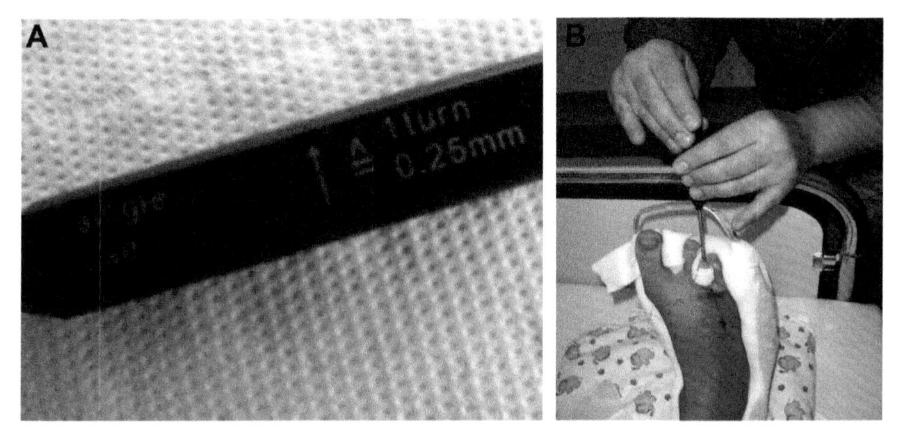

Fig. 25. In the distraction phase, the activator is working 0.25 mm corresponding to 1 turn every morning and evening (0.5 mm per day) (*A*, *B*).

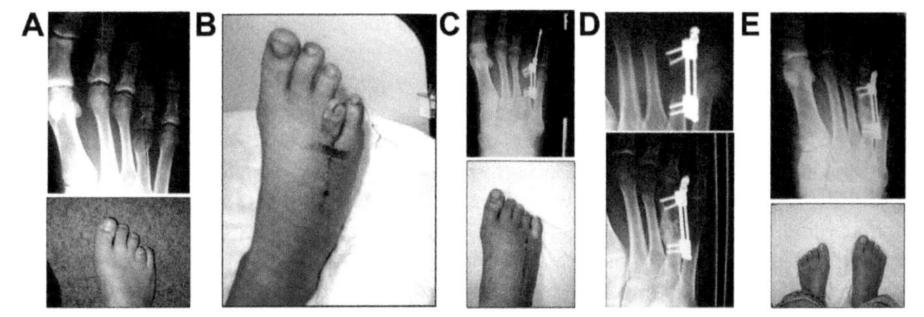

Fig. 26. The correction of brachymetatarsia of the fourth metatarsal bone on a 10-year-old female patient using an internal fixator. Preoperative situation (*A*), postoperatively in the resting phase to activate the regenerate preliminary stage (*B*), after callus distraction up to 12 mm over 24 days (*C*), neutralization phase over 90 days (*D*), remodeling phase and clinical result after 4 months (*E*).

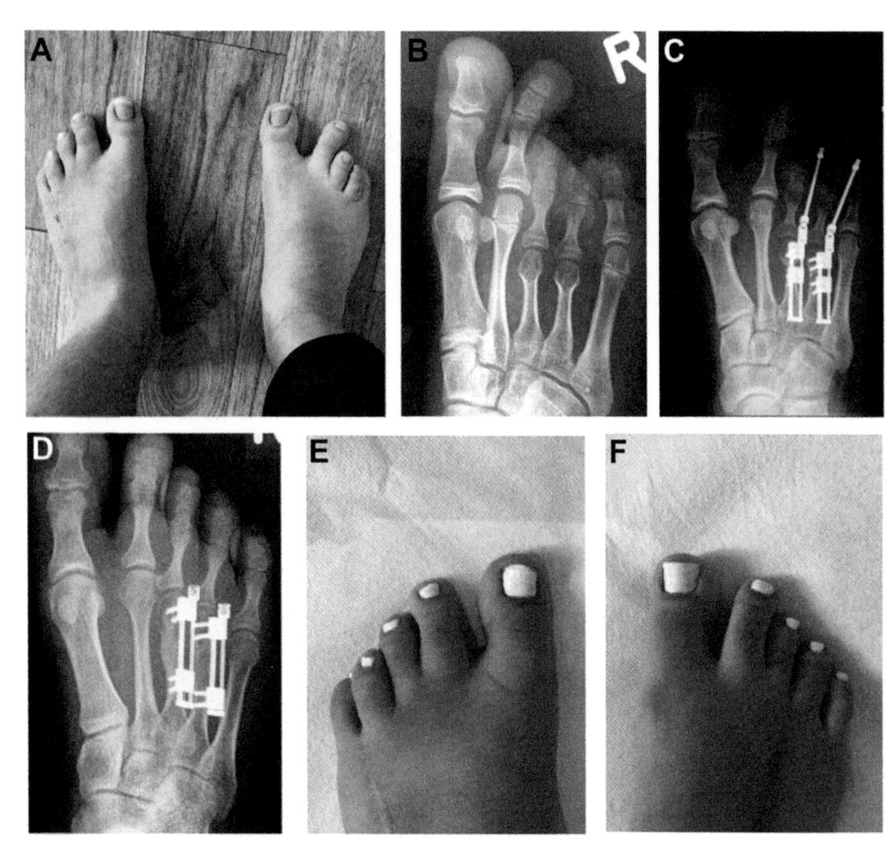

Fig. 27. The result 1 year after correction of brachymetatarsia of the fourth metatarsal bone left by callus distraction with internal fixator (*A*), the correction of bilateral brachymetatarsia of the third and fourth metatarsal bones right (*A, B*) by callus distraction with internal fixator (*C, D*) on a 14-year-old girl and the clinical result after 9 months (*E, F*).

the interdigital space is necessary, which later functions as a channel for the activator rod of the internal fixator. This is followed by preparation of the short and long extensor tendon. As well an arthrolysis of the metatarsophalangeal joint should always be carried out, as due to the lengthening of the metatarsal bone during callus distraction, there is always a significant compression on the joint with the risk of stiffness. The toe could deviate into a dorsal or less commonly plantar direction, so to avoid this phenomenon, the tension of the extensor tendon must be examined with a push-up and a traction test, and if necessary, a Z-plasty lengthening of the extensor tendon should be performed (**Figs. 19** and **20**).[2] The entire metatarsal bone from the head to proximal metaphyseal region is prepared and the internal fixator is positioned on the lateral side, while the activator rod is channeled through the interdigital skin incision. The internal fixator is generally used with the right cardanic for the right foot, and with the left cardanic for the left one. In the next step, the locked angle stable minifixator is fixed distally on epiphysis with 2.3 or 2.0 mm screws depending on the age of the patient and the volume of the bone. X-ray evaluation should be performed to check the correct position of the internal fixator on the metatarsal bone and final fixation of the minifixator distally and proximally with 2 screws each. Once the internal minifixator is positioned on the lateral side of the metatarsal bone, dorsal sawing of the osteotomy in the distal metaphyseal region can be carried out. Setting of the regenerate preliminary stage to 1 to 2 mm by turning the activator with the activator screwdriver followed by retrograde wound closure (see **Figs. 19** and **20**, **Figs. 21** and **22**). The interdigital skin incision remains open. If the toenail of the affected ray appears large enough, a strong thread is pulled through the toenail for traction of the affected ray. Application of a posterior lower leg plaster splint is shown in **Fig. 23**. After a 5-day rest period to activate the regenerate begins the distraction phase. It consists of a circular cast with callus distraction of 0.25 mm every morning and evening with an interval of 12 hours in-between, which corresponds to 0.5 mm per day. The toe of the affected ray is tensed with an orthograde thread extension by a special device in a carbon plate, which is attached to the sole inside the cast and prevents a significant compression and stiffness of the metatarsophalangeal joint as well as positions the toe in an orthograde alignment during the distraction phase (**Figs. 24** and **25**). After complete radiological reconstruction of the metatarsal parabola, the activator rod is disconnected from the minifixator, which remains in situ until bone consolidation, and is pulled out with special forceps during a second operation (see **Fig. 23**). Owing to the increased joint compression and tendon tension, especially for callus distraction more than 20 mm and depending on the extent of the deformity, once more a metatarsophalangeal joint (MTP) release and further extensor tendon lengthening or even augmentation of the short extensor tendon to the extended long one is required. Leading out a drainage through the interdigital skin incision is recommendable. During the neutralization phase, a posterior lower leg plaster splint has to be applied for 2 weeks, followed by a special shoe, that is, short walker with a hard shell insole and increased partial weight-bearing for 6 weeks until bone union is achieved. Thereafter, full weight-bearing in ready-made shoes with hard shell insoles. To avoid stiffness in the metatarsophalangeal joint during this period, a mobilization of the toe in the MTP by a physiotherapist and the patient itself with additional traction of this joint is important.[2] Temporary swelling, local redness, and hyperthermia on the dorsum of the foot during the neutralization phase are typical characteristics of the callus distraction, which causes localized hyperemia.[2,20] About 9 to 12 months after the first operation, once the remodeling phase has been finished and the metatarsal parabola is fully reconstructed by achieving the targeted length of the affected metatarsal bone, the internal fixator can be removed during a third operation (**Fig. 26**). This internal minifixator is a locked angle stable titanium fixator available in 2 sizes for metatarsal bone lengthening of 18 mm or 23 mm and is suitable for correction of all metatarsal bones (see **Figs. 3**, **12**, **15**, **16**, **22**, and **26**, **Fig. 27**).[2,11] There are few articles describing callus distraction with the use of nonlocking internal devices. Callus fracture and breakage of the internal device was reported as a disadvantage during the callus distraction, which we cannot confirm using a locking internal fixator.[47–49]

SUMMARY

For the correction of congenital brachymetatarsia, there are 3 main lengthening options available for each of the conditions associated with inherent complications. Over the recent years, callus distraction with an internal minifixator has become increasingly established in the European area because of the significantly improved aftercare and far superior stability of the locked angle stable titanium minifixator. This procedure is an excellent alternative to the gradual lengthening with callus distraction by external fixator systems, which has been rated as a standard procedure for the lengthening of large metatarsal longitudinal defects. For correction of shortened metatarsal bones of less than 10 mm, one-stage lengthening by interposition of an allogenic or autologous bone graft or lengthening osteotomy is still the option and presents good results in one operation procedure. To avoid harm to child's or adolescent's physical development through disturbed proprioception and because of a higher bone growth potential and elasticity of the soft tissue structures, the reconstruction of metatarsal alignment as well as metatarsal parabola should be carried out early, around 8 years of age. The advantages of callus distraction with an internal minifixator are the uncomplicated handling of the fixator during the distraction phase, its high stability and early increased weight-bearing in the distraction and neutralization phase as well as the remain of the locked angle stable fixator in situ under full weight-bearing during the remodeling phase. It is suitable for lengthening of all metatarsal bones by 18 or 23 mm and allows a distraction of up to 3 metatarsals simultaneously.

CLINICS CARE POINTS

- Preoperatively, a distinction between brachydactyly and brachymetatarsia is to consider or rather one should bear in mind the presence of both pathologies and make sure to differentiate these.
- To safely position the minifixator, it should preferably be inserted from lateral, which avoids soft tissue irritation and ensures a bicortical fixation of the screws.
- To avoid a dorsal or plantar deviation of the toe, it is necessary to review the need of an arthrolysis and/or an extensor tendon lengthening in the first or latest the second operation and to perform it where appropriate.
- During the postoperative course, a traction of the afflicted toe is mandatory either self-contained or with the help of a physiotherapist to avoid a contracture and stiffening of the operated foot ray and a deviation of the involved toe.
- If the reconstruction of brachymetatarsia is not performed in the childhood, the risk to develop a pseudarthrosis after a callus distraction of the metatarsal bone is strikingly increased and, by extension, the need of an additional operation with autologous spongiosa graft.

DISCLOSURE

The author has nothing to declare.

REFERENCES

1. Kim HT, Lee SH, Yoo CI, et al. The management of brachymetatarsia. J Bone Joint Surg Br 2003;85:683–90.
2. Klauser H, Mellerowicz H. The reconstruction of brachymetatarsia using an internal fixator - a new treatment concept. FuSpru 2009;7(1):22–30.
3. Hefti F. Malformations of the lower extremities. Orthopäde 2008;37(4):381–402.
4. Giannini S, Faldini S, Pagkrati S, et al. One-stage metatarsal lengthening by allograft interposition: a novel approach for congenital brachymetatarsia. Clin Orthop Relat Res 2010;468(7):1933–42.
5. Urano Y, Kobayashi A. Bone-lengthening for shortness of the fourth toe. J Bone Joint Surg Am 1978;60:91–3.
6. Magnan B, Bragantini A, Regis D, et al. Metatarsal lengthening by callotasis during the growth phase. J Bone Joint Surg Br 1995;77:602–7.

7. Marcinko DE, Rappaport MJ, Gordon S. Post-traumatic brachymetatarsia. J Foot Surg 1984;23(6):451–3.
8. Schimizzi A, Brage M. Brachymetatarsia. Foot Ancle Clin North Am 2004;9: 555–70.
9. Pisani G. Vorfußbedingte Zehendeformitäten. Missbildungen und Deformitäten der kleinen Zehen. In: Fußchirurgie. Stuttgart – New York: Georg Thieme Verlag; 1998. p. 340–1.
10. Barik S, Farr S. Brachymetacarpia and Brachymetatarsia: do we need to operate? EFORT Open Rev 2021;6:15–23.
11. Wingenfeld C, Arbab D, Abbara-Czardybon M. Treatment options for brachymetatarsia. Orthopäde 2013;42(1):30–7.
12. Skirving AP, Newmann JH. Elongation of the first metatarsal. J Pediatr Orthop 1983;3:508–10.
13. Davidson RS. Metatarsal lengthening. Foot Ankle Clin 2001;6:499–518.
14. Desai A, Lidder S, Armitage AR, et al. Brachymetatarsia of the fourth metatarsal, lengthening scarf osteotomy with bone graft. Orthop Rev (Pavia) 2013;5(3):e21.
15. McGlamry ED, Cooper CT. Brachymetatarsia: a surgical treatment. J Am Podiatric Med Assoc 1969;59:259–64.
16. Tabak B, Lefkowitz H, Steiner I. Metatarsal-slide lengthening without bone grafting. J Foot Surg 1986;25:50–3.
17. Dua RS. One-stage lengthening for congenitally short metatarsals. Foot 2004;14: 164–8.
18. Naoshige I, Watanabe A. A new surgical procedure for brachymetatarsia by a hydroxyapatite graft. Eur J Plast Surg 2013;36:41–4.
19. Shecaira AP, Fernandes RMP. Brachymetatarsia: one-stage versus two-stage procedures. Foot Ankle Clin 2019;24:677–87.
20. Lamm BM, Gourdine-Shaw MC. Problems, obstacles and complications of metatarsal lengthening for the treatment of brachymetatarsia. Clin Podiatr Med Surg 2010;27:561–82.
21. Kwon ST, Chung CY. Changes in blood flow during one stage lengthening of bone: an experimental study in rats. Scand J Plast Recon Surg Hand Surg 2000;34:109–12.
22. Ilizarov GA. Basic principles of transosseous compression and distraction osteosynthesis. Orthop Traumatol Protez 1971;32:7.
23. Mah KK, Beegle TR, Falknor DW. A reconstruction for short fourth metatarsal. J Am Podiatry Med Assoc 1983;73:196.
24. Shim JS, Park SJ. Treatment of brachymetatarsia by distraction osteogenesis. J Pediatr Orthop 2006;26:250–4.
25. Masada K, Fujita S, Fuji T, et al. Complications following metatarsal lengthening by callus distraction for brachymetatarsia. J Pediatr Orthop 1999;19:394–7.
26. Robinson JF, Ouzounian TJ. Brachymetatarsia: congenitally short third and fourth metatarsals treated by distraction lengthening – a case report and literature summery. Foot Ankle Int 1998;19(10):713–8.
27. Wilusz PM, Van P, Pupp GR. Complications associated with distraction osteogenesis for the reconstruction of brachymetatarsia: a review of five procedures. J Am Podiatric Med Assoc 2007;97(39):189–94.
28. Erdem M, Sen C, Eralp L, et al. Lengthening of short bones by distraction osteogenesis - results and complications. Int Orthop 2009;33(3):807–13.
29. Oh CW, Sharma R, Song HR, et al. Complications of distraction osteogenesis in short fourth metatarsals. J Pediatr Orthop 2003;23(4):84–487.

30. Masuda T, Matoh N, Nakajima T, et al. Treatment of Brachymetatarsia using a semicircular lengthener: 1-3 years results in 6 patients. Acta Orthop Scand 1995;66:43–6.
31. Song H-R, Oh C-W, Kyung H-S, et al. Fourth brachymetatarsia treated with distraction osteogenesis. Foot Ankle Int 2003;24:706–11.
32. Kim JS, Baek GH, Chung MS, et al. Multiple congenital brachymetatarsia. A one-stage combined shortening and lengthening procedure without iliac bone graft. J Bone Joint Surg Br 2004;86(7):1013–5.
33. Biggs EW, Brahm TB, Efron BL. Surgical correction of congenital hypoplastic metatarsals. J Am Podiatry Assoc 1979;69:241–4.
34. Baeck GH, Chung MS. The treatment of congenital brachymetatarsia by one-stage lengthening. J Bone Joint Surg Br 1998;80:1040–4.
35. McGlamry ED, Fenton CF. Brachymetatarsia. A case report. J Am Podiatr Med Assoc 1983;73(2):75–8.
36. Alter SA, Feinman B, Rosen RG. Chevron bone graft procedure for the correction of brachymetatarsia. J Foot Ankle Surg 1995;34:200–5.
37. Smolle E, Scheipl S, Leithner A, et al. Management of congenital fourth brachymetatarsia by additive autologous lengthening osteotomy (AALO): a case series. Foot Ankle Int 2015;36:325–9.
38. Mansur H, Meira RT, Gusmao L, et al. One-stage correction of multiple brachymetatarsia and hallux valgus with calcaneal autograft. Sci J Foot Ankle 2018;12(4): 342–6.
39. Waizy H, Polzer H, Schikora N, et al. One-stage metatarsal interposition lengthening with an autologous fibula graft for treatment of brachymetatarsia. Foot Ankle Spec 2009;12:330–5.
40. Fuiano M, Mosca M, Caravelli S. Callus distraction with external fixator for the treatment of congenital brachymetatarsia of the fourth ray. Foot Ankle Surg 2020;26:693–8.
41. Ruffer M, Heijens E, Pfeil J. Distraction lengthening for the fourth metatarsal with an intramedullary K-wire in brachymetatarsia. FussSprungg 2006;4:234–9.
42. Sher DM, Blyakher A, Krantzow M. A modified surgical technique for lengthening of a metatarsal using an external fixator. HSS J 2010;6:235–9.
43. Barbier D, Neretin A, Journeau P, et al. Gradual metatarsal lengthening by external fixation: a new classification of complications and a stable technique to minimize severe complications. Foot Ankle Int 2015;36:1369–77.
44. Wada A, Bensahel H, Takamura K, et al. Metatarsal lengthening by callus distraction for brachymetatarsia. J Pediatr Orthop B 2004;13:206–10.
45. Lee KB, Yang HK, Chung JY, et al. How to avoid complications of distraction osteogenesis for first brachymetatarsia. Acta Orthop 2009;80(2):220–5.
46. Levine SE, Davidson RS, Dormans JP. Distraction osteogenesis for congenital short lesser metatarsals. Foot Ankle Int 1995;16(4):196–200.
47. Klauser H. Lengthening of metatarsal bones by callus distraction. My medibook. Elearning & medical science; 2015. Available at: http://www.hfz-berlin.de/wp-content/uploads/2015/09/my_medibook.pdf. Accessed November 30, 2020.
48. Yamada N, Yasuda Y, Hashimoto N, et al. Use of internal callus distraction in the treatment of congenital brachymetatarsia. Br J Plast Surg 2005;58:1014–9.
49. Kitabata R, Sakamoto Y, Nagasao T, et al. Distraction osteogenesis for brachymetatarsia by using internal device. Plast Reconstr Surg Glob Open 2017;5(7): e1381.

The Treatment of Neglected Clubfoot

Anja C. Helmers, MD, PhD

KEYWORDS

- Neglected clubfoot • Severe disability • Ponseti method • Lambrinudi arthrodesis • Talectomy • Soft tissue release • Skin necrosis

KEY POINTS

- Choosing a treatment strategy depends on the age of the patient, the severity and rigidity of the deformity, and its previous treatment.
- In less-severe neglected clubfoot cases, the Ponseti method can lead to a complete correction of the deformity, making surgery avoidable.
- Preoperative application of the Ponseti method can improve the success in correcting the deformity of the neglected clubfoot.
- Postoperative treatment management in underdeveloped countries and the obligatory need of orthopedic technicians in clubfoot treatment are essential.
- The advantages of Lambrinudi arthrodesis compare with primary talectomy in foot function.

INTRODUCTION

A clubfoot is a severe 3-dimensional foot deformity. The causes can be congenital and developmental, syndromic, or neurologic. If the clubfoot remains untreated after birth, it is considered a neglected clubfoot with persistent hindfoot varus, equinus, forefoot adductus, serious inversion of the entire foot, and increased pronation in the midfoot and forefoot as well as hyperpronation of the first metatarsal (**Fig. 1**).

The center of these different individual components of a clubfoot is subtalar in the anterior aspect of the subtalar joint[1] and can be identified as the center of rotation and angulation (CORA) of the clubfoot. The soft tissue contraction, which is maximal between the navicular bone and the medial distal tibia, shapes the bone development that results in the deformity.[2] The navicular bone becomes wedge shaped, and the talus head becomes conical shaped.[2–4] The subtalar joint is held in plantar flexion, inversion, and adduction. The calcaneocuboid joint becomes oblique and medially subluxated.[3] Because of the inversion of the foot, the sole of the foot does not touch the ground, and the back of the foot is stressed from walking. The foot consequently develops a significant bursa to protect it (**Fig. 2**).

President of Doctors for Disabled-International. www.doctorsfordisabled-international.com.
EWK Spandau, Stadtrandstraße 555, Berlin 13589, Germany
E-mail address: anja.helmers@jsd.de

Foot Ankle Clin N Am 26 (2021) 705–725
https://doi.org/10.1016/j.fcl.2021.07.004

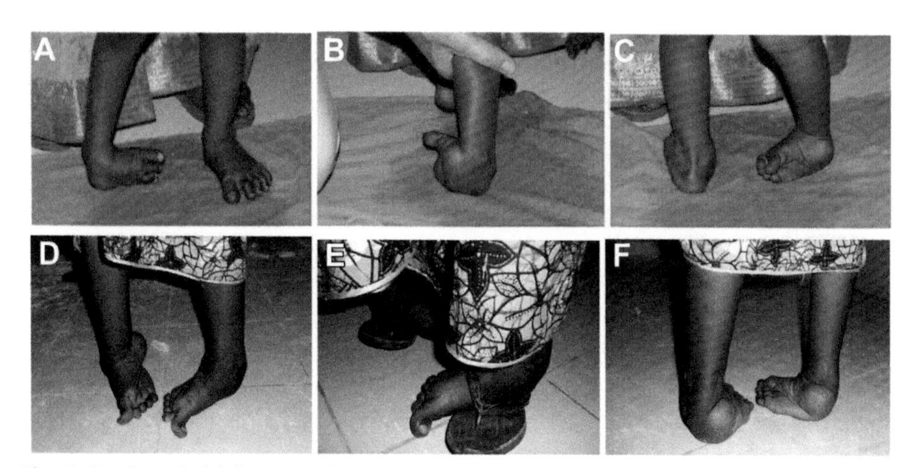

Fig. 1. Neglected clubfoot at 3 (*above*) and at 23 years of age (*below*).

A total of 80% of clubfeet worldwide are neglected clubfeet.[3] These untreated clubfeet are mainly observed in underdeveloped countries, as affected people in underfunded health systems have little or no access to medical care. The impact of an untreated clubfoot on the function of the foot is enormous and is associated with massive restrictions for the patient.

> *The neglected clubfoot, however, is one in which there has been no initial treatment or perhaps very inadequate and incomplete initial treatment. The deformity is made worse at the time the child starts to walk because weight- bearing takes place on the side or dorsum of the foot, exaggerating the abnormal shape and causing further deformation. The sole of the foot never experiences proper weight bearing, and it is impossible to wear normal shoes. A thickened callous and large bursa develop over the prominent weight bearing head of the talus on the dorsolateral side of the foot, often associated with deep fissures, which are vulnerable to breakdown and infection.*[3]

Currently, the standard treatment of infants' congenital clubfeet, regardless of the cause, is the Ponseti method, with very good primary correction results in more than 90% of cases.[5–7] Since 1996, this extremely effective treatment method has spread from Iowa, where it was developed, to the whole world. The Ponseti method is increasingly available in many underdeveloped countries, and investigators

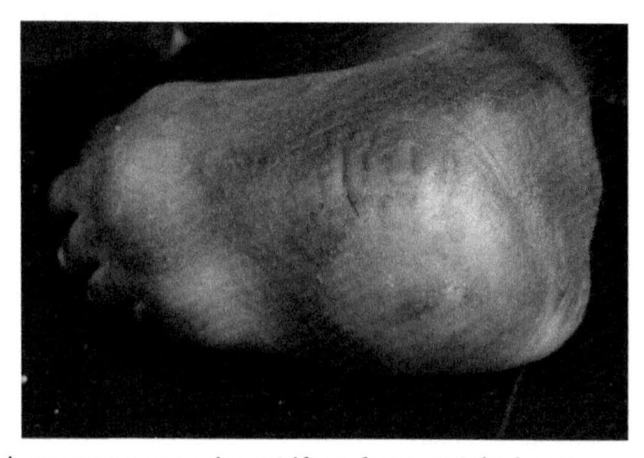

Fig. 2. Developed bursa to protect the midfoot from weight bearing.

describe good primary correction results even in almost 80% to 90% of older children with untreated clubfeet.[8–16]

One of the important projects to spread the Ponseti method in medically underserved countries is undoubtedly the Ponseti project in Uganda (Uganda Sustainable Clubfoot Care Project), supported by Shafique Pirani, which started in 1999.[16] With a funding concept, the cooperation of a university, and the involvement of responsible government authorities and comprehensible teaching material,[17] well-functioning Ponseti treatment centers can be set up, and local staff can be trained in applying the method. Involving the responsible health authorities is often necessary to maintain such projects independent of substantial support from abroad.

Additional organizations like CURE International have been founded to spread the Ponseti method. CURE India established as of today 324 different Ponseti treatment centers all over India. Their unique workshop in Delhi manufactures Steenbeek abduction splints and sends them to the treatment centers at low cost. The workforce of this workshop consists mainly of people with physical disabilities, thus contributing to an inclusive society (**Fig. 3**).

Unfortunately, by far, not all newborns with clubfoot have access to such institutions. Many parents with low income in hard-to-reach or crisis regions are not able to receive medical care at the necessary regular intervals.

With a neglected clubfoot, a person is unable to walk long distances and has reduced access to education or employment. As a result, patients are not only physically restricted but also socially discriminated[3] (**Fig. 4**).

GENERAL CONSIDERATION

If a clubfoot is left untreated, the chance of complete remodeling of the tarsal bones during therapy through the Ponseti method decreases after the age of 8, and the necessity of additive surgery for long-term, recurrence-free correction of these feet becomes increasingly more likely. Depending on age, severity, and degree of flexibility, there is progression from soft tissue surgery alone through a combination with midfoot osteotomies to arthrodesis.[3]

The neglected clubfoot is a challenge in foot surgery, as all 3 levels of the foot must be taken into account. A precise knowledge of the anatomy of the untreated clubfoot and its planes of movement is a basic requirement for surgical treatment. Already from the age of 4, a sole soft tissue surgery can often not lead to a long-term satisfactory result, making bony correction inevitable.[3] Experience has shown that the bones must be adjusted correctly in order to achieve long-term success. Many investigators prefer, which is also confirmed by the author's experience, to pretreat the neglected

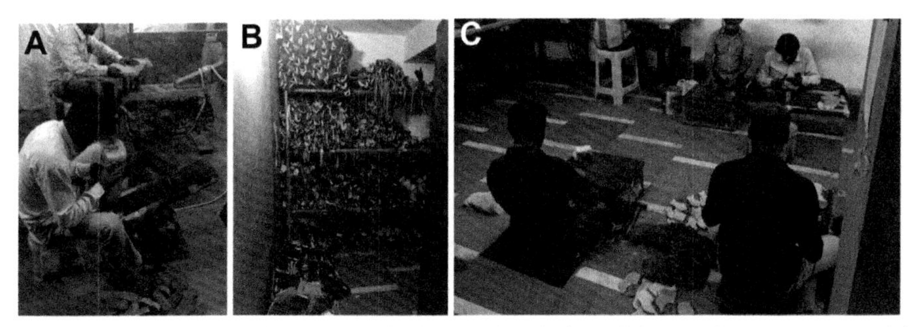

Fig. 3. (*A*) CURE India workshop in Delhi. (*B*) Handmade foot abduction brace mounting. (*C*) The workforce are mainly disabled people with Polio.

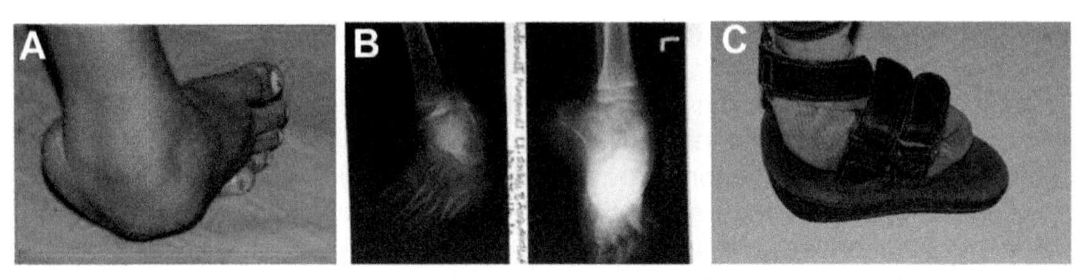

Fig. 4. Neglected clubfoot (*A*); X ray (*B*); special shoewear for an untreated clubfoot (*C*).

clubfoot with the Ponseti method[8–16] and subsequently carry out the surgical correction.[18]

The treatment of the neglected clubfoot is largely surgical, and there is no single surgical procedure that can resolve all clubfoot scenarios.[3]

The various options for surgical correction are tenotomy or open Achilles tendon lengthening, a dorsal, dorsomedial, or peritalar release, bony wedge removal, triple arthrodesis, or a complete talectomy. Under certain conditions, the correction of severely affected feet can even require an external fixator with a high rate of good results, low frequency of complications, and low incidence of recurrence.[19] Literature shows good results can be achieved in 70% to 90% of cases. The disadvantage of the Ilizarov fixator is the need for high-cost equipment and a long treatment time, up to 1 year in frame.[19]

When conducting an aid project abroad with a narrow time frame being confronted with severe or older neglected clubfeet, the therapeutic options are very limited. The talectomy and Lambrinudi arthrodesis are the best options in these cases. The Lambrinudi arthrodesis is a good procedure for long-term correction with good functional results in patients with untreated clubfeet older than 6 years because the talar dome is preserved.[3]

NEGLECTED CLUBFOOT TREATMENT WITH THE PONSETI METHOD

Since 1996, the Ponseti method has been a globally accepted therapy not only for infant clubfeet but also for older children with neglected clubfeet[8–16] or with pretreated clubfeet, including surgical treatment.[20,21] The author's experience when working in West Bengal and Kanyakumari districts in India and countries in Africa, such as Mali, South Sudan, and Togo, confirms this. In the opinion of many investigators, the complete primary correction of an untreated clubfoot through the Ponseti method is possible and achieved in close to 70% to 80% of cases.[8–16] Lourenço and Morcuende[8] describe complete corrections in 67% of patients at an average age of 3.9 years, and Spiegel and colleagues[10] describe complete corrections in 79% of patients at the age of 1 to 6 years. Gupta and colleagues[15] treated 154 clubfeet from 2003 to 2005 with primary correction more than 90% and only 10% needed secondary treatment (**Fig. 5**).

> *It should be noted however that a cast treatment of a child that is already walking takes longer, requiring more cast changes and thus using more material than an infant.*[3]

Affected children 1 year of age and older are immobilized for a longer time and often have to be laboriously transported or accommodations are needed. The time factor of the treatment plays a very important role and leads to increased logistical effort and additional costs for everyone involved. These insurmountable barriers have a strong negative impact on adherence.[3] At the same time, an increased risk of recurrence is

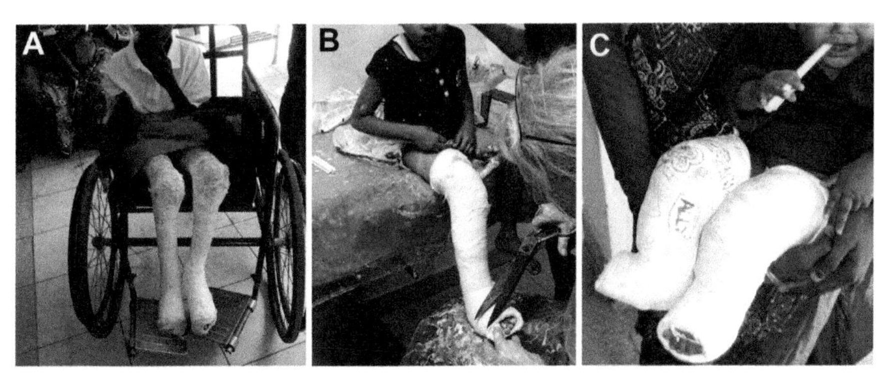

Fig. 5. Plaster (*A*), walking child (*B*), and infant (*C*).

to be expected in patients older than 8 years, as the remodeling of the bones decreases with age.[3]

In the case of an aid project abroad, the time on site is often limited to a few weeks, and a complete correction of an untreated clubfoot with the Ponseti method is difficult to achieve. It makes all the more sense to train local medical staff in the method during the stay while treating patients in need of surgery. This works particularly well when a team returns to the same location annually (**Fig. 6**).

With good practical experience, local staff can pretreat the children with the Ponseti method and correct them as much as possible before a surgery. Children and adolescents prepared in this way require significantly reduced surgical therapy with a lower risk of postoperative wound-healing disorders.[18]

The Ponseti method has additional advantages in structurally weak countries. The costs are significantly lower in relation to alternative therapy techniques. Only white plaster and cotton roll are required to prepare an untreated clubfoot for surgery or tenotomy of the Achilles tendon, which is required in more than 80%[10] or almost 100% in the case of an untreated clubfoot to correct the equinus foot.[3] It can be performed with a single scalpel under local anesthesia. The subsequently required abduction splint (Foot Abduction Brace [FAB]), which must be worn at night until the fourth birthday, can be made using simple materials available even in the poorest countries in the world. For this purpose, Steenbeek[22] has published exact building instructions on the "global help" Web site (**Fig. 7**).

In summary, the Ponseti method is a highly efficient, cost-effective method for treating clubfeet with an abundance of freely accessible learning material provided. It is also a good pretreatment for untreated clubfeet for subsequent surgical therapy in children[18] and in some cases for adolescents older than 12 years of age.[20,21]

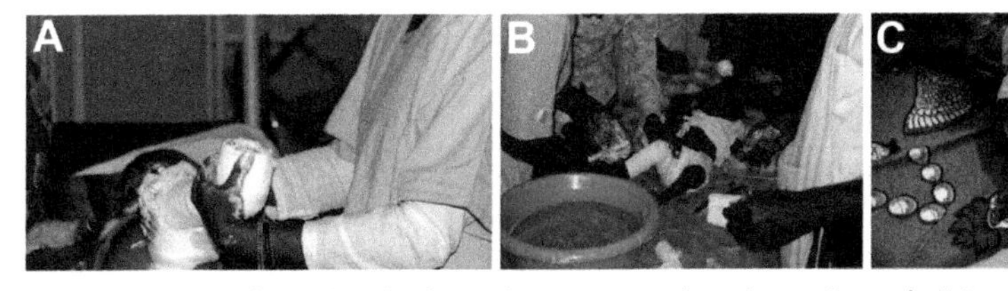

Fig. 6. (*A,B*) Teaching local physiotherapists and orthopedic technicians in the Ponseti method. (*C*) Preparing of an achilles tendon tenotomy in local anaesthesia.

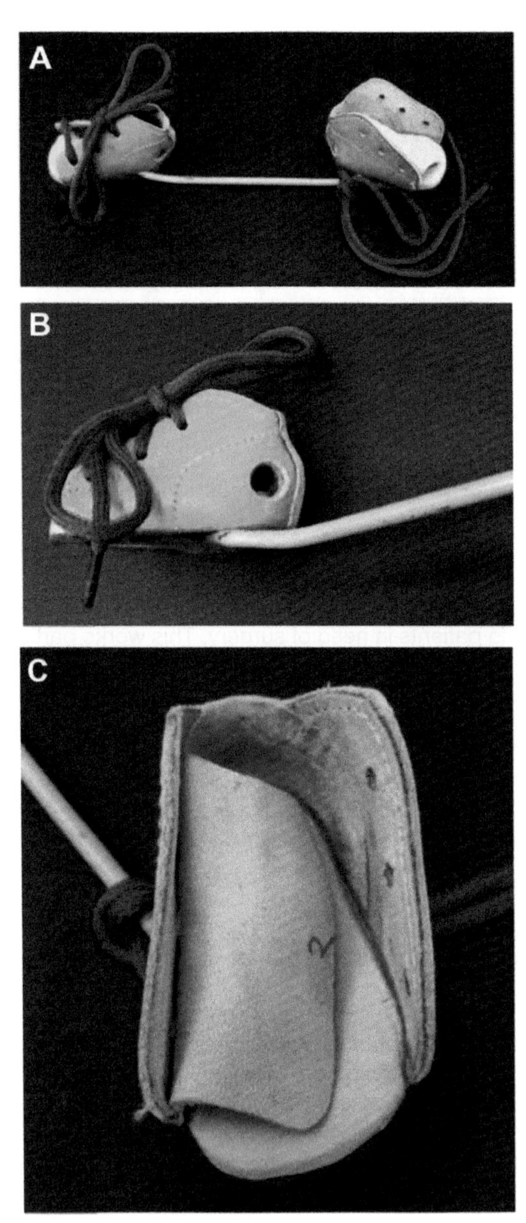

Fig. 7. (*A–C*) Steenbeek foot abduction brace.

SURGICAL TREATMENT ALGORITHM

Additional Soft Tissue Procedures Before Extensive Surgery

The pretreatment for a surgical intervention of an untreated clubfoot with the Ponseti method can be accelerated by detaching the plantar fascia percutaneously with an 18-gauge needle under short or local anesthesia. This procedure is also suitable in the case of clubfoot recurrence in a child that is already walking. Percutaneous needling of the plantar fascia saves the foot from a Steindler stripping,[23] whereby it must be opened surgically and has therewith the great advantage of being gentle on the surrounding tissue. The prick with a needle prevents the development of pronounced scars that would cause the foot to contract again as it grows. With this additive needling to the Ponseti treatment, a contracted cavus with a subsequently applied Ponseti cast in the first position can be corrected much faster. This experience is based on unpublished data from several aid projects in Chalsa/West Bengal (India) conducted between 2006 and 2015 with a constant treatment crew, including the author. There is no literature on plantar fascia needling, only on cutting the Achilles tendon with an 18- or 19-gauge needle.[24,25] One investigator recommends the combination of Ponseti method treatment, including open plantar fascia release (Steindler procedure), in neglected clubfoot in developing countries[26] (**Fig. 8**).

The plantar fascia is palpated in the patient's supine position holding the foot in dorsal extension. The needle is inserted through the skin at the calcaneal attachment in order to cut the tissue transversely with short, scratching movements. The yielding of the plantar cavity contracture is usually clearly noticeable. The flexor tendons of the musculi digitorum and hallucis longus are protected by moving the toes under the needling and thus checking for the muscle function. Once the plantar fascia has been cut (PFR), the metatarsus is stretched to the maximum while lifting the first ray, and the cavus is put into a well-molded Ponseti cast. In a short period, the cast can be changed to an increased corrective position of the foot every 3 to 4 days (regular 5–7 days). In the patient age group of children from 1 to 6 years and in exceptional cases also with older children, a complete correction of the untreated foot deformity can be achieved through this procedure only followed by a percutaneous tenotomy or an Achilles tendon extension to a three-point-technique[24–26] (**Fig. 9**).

In very rare cases, the above described method can lead to a complete correction even in older children within a shorter time period. Nogueira and colleagues[20] describe this possibility for surgically pretreated and untreated clubfoot up to 14 years with a long treatment period. The author successfully treated one 12-year-old patient with a soft clubfoot in 10 days (**Fig. 10**).

Patients up to 4 Years

If a complete correction is not achieved with the Ponseti method, an adapted surgical therapy should follow the cast treatment. For clubfeet in patients under 4 years of age, which can be passively corrected, a soft tissue procedure with a dorsomedial release or a more extensive peritalar release can lead to a complete correction.[27] This

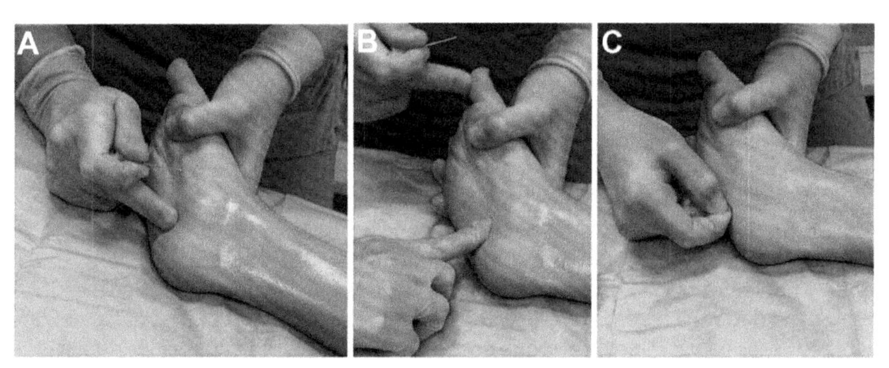

Fig. 8. Percutaneous plantar fascia needling: (*A*) investigation of the fascia; (*B*) separating the fascia from the flexor tendons; (*C*) needle sectioning.

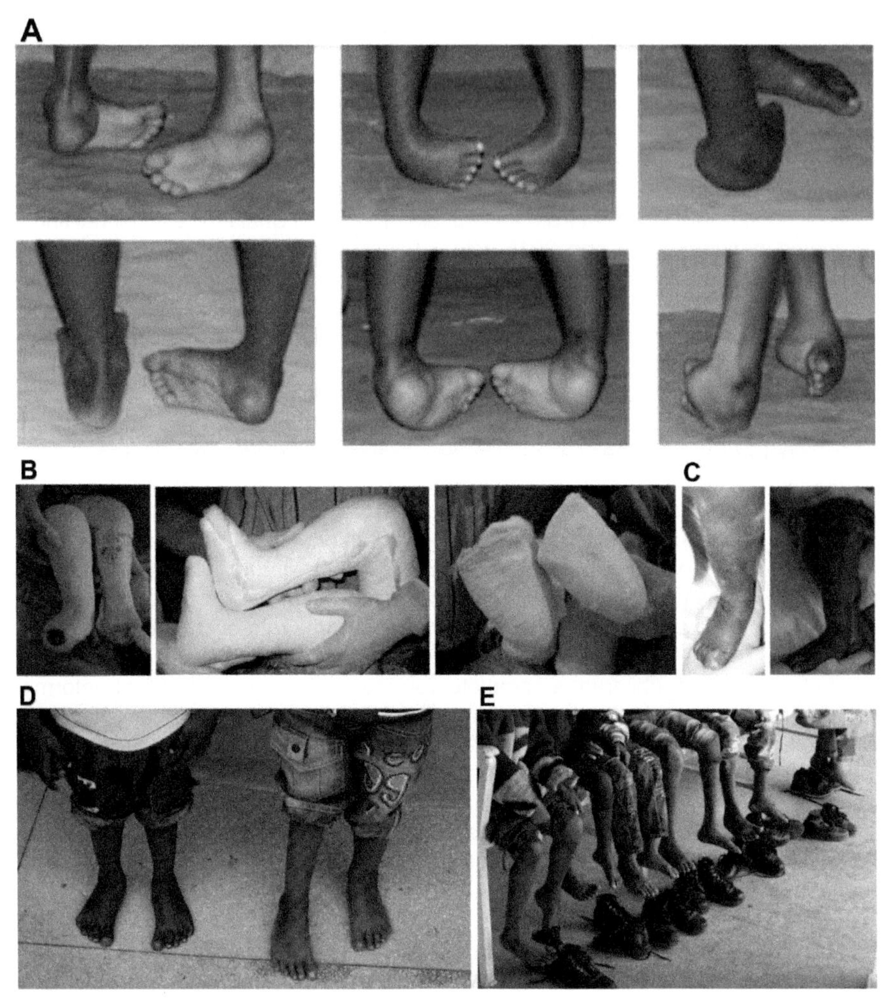

Fig. 9. (*A*) Children from 4 to 6 years of age with neglected clubfeet; (*B,C*) successfully treated within 14 days with the Ponseti method, needling of the plantar fascia and tenotomy shown in increasing abduction and dorsiflexion of the foot; (*D*) follow-up visit after 2 and (*E*) after 4 years.

procedure is particularly successful if the clubfeet have been pretreated with the Ponseti method. The Turco approach[28] and the Cincinnati approach[29] are available, the latter showing significantly better wound healing.[30] Under uncertain conditions without skilled postoperative treatment, the foot can be protected from relapse with a tibialis anterior tendon transfer[3] (**Figs. 11** and **12**).

Patients Between 4 and 6 Years of Age

If the children are older than 4 years of age or have not been pretreated with the Ponseti method, a correction of the bones must be added to the soft tissue management in most cases. The 2 possibilities here are the removal of a laterodorsal bone wedge (see third step) or the subtractive removal of a wedge from the anterior part of the calcaneus, the Lichtblau procedure,[31] or the wedge resection out of the calcaneocuboid joint, the Evans procedure.[3] The author prefers the laterodorsal wedge removal from the entire tarsus, as this takes better account of the CORA of the clubfoot (**Fig. 13**).

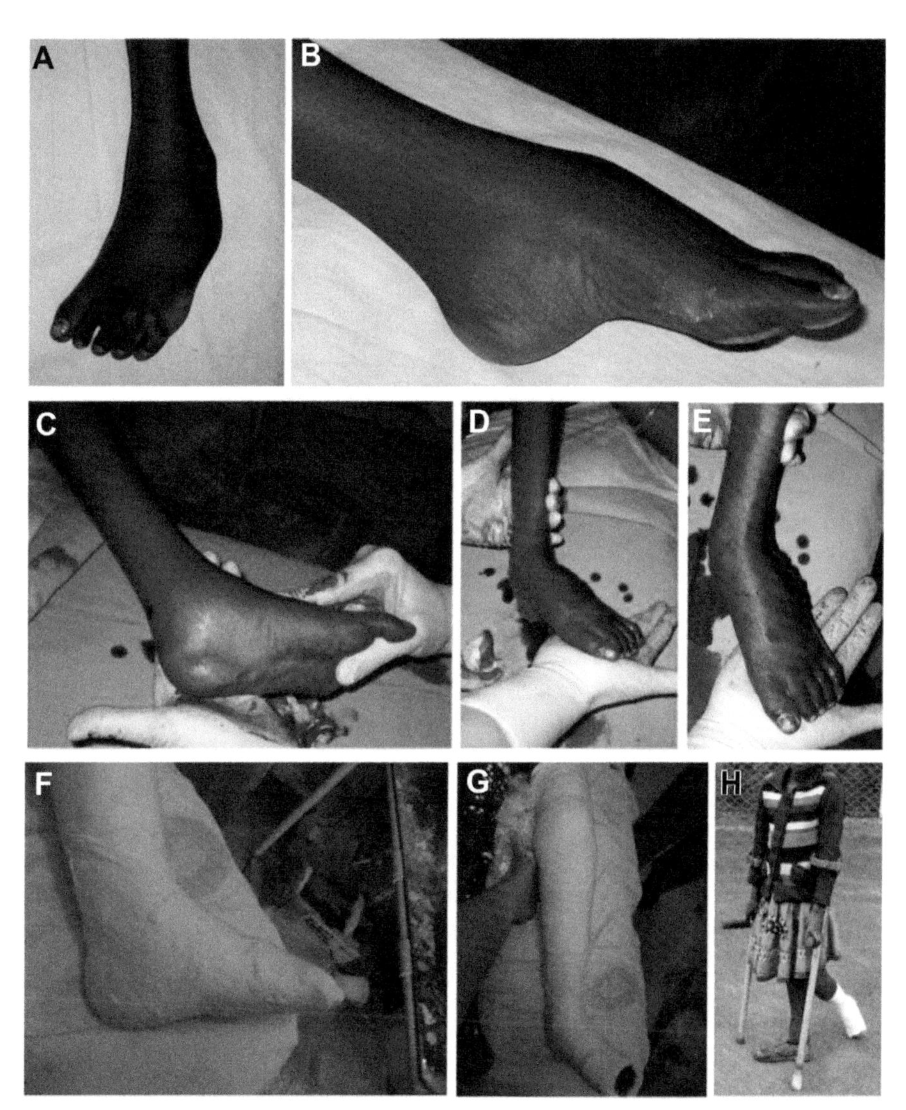

Fig. 10. (*A–H*) Chalsa/West Bengal, India 2015: girl 12 years of age, treated with the Ponseti method, plantar fascia needling, and Achiles Tendon Lengthening with a complete tenotomy.

Patients Older than 6 Years of Age (Lambrinudi Arthrodesis)

For children older than 6 years of age with neglected clubfeet without the possibility of treatment, the extent of the surgical intervention is significantly higher. In such cases, the Lambrinudi arthrodesis is a good method to achieve the complete correction of the untreated clubfoot while maintaining the mobility of the ankle joint.[32,33] This procedure was summarized by Penny[3] in his 2005 publication based on his 6 years of full-time experience in Uganda. Apart from that, there is hardly any literature on the treatment of untreated clubfoot through Lambrinudi arthrodesis.

Between 2006 and 2009, the author's team mainly performed talectomies for treating pronounced clubfeet in their aid project in West Bengal/India. This resulted in 2

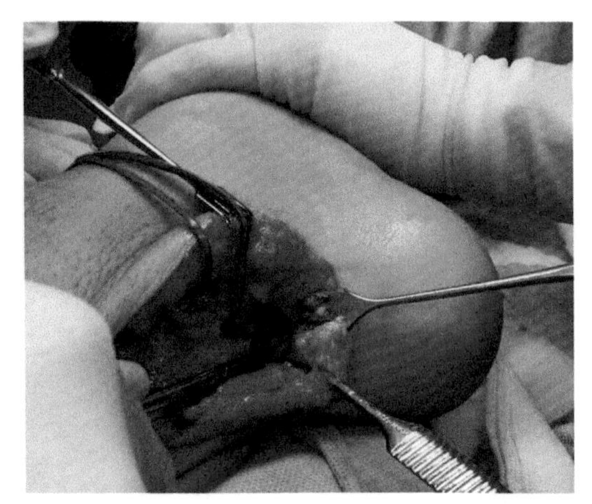

Fig. 11. Hindfoot capsule release for equinus correction + Achiles Tendon Lengthening Z-form.

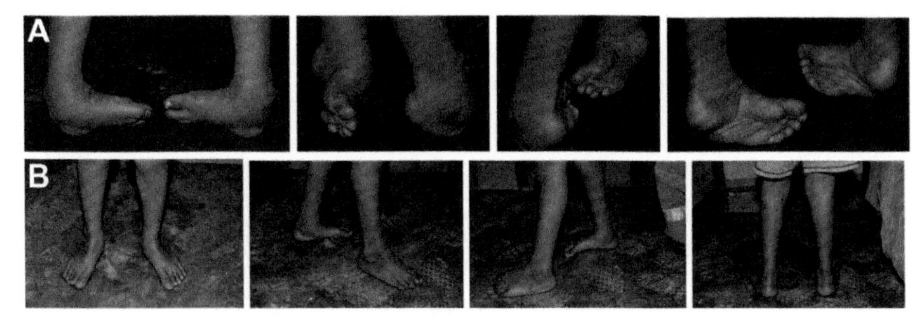

Fig. 12. (*A*, *B*) Preoperative and postoperative after dorsomedial release and 2 years after the surgical treatment.

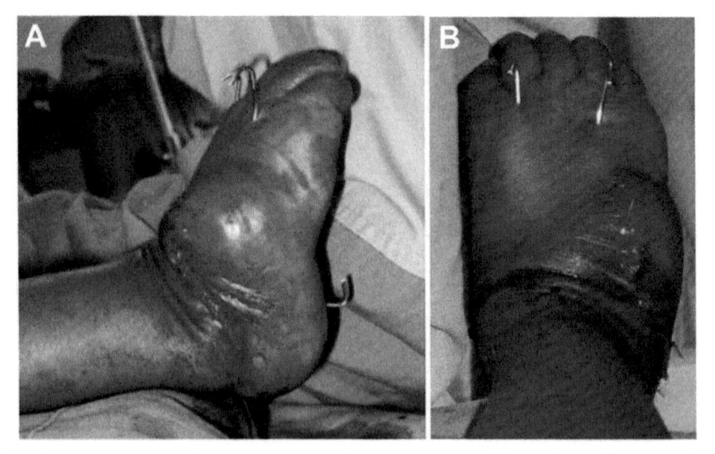

Fig. 13. (*A*, *B*) Boy 5 years of age, dorsomedial release, and lateral midfoot wedge.

extensive wound-healing disorders. In 2009, based on Penny's 6 years of full-time experience in Uganda, the author's team switched to correction with the Lambrinudi arthrodesis using a double incision and subsequently observed hardly any significant wound-healing disorders (described in **Figs. 14** and **15**).

The bone growth of the rear foot and metatarsus in younger children is not influenced by a Lambrinudi arthrodesis.[3]

The double incision allows for dorsal release with the Turco approach and arthrodesis via an Ollier approach.[3] The resulting intermediate skin bridge between the 2 incisions is the yardstick for the individual equinus correction of an untreated clubfoot.

The skin should only be slightly under tension, and skin color must be checked after opening the tourniquet. This prevents reduced blood flow leading to necrosis with superinfected wound-healing disorders, which are a difficult-to-treat complication, especially in countries with limited medical care. The necessary plastic surgery to treat these skin defects with exposed tendons is unavailable in many countries. In these cases, the risk of infection increases, and osteomyelitis might develop.

This procedure offers the advantage over the corresponding bony reduction of the foot to compensate for the often severe equinus foot at this level. With the triple arthrodesis according to Lambrinudi, the joint congruence of the talus dome to the distal tibial joint surface is preserved. This is not possible with the isolated talectomy, whereby the equinus foot correction is limited by the height of the talus (**Figs. 16** and **17**).

If the talus is completely removed and an equinus remains, further surgical options are limited. Additional bony reduction in the rearfoot like hindfoot area is no longer possible at this point, because otherwise the joint surfaces can no longer articulate with each other. With Lambrinudi arthrodesis, on the other hand, the bone can be further resected until the equinus is adequately balanced. This is achieved by

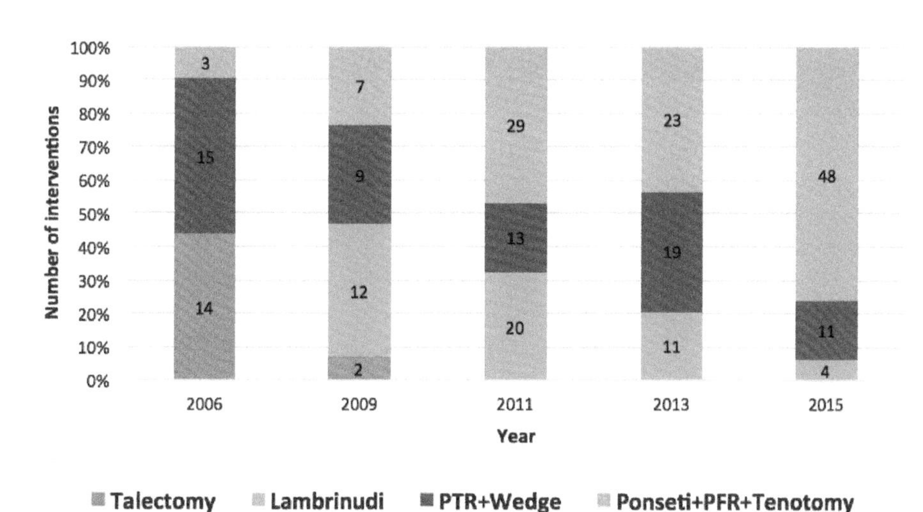

Fig. 14. The increase in cases pretreated with Ponseti method (*green*) as well as the switch from talectomy (*orange*) to Lambrinudi arthrodesis (*blue*). Patients treated with peritalar release and bony wedge have remained relatively constant (*violet*). *Data from* 173 patients with 245 neglected clubfeet aged between 1 and 9 years treated between 2006 and 2015 in India per method applied (unpublished).

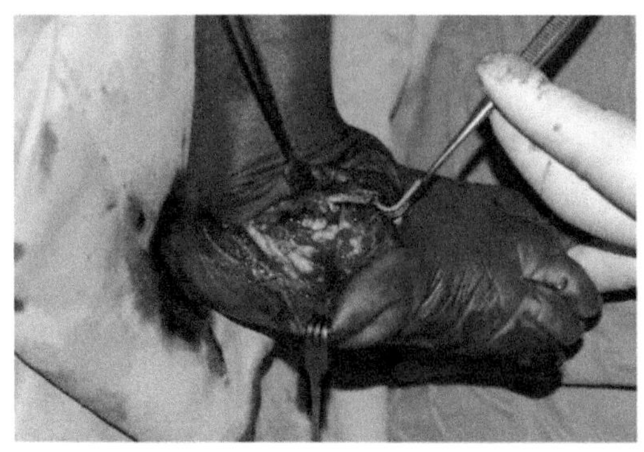

Fig. 15. Lambrinudi arthrodesis in an 8-year-old boy without Ponseti method pretreatment.

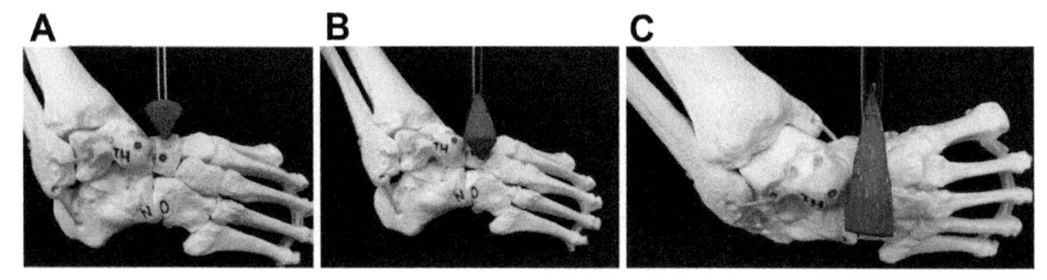

Fig. 16. (*A–C*) Two-dimensional wedge for midfoot equinus and adductus correction (Ponseti foot model; MD Orthopaedics/John Mitchell). If the dorsal or dorsomedial release does not provide sufficient equinus foot correction, the equinus is additionally corrected in the metatarsus.

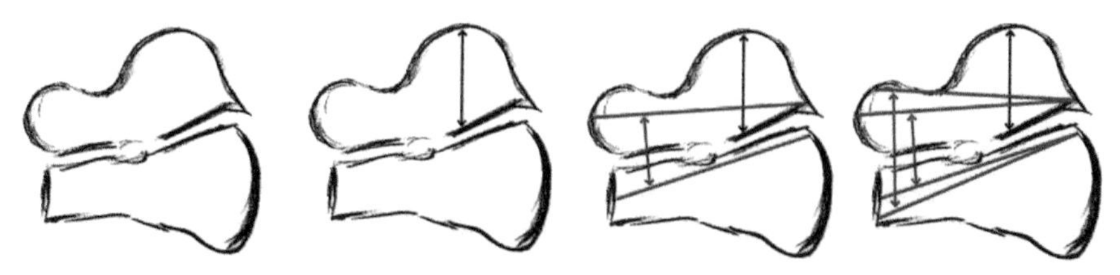

Fig. 17. (*A–D*) Talus height limits the equinus correction after its removal. Lambrinudi procedure offers more bone reduction options for equinus correction.

resection of a laterodorsal wedge of the upper surface of the calcaneus and/or the lower surface of the talus.

The Lambrinudi arthrodesis is combined with additional surgical procedures in untreated severe clubfeet in patients older than 6 years of age without pretreatment with the Ponseti method (**Fig. 18**).

FIRST STEP

The first step in the surgical treatment of an untreated clubfoot is the needling of the plantar fascia in the way described above. The often very shortened and rigid fascia supports the cavus as an important component of the clubfoot deformity. It can be performed with a simple 18-gauge injection needle or a beaver blade. Skin suture is not required when proceeding with an injection needle.

SECOND STEP

The needling is followed by a dorsal or dorsomedial soft tissue release. As an access route in combination with the Lambrinudi arthrodesis, the Turco approach is preferred with a longitudinal incision of approximately 8- to 10-cm medial to the Achilles tendon extending to the navicular bone (**Fig. 19**).

This access offers the advantage that the remaining skin bridge after the second skin incision described in step 3 acts as a reference for the lateral removal of the wedge by showing to what extent the bony correction has to be made. If the skin bridge is still under tension after lateral wedge removal (step 3) and triple arthrodesis (step 4), the skin can be additionally relieved with a bony resection. This approach reduces the risk of later suture dehiscence and wound-healing disorders.[3]

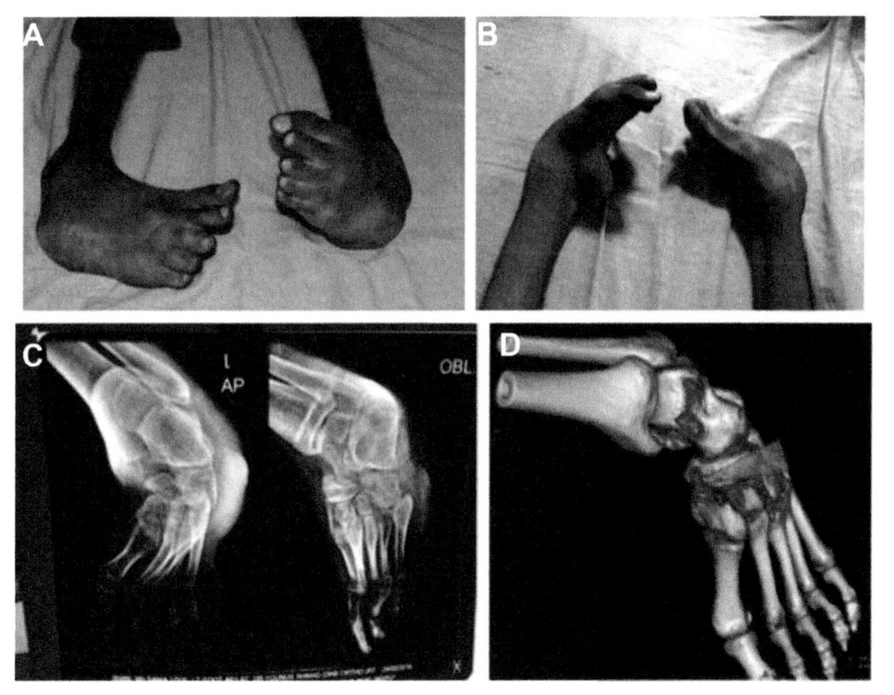

Fig. 18. Man, 18 years of age. (*A*, *B*) Congenital neglected clubfoot; (*C*) preoperative X ray; (*D*) plan for osteotomy.

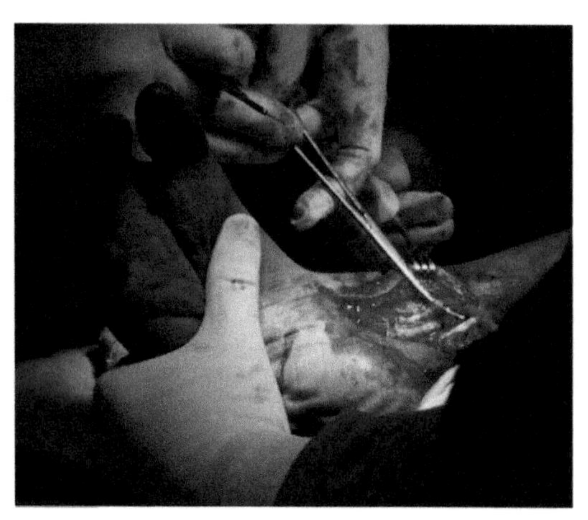

Fig. 19. Turco approach: Achiles Tendon Lengthening and dorsomedial release.

The peritendineum of the Achilles tendon is opened medially to prevent the tendon from sticking to the skin. The tendon is shown and extended in a Z-shape in a sagittal or frontal plane. The distal end is detached medially, and the proximal end is detached laterally in order to reduce the medial tension. After exposing the neurovascular bundle, the dorsal capsules of both ankle joints are opened to an extend that depends on the severity of the equinus. The dorsal portions of the stabilizing ligaments of the deltoid ligament and the ligamentum fibulotalare posterius are severed.[27] The interosseus ligament must be protected carefully.[3] In a very few cases, it is necessary to lengthen the tendons of the tibialis posterior, flexor hallucis, or digitorum longus muscles. As a standard, it can lead to severe overcorrection. The shortened tendons expand from the postsurgical cast treatment for 6 to 8 weeks, and the subsequent orthotic fitting of the surgically corrected foot for 6 to 12 months for older children and until the foot is outgrowing in younger children.[3]

THIRD STEP

In the third step, a curved skin incision, similar to the Ollier approach, is carried out below the lateral malleolus over the sinus tarsi on the dorsum of the foot. The often atrophic belly of the extensor digitorum brevis muscle is detached from the sinus tarsi with its tendinous attachment and dissected distally. The upper limit for the preparation is given by the long extensor tendon of the digit V, whereas the plantar limit is given by the peroneal tendons. With this preparation, the entire laterodorsal tarsus is bony, and the lower ankle is exposed. This gives an excellent overview of the center of the bony deformity of an untreated clubfoot. The CORA is located in the joint cross, formed by the head of the talus, the anterior part of the calcaneus, the cuboid bone, and the navicular bone. Depending on the severity and its rigidity in passive correction of the foot, an attempt can be made to preserve the talonavicular joint. In most cases, this is not possible with an untreated clubfoot. Nevertheless, the first saw cut can be made straight, thus maintaining the joint but complemented through the entire tarsus. The anatomically changed curvature of the untreated clubfoot must be taken into account in order to protect the plantar vessels. The second saw cut runs further distal, and the wedge shape is now determined. The saw blade is tilted distally and laterally at the same time. In this way, a wedge that is broadly based dorsally for the equinus

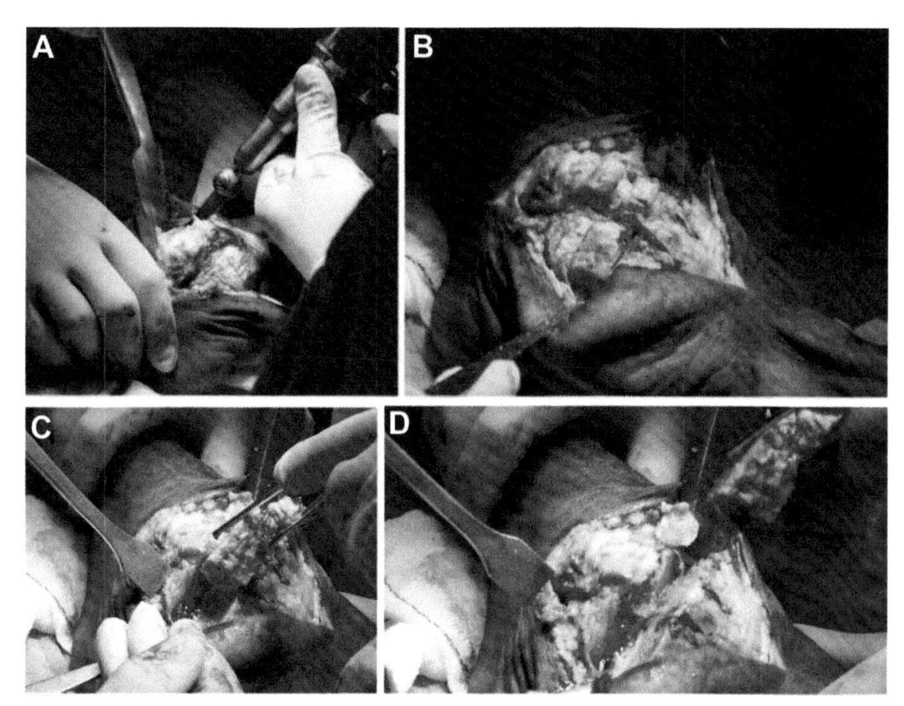

Fig. 20. (*A–D*) Man, 18 years of age; laterodorsal midfoot wedge removal.

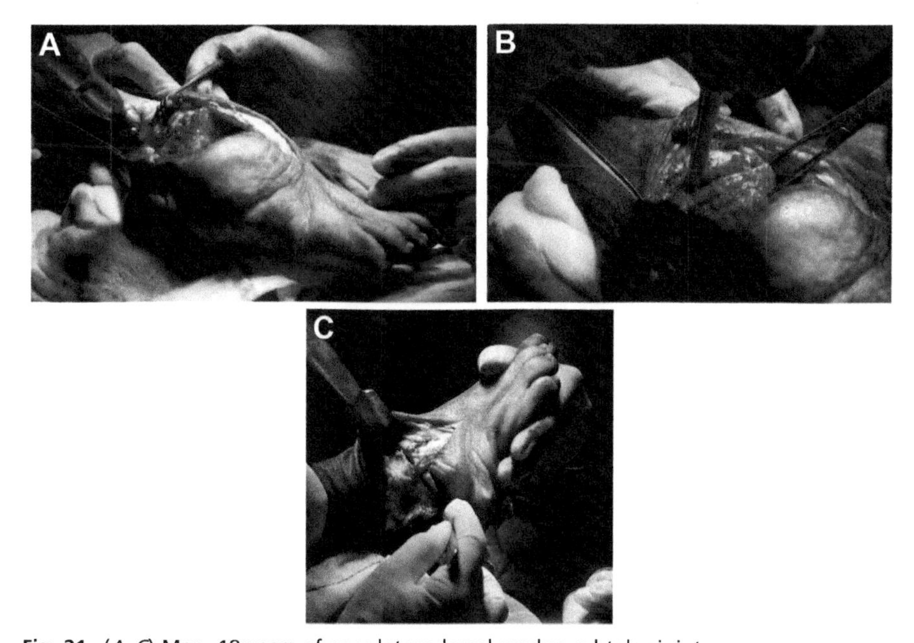

Fig. 21. (*A–C*) Man, 18 years of age; laterodorsal wedge subtalar joint.

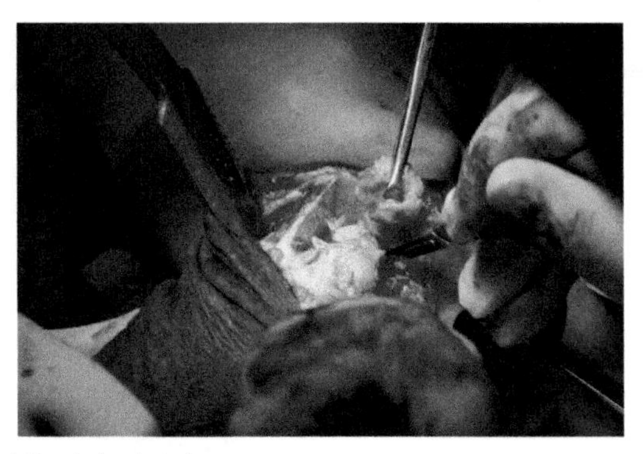

Fig. 22. Removal of the talar head.

correction and broadly based laterally for the adduction correction can be sawed (**Fig. 20**).

Both saw cuts are pointed medially and the insertion of the musculus tibialis posterior tendon on the navicular bone can be protected. The osteotomy gap is then closed provisionally, and the correction achieved is assessed. If the correction is not sufficient, more bone must be resected in the corresponding sawing directions. If a complete correction is still not successful, the talonavicular joint cannot be preserved, and a triple arthrodesis according to Lambrinudi has to be performed.

FOURTH STEP

For the triple arthrodesis according to Lambrinudi, another 2-dimensional wedge is removed for further osseous correction of the equinus and the hindfoot varus.[32,33] The saw cut for removing the wedge on the subtalar joint rises from the rear foot distally: on the talus in a dorsal direction to the dorsum of the foot and on the calcaneus in a plantar direction to the sole of the foot. At the same time, the saw blade is tilted accordingly for the lateral widening of the wedge. The equinus is corrected by widening the wedge distally, and the hindfoot varus is corrected by widening the wedge laterally (**Fig. 21**).

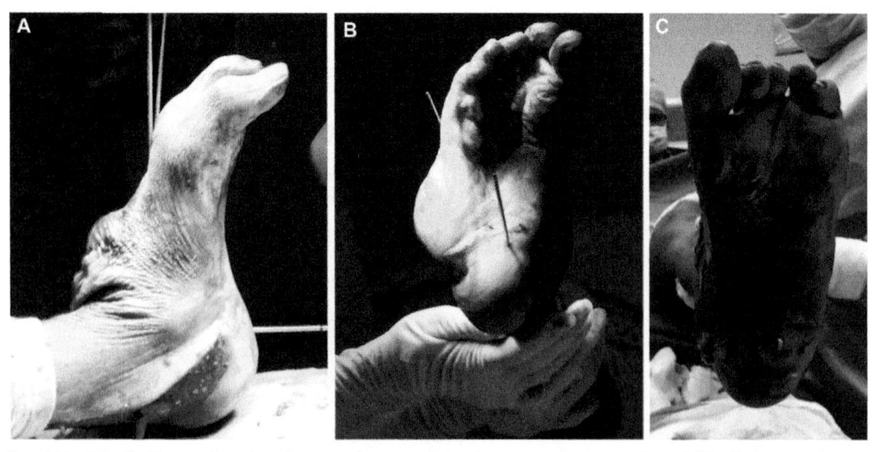

Fig. 23. (*A–C*) To maintain the equinus correction, a wire can be drilled from plantar through the calcaneus into the tibia.

All osteotomies from the middle and rear foot are closed, and the overall correction of the foot is assessed. In most cases, it becomes apparent at this point if a complete correction of the foot cannot be achieved without removing the talar head (**Fig. 22**).

If the foot is corrected adequately, the skin does not show high tension, and the blood circulation in the foot after opening the tourniquet is assured through the adequate bony correction. The osteosynthesis can be carried out with Kirschner wires. These are placed interdigital between digitorum II and III as well as between digitorum IV and V and anchored dorsally in the bones of the hindfoot in the talus and calcaneus. Because an image converter is often not available in lesser economically developed countries, the anchoring of the wires is controlled by checking for a hard resistance when drilling into the bone (**Fig. 23**).

This kind of middle and hindfoot correction of untreated clubfoot has the advantage that the talus dome with its joint surface can be maintained, articulating with the distal

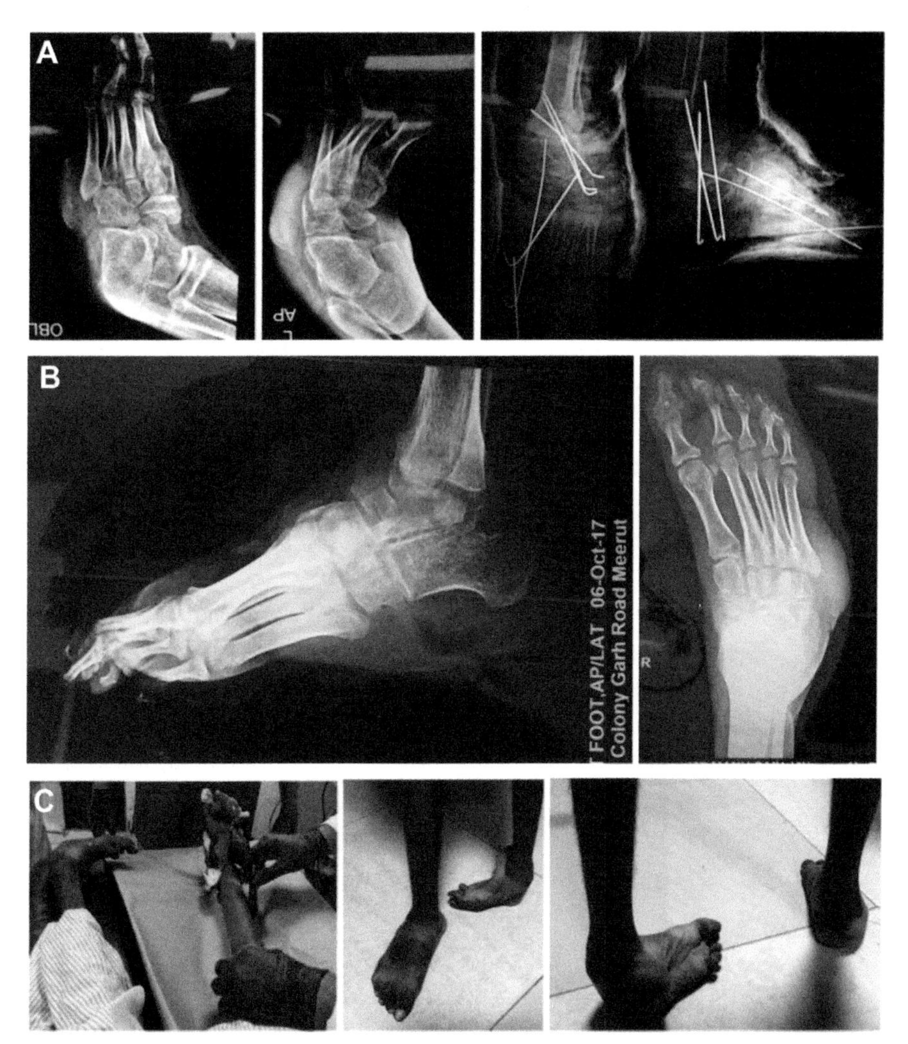

Fig. 24. Man, 18 years of age: (*A*) preoperative and postoperative X ray; (*B*) X ray after K-wire removal; (*C*) postoperative measurement for orthosis and follow-up after 1 year.

tibial joint surface, and the upper ankle remains functional. This is not possible with a talectomy.

FIFTH STEP

Once the laterodorsal wedge is removed from the tarsus and the rear- and midfoot osteotomy is closed with a wedge removal that rises distally and laterally, it is not uncommon to observe that the first metatarsal is still deeper in the plantar direction. This misalignment cannot be corrected adequately with the tarsal wedge or the connected triple arthrodesis (Lambrinudi). Without a correction of the first ray, full load-bearing of the foot then leads to a varisation of the rearfoot and a progressive load on the lateral edge of the foot. To make the correction perfect, an extension osteotomy of the first metatarsal must be performed for the hindfoot correction described above. A dorsally broadly based wedge is removed from the base of the first metatarsal, and the head is raised.[34] If the metatarsal I and metatarsal V are at the same level, the osteotomy is closed and fixed with a K-wire or a small dorsal clamp (**Fig. 24**).

When closing the skin, the bursa will not be resected on the lateral edge of the foot, as it regresses completely on its own. After suturing the skin, Betadine ointment is used for all wounds and wire entries, keeping the skin soft and elastic, preventing seam divergence (experience from the author's own operations).

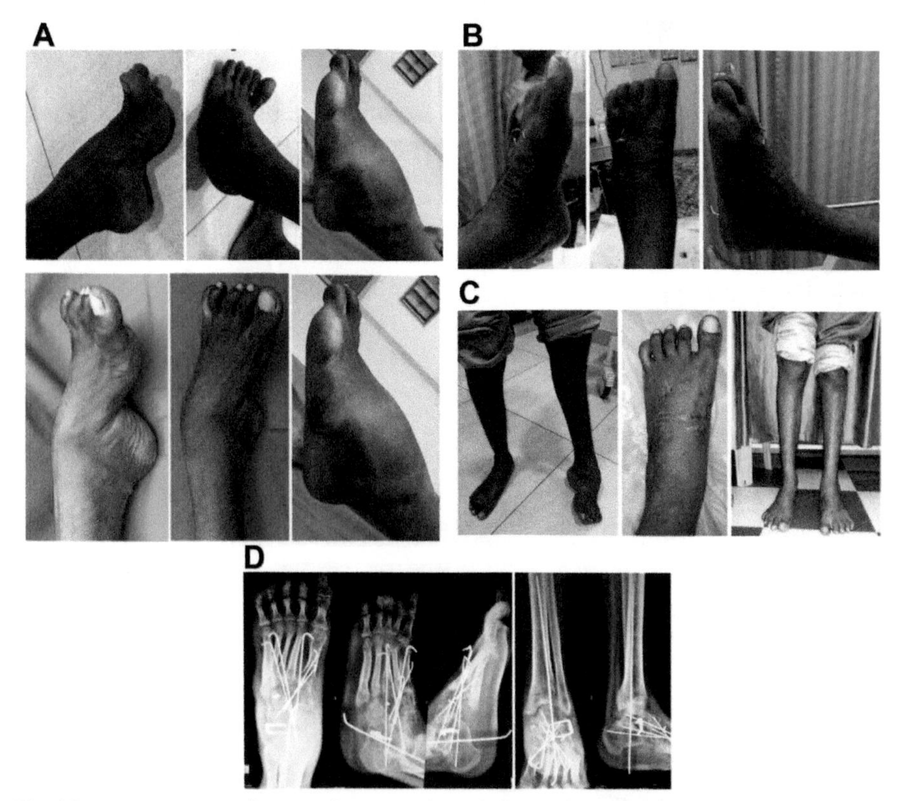

Fig. 25. Man, 21 years of age with a neurologic left clubfoot: (*A*) preoperative; (*B*) Lambrinudi triple arthrodesis and tibialis posterior muscle transfer; (*C*) preoperative and postoperative after 1 year in standing position; (*D*) X ray postoperative.

POSTOPERATIVE CARE

After the surgery, significant flexion of all toes is observed, which is caused by the strong corrective tension of the flexor tendons of the musculi flexor digitorum and hallucis longus as the tendon of the tibialis posterior muscle is also shortened. These tendons do not have to be lengthened in the Lambrinudi arthrodesis because, according to the author's experience, the tendons stretch and adjust correctly after the postoperative cast treatment. Avoiding lengthening of the tendons also protects the foot from overcorrection by stabilizing the foot postoperatively.

However, this does not necessarily hold for a neurologic or syndromic clubfoot. Here, the muscular imbalance is higher, and the operative therapy must adapt accordingly. Depending on the syndromic or neurologic dysfunction, tendons are transposed or lengthened. This often affects the tendons of the tibialis posterior and anterior muscles. The tendon of the tibialis posterior muscle can be transposed laterally by placing it on the lateral cuneiform bone through the interosseous membrane. The same applies to the tendon of the tibialis anterior muscle. If there is significant functional adduction in the swing phase of walking, the tendon can be moved from medial to lateral to the cuneiform laterale (**Fig. 25**).

SUMMARY

Clearly, the treatment with the Ponseti method is getting functionally better results for a clubfoot than surgical treatments.[35] With restricted time available, as it is often the case in aid projects, the Lambrinudi arthrodesis offers several advantages for severe and rigid neglected clubfeet. It has great potential for correction and can be adapted individually as described in the 5 steps above:

Its key step is the additive equinus correction with removal of the dorsolateral wedge of the tarsal bone.

Despite significant bony wedges being removed, the correction of the adductus and hindfoot varus increases the length of the foot. The valley dome is retained and allows the foot to roll over. The untreated clubfoot is a foot surgical challenge that has to generate a complete and long-lasting corrective result for the affected person. Therefore, the great corrective potential and the well-preserved function make the Lambrinudi arthrodesis an important surgical procedure for untreated clubfoot independent of patients age, even under precarious treatment conditions.

CLINICS CARE POINTS

Key Rules in Treatment of Neglected Clubfoot

- Train local staff in using the Ponseti method during a foreign deployment.
- Prepare surgical interventions with pretreatment via Ponseti method at all times.
- Treat patients with neglected clubfeet according to the following age-specific treatment algorithm:

Age-specific Therapy Algorithm

Children under the age of 6

The neglected clubfeet can often be fully corrected within 14 days by using the Ponseti method, needling of the plantar fascia, and tenotomy of the Achilles tendon. In cases whereby full correction cannot be achieved, a dorsal release and possibly a laterodorsal wedge osteotomy can be performed additionally.

Children aged 6 to 12

If the time frame of therapy is wide enough, a treatment using the Ponseti method can be started, followed by surgery using Achilles tendon lengthening, dorsal release, and laterodorsal wedge osteotomy. Should these surgical methods not lead to sufficient correction, an arthrodesis of the lower ankle (Lambrinudi arthrodesis) is recommended.

Adolescents aged 12 and above

The same procedure as with children aged 6 to 12 can be applied; however, in most cases, a Lambrinudi triple arthrodesis will be necessary. This method is preferable to performing a talectomy, as it preserves the upper ankle joint in its form, thus leading to better foot function.

- Use orthopedic splints in correction for nighttime until the feet are fully grown.
- Adolescent patients should use orthopedic splints for 12 months after surgery.
- A dynamic ankle and foot orthosis should be worn daily for 12 to 24 months.

DISCLOSURE

The author has no financial relationships or conflicts related to this work.

REFERENCES

1. Staheli L, Ponseti I. Clubfoot: Ponseti management, Global HELP Organization; 2009. 3 rd Edition.
2. Ippolito E, Ponseti IV. Congenital clubfoot in the human fetus: a histological study. J Bone Joint Surg Am 1980;62(1):8–22.
3. Norgrove Penny J. The neglected clubfoot. Tech Orthop 2005;20(2):153–66.
4. Pirani S, Zeznik L, Hodges D. Magnetic resonance imaging study of the congenital clubfoot treated with the Ponseti method. J Pediatr Orthop 2001;21(6):719–26.
5. Ponseti IV, Smoley EN. Congenital clubfoot: the results of treatment. J Bone Joint Surg 1963;45A:22261–75.
6. Cooper DM, Dietz FR. Treatment of idiopathic club foot: a thirty-year follow-up note. J Bone Joint Surg Am 1995;77-A:1477–89.
7. Ponseti IV. Congenital clubfoot: fundamentals of treatment. New York (NY): Oxford University Press; 1996.
8. Lourenço AF, Morcuende JA. A Morcuende correction of neglected idiopathic clubfoot by the Ponseti method. J Bone Joint Surg Br 2007;89(3):378–81.
9. Herzenberg JE, Frick SL, Bor N, et al. Ponseti management of clubfoot in older infants. Clin Orthop Relat Res 2006;444:224–8.
10. Spiegel D a, Shrestha OP, Sitoula P, et al. Ponseti method for untreated idiopathic clubfeet in Nepalese patients from 1 to 6 years of age. Clin Orthop Relat Res 2009;467(5):1164–70.
11. Ferreira GF, Stéfani KC, Haje DP, et al. The Ponseti method in children with clubfoot after walking age - systematic review and metanalysis of observational studies. PLoS One 2018;13(11):e0207153.
12. Haje DP, Canto SJ, Kumar R, et al. Ponseti method after walking age – a multicentric study of 429 feet. Iowa Orthop J 2020;40(2):1–12.
13. Nogueira MP, Pereira JC, Duarte PS, et al. Ponseti Brasil: a national program to eradicate neglected clubfoot - preliminary results. Iowa Orthop J 2011;31:43–8.
14. Khan SA, Kumar A. Ponseti's manipulation in neglected clubfoot in children more than 7 years of age: a prospective evaluation of 25 feet with long-term follow-up. J Pediatr Orthop B 2010;19(5):385–9.
15. Gupta A, Singh S, Patel P, et al. Evaluation of the utility of the Ponseti method of correction of clubfoot deformity in a developing nation. Int Orthop 2008;32(1):75–9.

16. Pirani S, Naddumba E, Mathias R, et al. Towards effective Ponseti clubfoot care: the Uganda sustainable clubfoot care project. Clin Orthop Relat Res 2009;467(5): 1154–63.
17. Staheli L. Help-Ponseti Uganda, Global HELP Organization; 2008.
18. Morcuende JA, Dolan LA, Dietz FR, et al. Radical reduction in the rate of extensive corrective surgery for clubfoot using the Ponseti method. Pediatrics 2004; 113:376–80.
19. Fernandes RM, Mendes MD, Amorim R, et al. Surgical treatment of neglected clubfoot using external fixator. Rev Bras Ortop 2016;51(5):501–8.
20. Nogueira MP, Ey Batlle AM, Alves CG. Is it possible to treat recurrent clubfoot with the Ponseti technique after posteromedial release?: a preliminary study. Clin Orthop Relat Res 2009;467(5):1298–305.
21. Ferreira GF, Stéfani KC, Haje DP, et al. The Ponseti method in children with clubfoot after walking age - Systematic review and metanalysis of observational studies. PLoS One 2018;13(11).
22. Steenbeck M, Book O. Steenbeck Brace for Clubfoot, Global HELP Organization; 2009. 2 nd Edition.
23. Steindler A. Release of the plantar fascia soft tissue for cavus deformity of the foot. Surg Gynecol Obstet 1917;612–5.
24. Minkowitz B, Finkelstein BI, Bleicher M. Percutaneous tendo-Achilles lengthening with a large-gauge needle: a modification of the Ponseti technique for correction of idiopathic clubfoot. Foot Ankle Surg 2004;43(4):263–5.
25. Evans A, Chowdhury M, Rana S, et al. 'Fast cast' and 'needle tenotomy' protocols with the Ponseti method to improve clubfoot management in Bangladesh. J Foot Ankle Res 2017;10:49.
26. Sengupta A. The management of congenital talipes equinovarus in developing countries. Int Orthop 1987;11:183–7.
27. McKay DW. New concept and approach to club-foot treatment: section I - principles and morbid anatomy. J Pediatr Orthop 1982;2:347–56.
28. Turco VJ. Surgical correction of the resistant clubfoot. One stage posteromedial release with internal fixation: a preliminary report. J Bone Joint Surg 1971;53:477–97.
29. Crawford AH, Marxen JL, Osterfeld DL. The Cincinnati incision: a comprehensive approach for surgical procedures of the foot and ankle in childhood. J Bone Joint Surg Am 1982;64(9):1355–8.
30. Hsu WK, Bhatia NN, Raskin A, et al. Wound complications from idiopathic clubfoot surgery: a comparison of the modified Turco and the Cincinnati treatment methods. J Pediatr Orthop 2007;27(3):329–32.
31. Lichtblau S. A medial and lateral release operation for clubfoot. J Bone Joint Surg (Am) 1973;55:1377–84.
32. Lambrinudi C. New operation on drop foot. Br J Surg 1927;15:193.
33. Döderlein L, Wenz W, Schneider U. Fußdeformitäten: Der Klumpfuß. Triple- und Lambrinudi-Arthrodese. Springer Verlag Berlin 1999. p. 212-19.
34. Mubarak SJ, Van Valin SE. Osteotomies of the foot for cavus deformities in children. J Pediatr Orthop 2009;29(3):294–9.
35. Ippolito E, Farsetti P, Caterini R, et al. Long-term comparative results in patients with congenital clubfoot treated with two different protocols. J Bone Joint Surg Am 2003;85(7):1286–94.

An Approach to the Management of Severe Clubfoot Deformities on Global Humanitarian Programs

The Role of Talectomy

Mark S. Myerson, MD[a,b,*], Davi P. Haje, MD[c]

KEYWORDS

- Clubfoot • Talectomy • Humanitarian • Recurrent clubfoot • Untreated clubfoot • Neglected clubfoot • Ponseti • Triple arthrodesis

KEY POINTS

- Provided some range of motion is present in the ankle joint correction of severe deformity can be accomplished with a triple arthrodesis and supplemented by appropriate soft tissue releases and tendon transfers to balance the foot as necessary.
- In the presence of a flat top talus and an equinus deformity following multiple prior surgeries, regaining dorsiflexion is difficult and one should consider an anterior tibial closing wedge osteotomy with additional procedures to correct multiplanar deformity.
- A talectomy is a useful procedure to correct a very rigid foot and ankle, particularly when alternative methods such as Ilizarov fixation are not feasible. This is ideally performed bilaterally.
- Talectomy is a very effective procedure to correct any deformity but may require a supplemental closing wedge of the calcaneocuboid joint to correct adduction.
- Talectomy can be performed in younger patients without any arthrodesis but in the older patient, a tibiocalcaneal and tibionavicular arthrodesis are useful to improve stability.

INTRODUCTION

The approach to treatment of severe untreated or recurrent congenital talipes equinovarus (CTEV) deformities is very different in the world where patients are mobile, have access to repeated return visits for follow-up treatment, and where more sophisticated options for gradual correction with external fixation are available.[1–4] Although the Ponseti treatment has been successfully applied to untreated deformity even in older

[a] Orthopedic Surgery, University of Colorado; [b] Steps2Walk; [c] Centro Clinico Orthopectus e IGESDF, SMHN Bloco A Ed. Clínicas, Sala 804-806, Brasília, DF 70710-904, Brazil
* Corresponding author. Orthopedic Surgery, University of Colorado.
E-mail address: mark4feet@gmail.com

Foot Ankle Clin N Am 26 (2021) 727–745
https://doi.org/10.1016/j.fcl.2021.07.005

children and young adults, some of these patients do not have the ability to return from rural regions for repeated casting and bracing after this treatment.[1,5] The Ponseti treatment nowadays is widely used in different low or middle-income countries for neglected clubfoot treatment. A multicenter study performed by 15 different centers of 8 countries with 429 neglected clubfeet (median age of 3 years and maximum of 30 years) reported that the Ponseti method was able to correct the deformity in 87%.[6] During the last 10 years, there have been increasing numbers of reports of neglected clubfoot treatment with the Ponseti method. **Table 1** shows a literature review of treatments for the neglected clubfoot.

The Ponseti method has been used regularly for treating relapses, residual deformities, and neglected clubfoot in children and adolescents.[16,17] Talectomy has been reported for clubfoot treatment in children and adults with a neglected clubfoot, especially associated with syndromes or nonidiopathic deformity associated with arthrogryposis multiplex congenita and myelomeningocele.[14,18] However, the Ponseti method has become the first line of treatment chosen in many centers even for those syndrome-associated feet in the first year of life.[15] Matar and colleagues[15] reported 82% of good results after treating syndrome-associated CTEV using the Ponseti method at a mean age of 6.1 weeks (range, 2–17 weeks). The treatment of syndromic or nonidiopathic clubfeet in older children of a walking age still remains a challenge. Letts and Davidson reported that 71% of the neglected clubfoot syndrome deformities had average or good results after talectomy at a mean age of 6 years (range, 1–15 years).[10] Trumble and colleagues[9] reported talectomy treatment for myelodysplasia in patients with a maximum age of 7 years. Although the coauthor has a nonpublished series of 10 syndromic-related neglected clubfeet treated with the Ponseti method (mean age, 7 years; range, 1 year and 2 months to 14 years and 7 months) (**Fig. 1**), there is only one report in the literature about this treatment method in walking age children. Golanski and colleagues[19] reported the application of the Ponseti method in a case of neglected clubfoot in a 4-year and 9-month-old boy with DiGeorge syndrome. De Mulder and colleagues[20] did a systematic review in 2018 about the treatment of nonidiopathic clubfeet with the Ponseti method and found articles that reported treatment at a maximum age of 2.8 months.

For treatment, talectomy may be the only option to treat certain neglected clubfoot deformities during humanitarian programs[1] and it may still have to be used as a salvage procedure used in modern foot surgery.[21] In feet with associated fixed equinus, the Lambrinudi arthrodeis is an option.[22] The spectrum of treatment of these recurrent or untreated deformities in children and adults is tremendous, ranging from minor procedures such as an anterior tibial tendon transfer, tendon transfers with or without osteotomy, to arthrodesis or even talectomy. The goal of treatment for these severe deformities is to obtain a plantigrade foot with no likelihood for recurrent deformity. Our extensive experience with these deformities has been on global humanitarian programs where we have very limited resources, a lack of availability of implants, and where the needs of patients are quite different from those which we as surgeons are accustomed to in the western world.

PONSETI VERSUS TALECTOMY

This setting will affect decision-making since resorting to a Ponseti treatment is frequently not possible when local surgeons do not have expertise in the Ponseti technique, and prolonged treatments with external fixation are not practical for these patients. Smythe and colleagues[23] reported that there is a lack of trained doctors to provide clubfoot treatment in Africa and there is no standard training. Various options

Table 1
Literature review about neglected clubfoot treatment

Author	Country	Year	Treatment Method	Journal
Zuniga	Honduras	1959	Extensive surgery	Rev Med Hond
Bartknowiak	Polonia	1961	Extensive surgery (Talectomy)	Chir Narzadow Ruchu Ortop Pol
Grassi and Murari	Italy	1967	Extensive surgery	Arch Chir Organi
Bartolomei and Vuono	Brazil	1971	Extensive surgery (Talectomy)	Rev Bras Ortop
Herold and Torok	Israel	1973	Extensive surgery	J Bone Joint Surg Am
Yadav	India	1981	Extensive surgery	Int Orthop
Napoli et al	Brazil	1982	Extensive surgery (Talectomy)	Actualities Med Chir Pred
Cooper and Capello[7]	EUA	1985	Extensive surgery (Talectomy)	Clin Orthop Relat Res
Hsu et al.[8]	Hong Kong	1985	Extensive surgery (Talectomy)	J Bone Joint Surg Am
Trumble[9]	EUA	1985	Extensive surgery (Talectomy)	J Bone Joint Surg Am
Grill and Franke	Austria	1987	External Fixator (Ilizarov)	J Bone Joint Surg Br
Sølund K	Denmark	1991	Extensive surgery (Talectomy)	Acta Orthop Scand
Santos et al.	Brazil	1992	Extensive surgery (Talectomy)	Rev Bras Ortop
Salomão et al.	Brazil	1993	Extensive surgery (Talectomy)	Rev Bras Ortop
de la Huerta	Mexico	1994	External fixator (Ilizarov)	Clin Orthop Relat Res
Sobel et al.	EUA	1996	Extensive surgery	J Foot Ankle Surg
D'Souza et al.	India	1996	Extensive surgery	J Postgrad Med
el-Tayeby	Egypt	1998	Extensive surgery	J Foot Ankle Surg
Lejman et al.	Polonia	1998	External fixator (Ilizarov)	Chir Narzadow Ruchu Ortop Pol.
D'Souza et al.	India	1998	Extensive surgery (Talectomy)	J Pediatr Orthop
Ferreira et al.	Brazil	1999	External fixator (Ilizarov)	Rev Bras Ortop
Letts and Davidson[10]	Canada	1999	Extensive surgery (talectomy)	Am J Orthop
El Barbary et al.	Egypt	2004	External fixator (Ilizarov)	Int Orthop
Yalçin et al.	Turkey	2005	Extensive surgery (talectomy)	Acta Orthop Traumatol Turc

(*continued on next page*)

Table 1
(continued)

Author	Country	Year	Treatment Method	Journal
Rosselli et al.	Colombia	2005	Extensive surgery	J Pediatr Orthop
Ferreira et al.[11]	Brazil	2006	External fixator (Ilizarov)	Foot Ankle Int
Khan and Chinoy	Pakistan	2006	Extensive surgery	J Foot Ankle Surg
Lourenço and Morcuende	Brazil	2007	Ponseti method	J Bone Joint Surg Br
Reize and Ulrich	Switzerland	2007	Extensive surgery	J Pediatr Orthop B
Spiegel et al.	Nepal	2009	Ponseti method	Clin Orthop Relat Res
Purushothamdas et al.	UK	2009	Extensive surgery	J Pediatr Orthop B
Khan and Kumar[12]	India	2010	Ponseti method	J Pediatr Orthop B
Lui TH	China	2010	Extensive surgery	Arch Orthop Trauma Surg
Tripathy et al.	India	2011	External fixator (Ilizarov)	J Pediatr Orthop B
Faldini	Italy	2013	Extensive surgery	Clin Orthop Relat Res
Banskota et al.	Nepal	2013	Ponseti method	Bone Joint J
Khanfour	Egypt	2013	External fixator (Ilizarov)	J Pediatr Orthop B
Haje DP[13]	Brazil	2013	Ponseti method	JBJS Case Connect
Ayana et al.	Ethiopia	2014	Ponseti method	Acta Orthop
Lohia et al.	India	2014	External fixator + extensive surgery	Foot Ankle Surg
Akinci and Akalin	Turkey	2015	Extensive surgery	Acta Orthop Traumatol Turc
El-Sherbiny and Omran	Egypt	2015	Extensive surgery (talectomy)	J Foot Ankle Surg
Chotigavanichaya et al.	Thailand	2015	Extensive surgery (talectomy)	J Med Assoc Thai
Faizan et al.	India	2015	Ponseti method	J Foot Ankle Surg
Sinha et al.	India	2016	Ponseti method	Indian J Orthop
Faldini et al.	Italy	2016	Extensive surgery	Musculoskelet Surg
Fernandes et al.	Brazil	2016	External fixator (Ilizarov)	Rev Bras Ortop
Bashi et al.	Iran	2016	Ponseti method	J Pediatr Orthop B

Adegbehingbe et al.	Nigeria	2017	Ponseti method	World J Orthop
Machida et al.[14]	Japan	2017	Extensive surgery	J Orthop Sci
Matar et al.[15]	UK	2018	Extensive surgery (talectomy)	J Pediatr Orthop B
Mehtani et al.	India	2018	Ponseti method	J Pediatr Orthop B
Ajmera	India	2019	External fixator (Ilizarov)	J Pediatr Orthop B
Jamil et al.	India	2019	Ponseti method	J Liaquat Uni Med Health Sci
Haje et al[6]	Multi-Centric	2020	Ponseti method	Iowa Orthop J

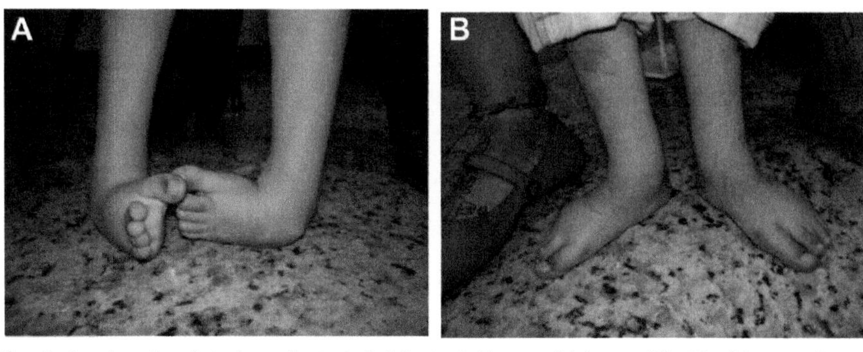

Fig. 1. Syndromic-related neglected clubfeet. A 5-year-old boy with Moebius syndrome before (*A*) and after the Ponseti treatment method (*B*).

that we have considered are to train orthopedic surgeons in these regions with the Ponseti method,[24–26] or to teach them how to perform procedures associated with talectomy. Moreover, the age limit for starting the Ponseti technique is not predictable, and the older cases published up to now are patients in their late twenties.[6,13] In underserved countries, there are adult patients with neglected CTEV that have limited access to surgical centers or there are no trained surgeons to treat surgically those cases with external fixator or extensive surgery including talectomy.[26] One advantage of using the Ponseti method in medical centers of these underserved regions of the world is that the treatment can be performed in an outpatient clinic, even when there is a need for percutaneous Achilles tenotomy, with low cost, nor any need for implants or extensive surgery. **Fig. 2** shows an example of a 24-year-old male with bilateral neglected CTEV where all the treatment was performed on an outpatient basis, and needed only sedation before the last cast to perform the percutaneous Achilles tenotomy and manipulate the feet in dorsiflexion.

These deformities are so variable that a simplistic algorithm for surgical treatment is not possible, especially when we are treating a foot with residual deformity after previous surgical treatment(s) or a relapsed case after surgery or surgeries. The results of treatment of these severe deformities that have been treated surgically previously, and for some patients with multiple interventions have a less predictable outcome with the Ponseti treatment and hence talectomy remains an option. There are those with a fixed equinus and no dorsiflexion of the ankle because of a flat top talus. Addressing the foot alone will not correct the deformity and in these children, an anterior closing wedge osteotomy of the tibia is required in addition to triplanar correction of the foot. In patients with some range of motion of the ankle but an equinus deformity, it may be very difficult to regain dorsiflexion because of severe scarring of the Achilles tendon, which may even be adherent to the skin (**Fig. 3**).

In some attempts to correct the equinus deformity, it is possible to have a limited dorsiflexion because of anterior tibiotalar impingement. Provided that some ankle range of motion is present, most deformities of the foot no matter how severe can be corrected with a combination of osteotomies, tendon transfers or arthrodesis, and a triple arthrodesis would be the procedure of choice. For rigid severe deformities of the foot and ankle in children with syndromic deformities and those who have undergone prior surgery(ies) and in particular where no motion whatsoever is present, talectomy is preferable. The indications for talectomy in the setting of an untreated or recurrent club foot deformity are nowadays uncommon and rarely necessary with the use of modern external fixation techniques.[21] As noted, however, this is not a

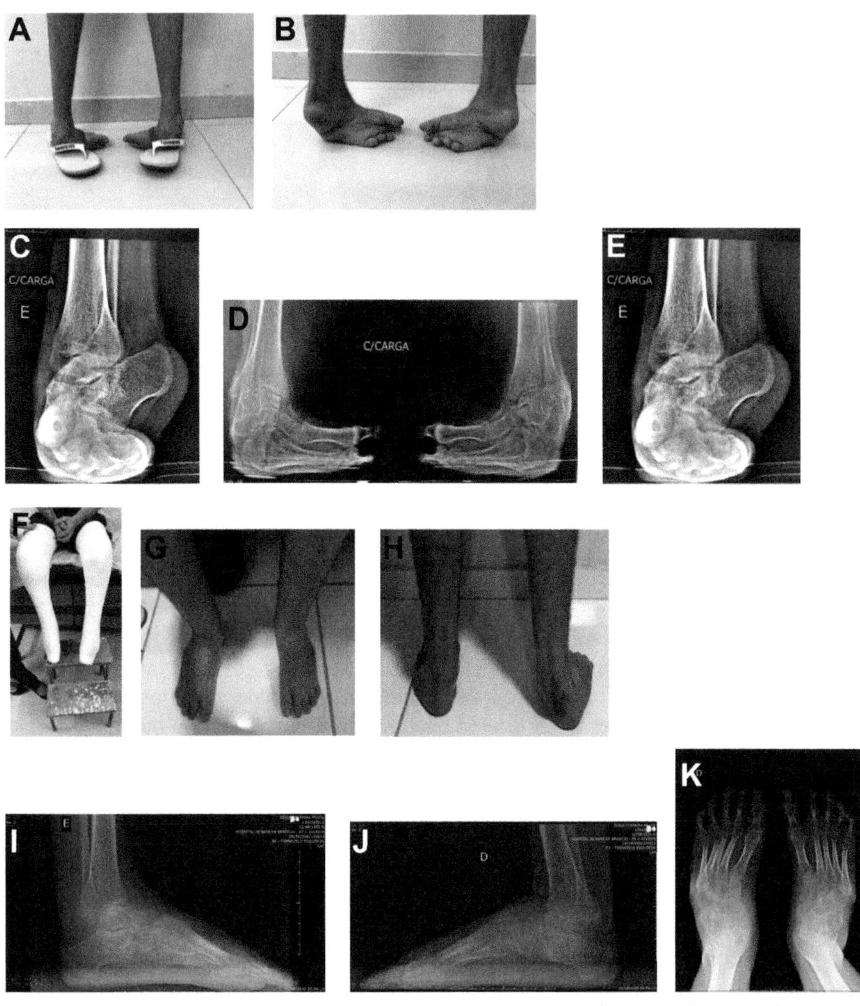

Fig. 2. A 24-year-old with bilateral neglected idiopathic clubfoot (*A–E*), treated with the Ponseti method. In total, 8 casts were applied, the fifth cast is illustrated (*F*) with a good clinical (*G, H*) and radiologic outcome (*I–K*).

treatment option for our patients in rural settings where continuous monitoring of fixation or serial casting is necessary and often there is not a surgeon with expertise in those devices or the Ponseti method. Moreover, the use of external fixators and extensive surgeries involve severe scarring, which lead to joint rigidity, residual pain and deformity, and an eventual need for future arthrodesis because of degenerative changes.[7] For this reason where we feel it is necessary, we may add a tibiocalcaneal (TC) and a tibionavicular (TN) arthrodesis to the talectomy in selected cases.

Ferreira and colleagues[11] reported spontaneous ankylosis of the ankle in 73.7% of cases, 50% recurrence, and a need for arthrodesis in 23.7% of their neglected clubfoot patients treated with the use of external fixator. Joint mobility was reported as functional in neglected clubfoot cases treated with the Ponseti method although there was not enough residual pain (secondary to joint degeneration) that could justify arthrodesis. However, the reported adult patients were few and had not enough

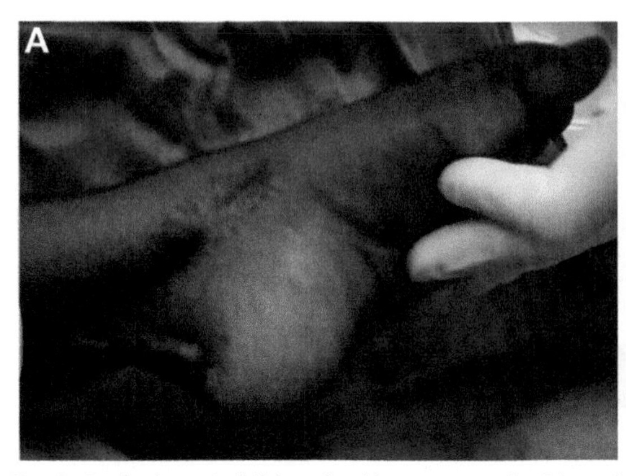

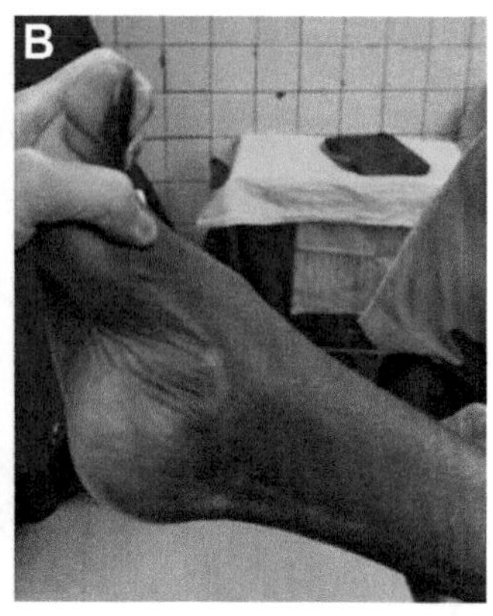

Fig. 3. Both these 2 children had been treated with multiple surgeries with severe scarring of the foot and ankle and adherence of the Achilles tendon to the skin with no range of motion whatsoever in the foot nor ankle.

follow-up.[12,13,27,28] Another point is that if the Ponseti method cannot fully correct the recurrent or neglected clubfoot, it can decrease the extent of subsequent surgery, avoiding talectomy.

Patient Evaluation

Decision-making is based on the mobility of the foot and ankle, the presence of scarring from prior surgeries, the presence of bilateral deformity, and the overall needs of the patient. These feet are already small, therefore, anything other than gradual correction with external fixation or Ponseti method will further reduce the foot size, as lateral shortening is always safer and easier than medial lengthening. One has to anticipate a significant leg length discrepancy after talectomy which averages 2.5 cm, and approximately 3 cm if a TC arthrodesis is performed. For this reason, a unilateral talectomy must be a last resort. If bilateral deformities are present, this decision-making is easier as both limbs will be shorter, and leg length discrepancy will not be a concern.[10] If some albeit limited ankle range of motion is present and the foot can be passively corrected into neutral, a talectomy is not indicated because a triple arthrodesis combined with tendon transfers and additional osteotomies can be performed regardless of the magnitude of deformity. If a flat top talus is present in the child associated with a fixed equinus deformity and limited dorsiflexion, it is quite reasonable to perform an anterior closing wedge osteotomy of the distal tibia to regain dorsiflexion, which is similar to the procedure of anterior distal tibial epiphysiodesis performed in children with residual or recurrent equinus deformity.[29] Therefore, it is the magnitude of the equinus deformity, the associated soft tissue scarring or contracture, and the possibility of ischemia with an attempt of correction with alternative methods that will determine the need for a talectomy. Scarring can be quite daunting and will limit the ability to use the Ponseti method as well as perform a revision with additional soft tissue release procedures, and if so, one may need to be versatile with the use of skin Z-plasty due to the medial contracture.

Bear in mind that active dorsiflexion will rarely be present in these very severe equinovarus deformities. It is rare that any of the extensor muscles of the foot are functional, and following any procedure whether arthrodesis (triple, tibiotalocalcaneal [TTC] or pantalar), although the hindfoot position may be recovered from equinus to neutral, no active dorsiflexor is present, and a static and dynamic equinus of the midfoot or forefoot may persist. Equinus of the forefoot is usually not fixed but dynamic following correction of the ankle and hindfoot, and generally the foot can be passively pushed up into a neutral position. However, the forefoot will drop back down into equinus. In such cases, a tendon transfer can be used as a dynamic or static force to help correcting the mid and forefoot equinus.[30] The same philosophy of muscle rebalancing will apply to correcting the deformity in the midfoot. This is difficult to determine preoperatively due to rigidity of the contracture, but an effort should be made to try to carefully examine the foot for function of various muscles as these will determine the need for a tendon transfer.

Transfer of the posterior tibial tendon is indicated if one can demonstrate that some posterior tibial muscle function remains, in which case the tendon can be transferred through the interosseous membrane to the dorsum of the foot to provide some degree of active dorsiflexion or at least to change its deforming force into a static dorsiflexion power. A tendon transfer is very difficult to perform in feet that have undergone a few prior surgeries. If there is little identifiable posterior tibial tendon, a tenotomy is more useful. If there is no functioning muscle (either the anterior or posterior tibial, or the peroneus brevis and or longus) to consider for a tendon transfer to increase dorsiflexion, then a tenodesis should be considered using one of the extensor tendons, generally the extensor digitorum longus (**Table 2**).

Talectomy

Talectomy is not by any means a physiologic procedure, but because of the ankylosis (or an incongruent joint) that it creates between the tibia and calcaneus and the ability to accept full bodyweight, it is a very reasonable procedure despite the limb shortening.[7] Most patients are free of pain, fairly functional, and ambulate satisfactorily. Another option is to correct the deformity gradually with an external fixator, which does maintain limb length; however, the foot is no more functional following correction of the deformity since rigidity persists. A talectomy should only be performed with very specific indications, and although always associated with severe foot deformity, a rigid ankle often associated with a flat top talus is invariably present.

Talectomy is rarely performed as an isolated procedure, as this will only correct a severe equinus deformity of the ankle and hindfoot, and to a lesser extent the changes in the transverse tarsal joint. Frequently, the adduction deformity of the Chopart joints is too severe to permit correction without an additional procedure that abducts the foot at the apex of the deformity, usually the calcaneocuboid joint. In addition to the

Table 2
Summary of treatment indications after patient evaluation

Patient Deformity or Dysfunction	Treatment Indication
Unilateral	Talectomy
Bilateral	Ponseti method or external fixator
Fixed equinus and flat top talus	Anterior closing wedge osteotomy of the distal tibia
Equinus deformity with weak or none ankle dorsiflexion without multiple previous surgery or rigidity	Posterior tibial tendon or extensor tendor transfer
Deformity can be mostly passively corrected into neutral	Triple arthrodesis combined with tendon transfers and additional osteotomies
Scarring with medial contracture	Skin Z-plasty and soft tissue release

talectomy and calcaneocuboid wedge arthrodesis, there are further procedures that must be considered to correct any residual adduction or equinus deformity of the midfoot and forefoot, as well as balance the soft tissue contracture. These could involve a transfer of the posterior tibial tendon, the anterior tibial tendon, or the peroneus longus to the peroneus brevis. Rarely, the deformity is in the ankle *and* hindfoot, and there is no severe midfoot deformity. In these cases, correction of the equinus deformity and the hindfoot varus can be addressed with a TTC arthrodesis. El-Sherbini et al. reported that along with talectomy in children and adults, calcaneal osteotomy with a laterally based wedge was performed in 42% of feet, and calcaneocuboid fusion in 16%. Despite these additional procedures, 16% had residual forefoot.

A decision will need to be made preoperatively and then again intraoperatively as to whether or not an isolated talectomy will be performed, or whether this will be performed in conjunction with a TC, or a TC and TN arthrodesis.[31] In general, a talectomy without arthrodesis is preferred as the residual motion is generally painless. The decision is based on stability of the hindfoot after temporary pin fixation, and the age of the patient, as it is very rare that an arthrodesis is necessary in childhood or even in adolescence. The range of motion after a talectomy is generally not significant, but it does improve function. Nicomedez and colleagues[32] reported that TC fusion may improve the function and the pain symptoms of arthrogrypotic pediatric patients, but it can lead to early degenerative arthritis of the adjacent joints.

Technique

We have found that the anterolateral approach for performing an isolated talectomy is the most versatile, as one has the opportunity to obtain a complete lateral exposure, extending the incision distally to include the calcaneocuboid joint and the peroneal tendons as necessary. This extensile approach permits a complete removal of the talus successfully (**Fig. 4**).

One has to always consider the potential for skin complications with any approach to correction of these very severe deformities, but a laterally based incision is not likely to lead to problems as a result of decompression of the soft tissue contracture after the talectomy. The extensile lateral approach has to be long, commencing behind the fibula toward the fifth metatarsal. One can either leave the fibula intact or remove the distal 2 cm for visualization. The main advantage of the transfibular approach is easy visualization and removal of the talus, and molding of the tibia and calcaneus for an arthrodesis. It is also easy to mold the anterior tibia and the navicular to include a TN arthrodesis. Most importantly, access to the lateral foot for a wedge resection of the calcaneocuboid joint can be performed with an extensile approach.

When considering a talectomy without arthrodesis, one can consider an anterior approach to the ankle. This is more useful for deformities that are predominantly locked in equinus, without midfoot adductus caused by a rigid contracture medially and which does not necessitate any additional procedures. By removing the talus from the anterior approach, both malleoli can be left intact, which may serve to provide some stability to the periarticular tissues as the calcaneus gradually scars into position. Occasionally, the anterior approach may lead to impingement between the margins of the malleolus and either the calcaneus or navicular medially and less laterally. If this is the case, a subsequent secondary procedure may need to be performed with an ostectomy of the offending bone causing the impingement. The one disadvantage of approaching a talectomy anteriorly is that it is not as easy to remove the talus as through a lateral approach as the talus has to be cut into pieces with an osteotome and then gradually removed (**Fig. 5**).

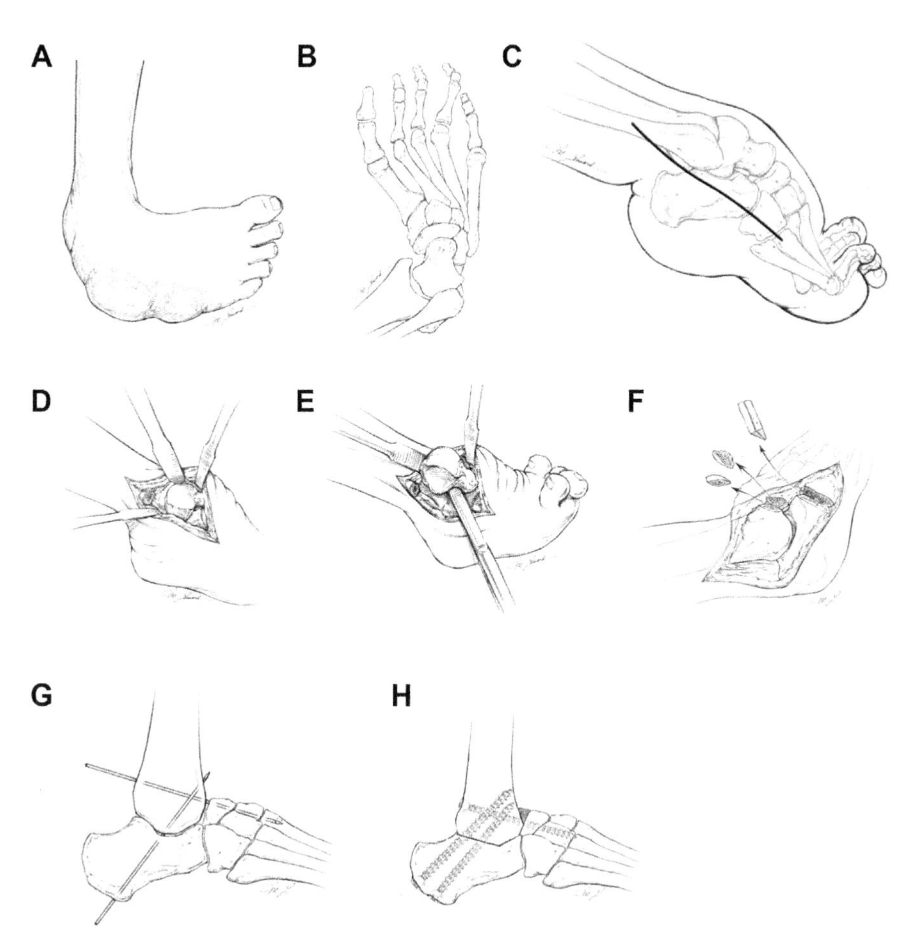

Fig. 4. The sequence of steps for the talectomy is illustrated in a very typical foot with severe rigid equinovarus, weight-bearing on the dorsal surface of the foot noted by hypertrophy of the dorsolateral skin (*A*). It is not just the magnitude of the deformity of the foot that determines the need for talectomy but the fixed rigid deformity of the ankle in equinus (*B*). Following an extensile lateral approach, the talus is exposed with or without removing the distal 2 cm of the fibula (*C–E*). Often, additional wedges need to be removed, one from the calcaneocuboid joint, and the other from the anterior tibia and dorsal surface of the navicular (*F*). Provisional fixation is performed with cannulated guide pins if available (*G*) and the screw fixation is demonstrated after molding the tibia to the calcaneus and inserting bone graft as noted between the tibia and calcaneus (*H*).

Thick skin flaps should be maintained. If one is certain that a TC arthrodesis will be performed, then the distal fibula can be resected to gain access to the talectomy and preparation of the joint surfaces. All the ligaments and capsules connecting the talus to the adjoining bones are divided, trying to avoid any injury to the articular surfaces, particularly in children. The anterior talofibular ligament is first to cut followed by the calcaneofibular ligament which should be detached as much as possible off the fibula so as to reattach it at the completion of the procedure if there is any coronal plane instability. It is generally not possible to maximally invert the foot and expose the talus without cutting the calcaneofibular ligament. The main ligament that anchors the talus

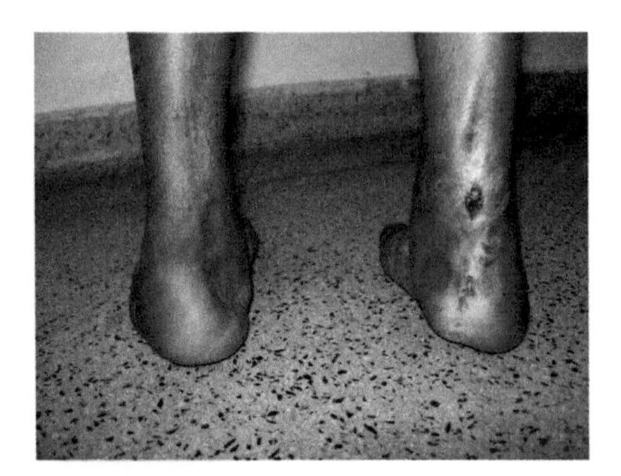

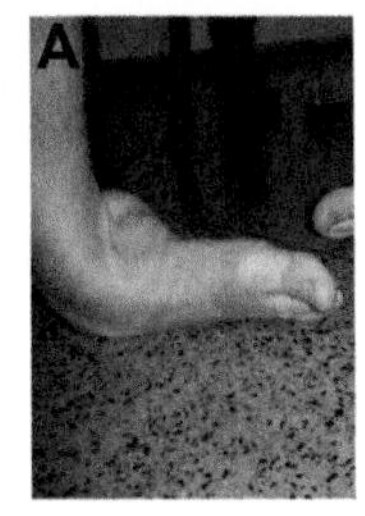

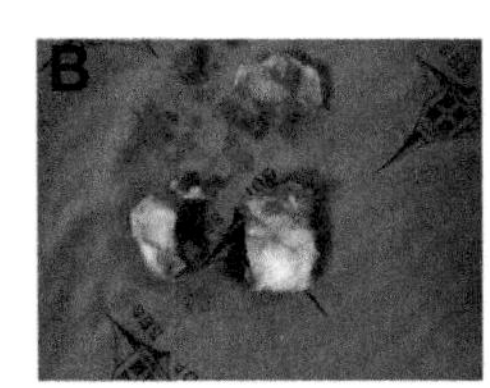

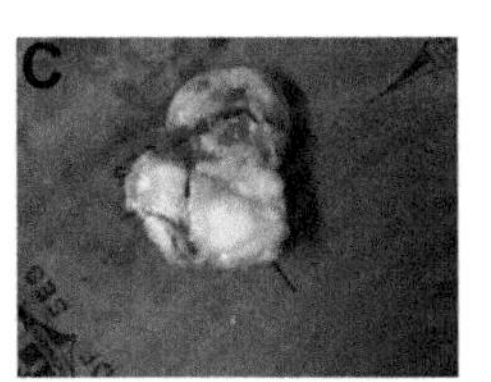

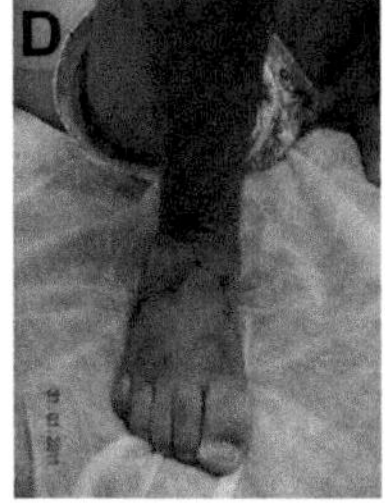

Fig. 5. A 13-year-old girl (*A*) with diplegic cerebral palsy was treated with talectomy through combined incisions, but the talus could not be removed until it was cut in pieces with a saw (*B*), here demonstrated in 3 pieces and then assembled back (*C*). The final position of the foot in the early recovery period is shown (*D*).

is the talocalcaneal interosseous ligament, which is easier to cut from the lateral approach thereby freeing up lateral attachments and subsequently dislocating the foot to remove the talus. This is not as easy if an anterior approach is used. After freeing up the lateral ligaments, the foot can be manipulated into more equinus and varus and by holding the talus with a large towel clamp, the medial capsule of the subtalar joint and the deep portion of the deltoid ligament, as well as the posterior ankle and posteromedial calcaneal capsule, are cut. A posterior capsulotomy is easier to perform under direct vision noting, however, the position of the flexor hallucis longus and the neurovascular bundle posteromedially. It is important to remove the entire talus and not leave any small bone fragments behind, which can lead to secondary deformity (**Fig. 6**). According to Hsu and colleagues,[32] the most common technical errors were incomplete removal of the talus and incorrect positioning of the calcaneus in the ankle mortise.

The foot should now be quite mobile and can easily reach a neutral position without any residual equinus or adductovarus. By manipulation, the foot is positioned under the tibia ensuring that there is no residual equinus nor any tension in the posterior ankle capsule. Division of the anterior inferior tibiofibular ligament in the syndesmosis has been described to widen the ankle mortise and more easily fit the calcaneus underneath the tibia but we do not have experience with this step.[33] It is essential that the foot is positioned correctly, and it should be translated slightly posteriorly under the tibia. Adequate posterior capsular release needs to be performed to move the foot posteriorly. At times this requires additional release as well as tenotomy of the Achilles tendon if contracture still presents. As the foot is moved posteriorly, the tip of the medial malleolus will be immediately adjacent to the navicular and the tip of the fibula

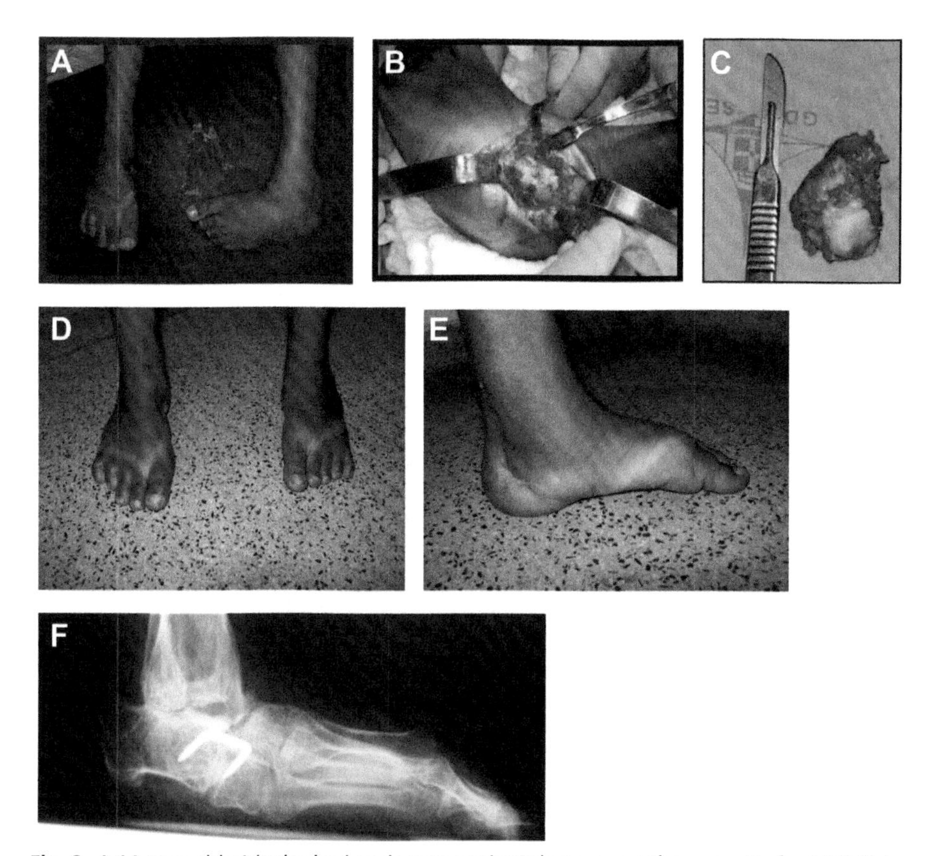

Fig. 6. A 14-year-old girl who had undergone prior talectomy on the opposite foot (*A*). Talectomy was performed resecting the bone in one piece (*B, C*). The final outcome with a well-aligned foot is shown (*D, E*) including a closing wedge calcaneocuboid arthrodesis (*F*).

just posterior to the calcaneocuboid joint. The goal is to provide a long lever to the foot by shifting the foot posteriorly to give a mechanical advantage to the gastrocnemius-soleus.[34] Once positioned, the foot is fixed to the tibia with two 3 mm Steinman pins. If any impingement occurs between the calcaneus and the fibula and prevents correction, one can remove the tip of the fibula or the medial malleolus to decrease the jamming. Occasionally, the tibia will abut against the navicular with the posterior shift of the calcaneus but in a child, an arthrodesis should be avoided, and to regain a neutral position, the anterior tibia can be shaved with an ostectomy to permit slightly more posterior translation. Slight dorsiflexion and plantarflexion may be possible despite the ankylosis and can provide some function (**Fig. 7**).

Dorsiflexion may not be possible because the anterior tibia is impinging against the navicular. The same may occur because of a medially rotated navicular where it is impinging against the medial malleolus. In either of these situations, one has to trim the anterior distal tibia, or the dorsal and medial navicular, or to resect the entire navicular bone to gain dorsiflexion. Both these procedures are necessary if one is performing a TN arthrodesis. The latter procedure is only occasionally necessary in conjunction with a TC arthrodesis when the foot is grossly unstable under the ankle. The distal cut can be extended medially to include the navicular as one cut if a TN arthrodesis is going to be considered. Once the calcaneocuboid wedge has been

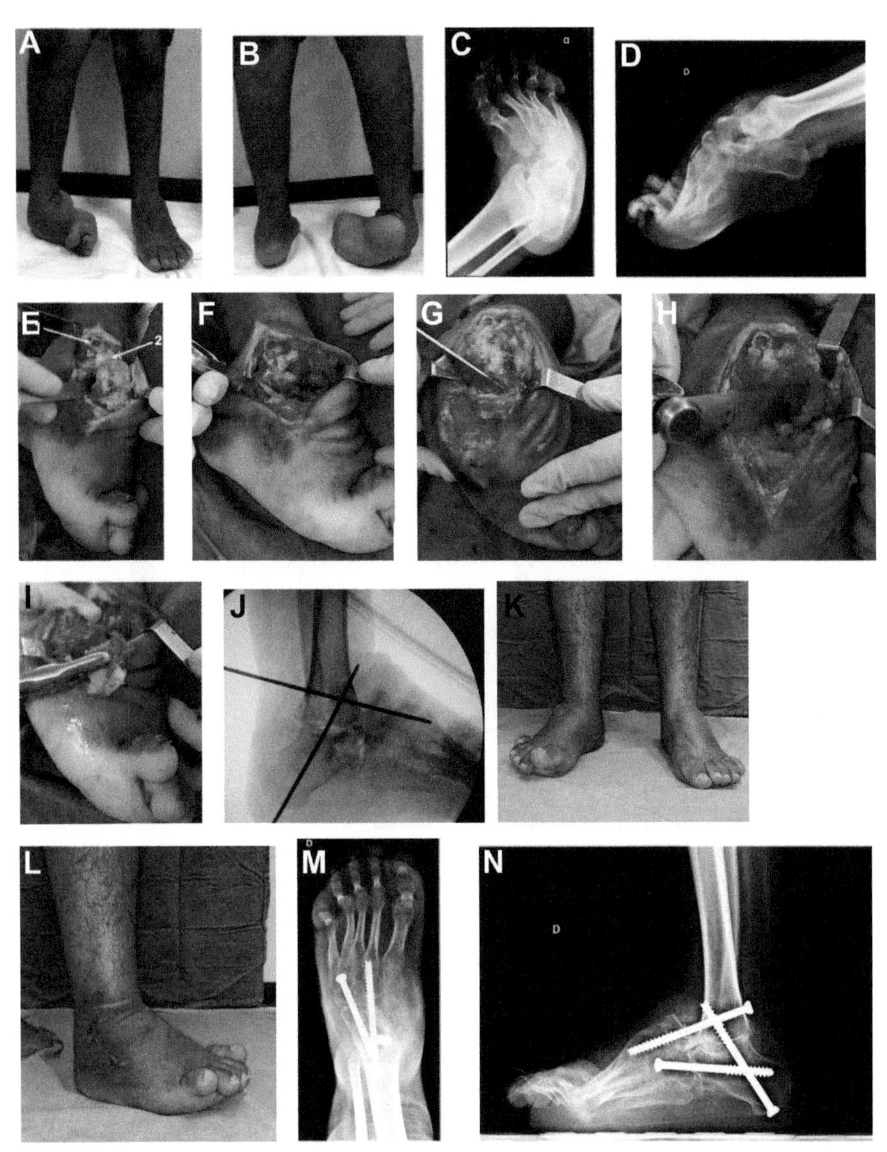

Fig. 7. A 16-year-old patient with a fixed and rigid equinovarus deformity with no motion in either the ankle or foot (*A–D*). Note the ostectomy of the terminal fibula (*E, 1*) and the articular surface of the distal tibia (*E, 2*), with the osteotome perforating through the interosseous ligament to lever out the talus (*E*). Saw cuts were made on the articular surface of the calcaneus, the tibia across to and including the medial malleolus, and then finally the anterior aspect of the tibia where it would articulate with the navicular (*F–H*). A wedge was removed from the calcaneocuboid joint followed by provisional fixation of the foot (*I, J*). The final clinical and radiographic appearance of the foot 5 months after surgery is demonstrated. Note that there is very little limb length inequality as a result of prior surgery on the contralateral foot (*K–N*).

removed, the foot should now assume a perfectly neutral position. Before completing the tendon transfer dorsally, the hindfoot is fixed to the tibia using two or three 3 mm pins. The one is introduced from the posterior and inferior calcaneus causing through the anterior cortex of the distal tibia, and the second is inserted vertically through the calcaneus into the tibia.

If persistent adductus is present after the talectomy, then the incision is extended more distally to the base of the fifth metatarsal, and a large wedge removed from the calcaneocuboid joint (**Fig. 8**).

Additional Procedures

Tenodesis

An equinus deformity of the forefoot may still persist after the talectomy, and if present, it is helpful to stabilize the deformity with a tenodesis using the extensor tendons. A 2 cm incision is made over the midfoot, and the longus extensor tendons to the second, third, and fourth toes are cut, sutured together, and inserted into the midfoot using either an interference screw, a suture anchor, or a soft tissue bolster on the plantar surface of the foot. In children, we prefer to use a padded bolster and not a suture button, which can cause necrosis of the skin. A 4-mm drill through the lateral cuneiform is made, and the tendons are passed through to the plantar surface. A useful technique to pass the tendon is to insert a guide pin through the cuneiform, hold the guide pin with a clamp below the foot, and then drill through the bone. Using a #15 blade, a small skin incision is made over the guide pin, then a metallic suction tip is passed over the guide pin from plantar to dorsal, and pushed out dorsally[33] The suture attaching the tendons is then inserted into the suction, which is then pulled out into the drill hole through to the plantar surface. The foot is then positioned in neutral and the sutures tied over a soft tissue bolster. We use the rubber stopper from a 30 mL syringe, which is perforated twice with a small clamp, and the sutures are passed through the rubber stopper and a soft tissue bolster is inserted between the stopper and the skin and then again over the stopper to prevent the suture from cutting through the rubber, thereby losing tension. In children, it is useful to reinforce this with a 2.0 absorbable suture through the dorsal bone and into the tendon. The bone may be too hard to accomplish

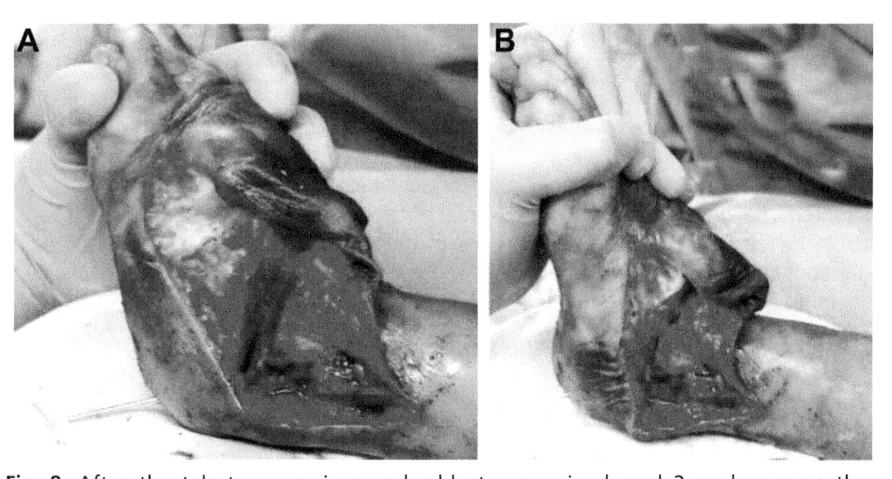

Fig. 8. After the talectomy equinus and adductus remained, and 2 wedges were then removed, one from the anterior tibia and the second from the calcaneocuboid joint (*A*) resulting in a plantigrade foot (*B*).

this in the adult, in which case, small holes are made with a 1.6 mm K wire, or a suture anchor can be inserted into the cuneiform directly. If a suture anchor is used, one should ensure that this does not pull out with very vigorous tension on the suture.

Equinus correction

Talectomy without arthrodesis will provide sufficient laxity of the soft tissue contracture to permit correction of the equinus and various associated deformities. Occasionally, however, an Achilles tenotomy needs to be performed simultaneously and only needs to be performed at the completion of the talectomy if equinus deformity persists. The tendon can easily be reached posterolaterally, grasped with a curved clamp and cut with the blade moving from outside to inside to avoid inadvertently cutting the skin. After the talectomy, regardless of whether it is performed with or without an arthrodesis, it is useful to shorten the peroneal tendons. The peroneal muscles will not function if the tendons are left alone due to considerable laxity after reduction of the foot, and one may want to restore muscle balance by shortening the tendons as necessary. Certainly, the peroneus brevis should be tightened, and a transfer of the peroneus longus to the brevis can also be considered. All the 15 arthrogrypotic feet that underwent talectomy by Hsu and colleagues had mild residual adduction of the forefoot and marked stiffness of the hindfoot, 40% had residual equinus at the ankle and 47% developed spontaneous bony ankylosis in the tibiotarsal joint.

Tibialis posterior transfer

Talectomy will correct most of the equinus deformity and some of the adductovarus deformity but is occasionally not sufficient to decompress the deformity and additional procedures must be considered. The simplest would be to transfer the posterior tibial tendon, which ensures that recurrent adductovarus deformity does not occur, and also may help provide an active dorsiflexor albeit weak, to the foot. It is rare that the extensor muscles are functional. If one is not able to perform a transfer of the posterior tibial tendon, a tenotomy of the tendon will need to be performed. Harvesting the tendon may not be easy because of prior scarring if a posteromedial incision has been used in early childhood. As it is never clear what has been previously performed, we initiate the incision at the level of the medial malleolus and try to find the posterior tibial tendon in its sheath which is opened. The tendon is usually firmly adherent to the posterior aspect of the medial malleolus and a smooth small clamp is inserted underneath the tendon to visualize it. From here, one can work distally by opening the sheath as far as possible distally. Because of scarring, one may not be able to harvest the entire tendon, but it is essential to attempt to obtain as long a piece of tendon possible for the interosseous transfer. If so, the distal 2 or 3 cm may have to be shaped and narrowed knowing that this is predominantly scar tissue. Once the tendon has been dissected free and sutured, one should take note of any persistent adduction contracture. In cases where on examination one is certain that either the anterior tibial or extensor tendon function is present, then these can be considered for use as an active transfer in combination with the talectomy.

Peroneal tendons transfer

Essentially, the foot must be balanced so that recurrent deformity of the midfoot and forefoot are less likely to occur. Bear in mind that the peroneal tendons are also not likely to be functioning in these advanced cases but one can perform a longus to brevis transfer in an effort to aid eversion and balance of the hindfoot. This transfer should not be considered, however, if the peroneal muscles are functioning strongly and the posterior and anterior tibial tendons are scarred, or the muscles dysfunctional.

At this stage, one should check the alignment of the toes since a flexion contracture may now be present. To some extent, this will always occur because of the pre-existing equinus deformity, and as the foot is dorsiflexed, the long flexor tendons are contracted. As passive dorsiflexion of the toes of 45° is desirable, the contracture may be decompressed by virtue of the talectomy in which case nothing needs to be performed. As these muscles may still be functional, if there are residual flexion contractures after the talectomy, one can consider a lengthening at the musculotendinous junction or through the tendon depending on the magnitude of the contracture. If severe scarring is present posteromedially, then lengthening is not necessary and tenotomies can be performed. If so, we find it easier to perform the tenotomy of the flexor hallucis longus looking through the ankle from posterior to anterior under direct vision. Needless to state, make sure that one is grasping the flexor tendon and not the tibial nerve.

At the completion of the aforementioned procedures, the tourniquet must be left down to ensure adequate circulation to the foot. This is frequently compromised because of the magnitude of the deformity, the inevitable traction on the neurovascular bundle, hypoplasia of the dorsalis pedis artery, or prior scarring around the posteromedial ankle from prior surgeries. If perfusion does not return immediately, apply warm moist cloths to the foot and ankle and wait 10 minutes. It is also useful to drop the foot down slightly off the side of the table to a dependent position. If circulation does not improve after 10 minutes, we recommend applying nitroglycerin paste (Nitro-Bid). This promotes vasodilatation and may sufficiently improve venous return such that the ischemia is resolved. If not, use a Doppler to mark out the tibial artery, and if there is an appreciable change at the level of the ankle, open posteromedially and perform a complete tarsal tunnel release. When releasing the tibial nerve and artery, it is important to trace the bundle distally beyond its bifurcation to the medial and lateral branches as the flexor retinaculum may be constricting either or both vessels.

DISCLOSURE

The authors have nothing to disclose.

REFERENCES

1. Li S, Myerson MS. Managing severe foot and ankle deformities in global humanitarian programs. Foot Ankle Clin 2020;25(2):183–203.
2. Dobbs MB, Morcuende JA, Gurnett CA, et al. Treatment of idiopathic clubfoot: an historical review. Iowa Orthop J 2000;20:59–64.
3. Radler C, Mindler GT. Treatment of severe recurrent clubfoot. Foot Ankle Clin 2015;20(4):563–86.
4. Thomas HM, Sangiorgio SN, Ebramzadeh E, et al. Relapse rates in patients with clubfoot treated using the ponseti method increase with time: a systematic review. JBJS Rev 2019;7(5):e6.
5. Eidelman M, Kotlarsky P, Herzenberg JE. Treatment of relapsed, residual and neglected clubfoot: adjunctive surgery. J Child Orthop 2019;13(3):293–303.
6. Haje DP, Canto SJ, Kumar R, et al. Ponseti method after walking age – a multicentric study of 429 feet. Iowa Orthop J 2020;40(2):1–11.
7. Cooper RR, Capello W. Talectomy. A long-term follow-up evaluation. Clin Orthop Relat Res 1985;201:32–5.
8. Hsu LC, Jaffray D, Leong JC. Talectomy for club foot in arthrogryposis. J Bone Joint Surg Br 1984;66(5):694–6.

9. Trumble T, Banta JV, Raycroft JF, et al. Talectomy for equinovarus deformity in myelodysplasia. J Bone Joint Surg Am 1985;67(1):21–9.
10. Letts M, Davidson D. The role of bilateral talectomy in the management of bilateral rigid clubfeet. Am J Orthop (Belle Mead NJ) 1999;28(2):106–10.
11. Ferreira RC, Costo MT, Frizzo GG, et al. Correction of neglected clubfoot using the Ilizarov external fixator. Foot Ankle Int 2006;27(4):266–73.
12. Khan SA, Kumar A. Ponseti's manipulation in neglected clubfoot in children more than 7 years of age: a prospective evaluation of 25 feet with long-term follow-up. J Pediatr Orthop B 2010;19(5):385–9.
13. Haje DP. Neglected idiopathic club foot successfully treated by the Ponseti method: a case report of an adult patient who started treatment at 26 old. J Orthop Case Rep 2020;10(4):74–7.
14. Machida J, Inaba Y, Nakamura N. Management of foot deformity in children. J Orthop Sci 2017;22(2):175–83.
15. Matar HE, Makki D, Garg NK. Treatment of syndrome-associated congenital talipes equinovarus using the Ponseti method: 4-12 years of follow-up. J Pediatr Orthop B 2018;27(1):56–60.
16. Nogueira MP, Ey Batlle AM, Alves CG. Is it possible to treat recurrent clubfoot with the Ponseti technique after posteromedial release?: a preliminary study. Clin Orthop Relat Res 2009;467(5):1298–305.
17. Dragoni M, Farsetti P, Vena G, et al. Ponseti treatment of rigid residual deformity in congenital clubfoot after walking age. J Bone Joint Surg Am 2016;98(20): 1706–12.
18. El-Sherbini MH, Omran AA. Midterm follow-up of talectomy for severe rigid equinovarus feet. J Foot Ankle Surg 2015;54(6):1093–8.
19. Golański G, Niedzielski KR. [Application of Ponseti method in case of neglected talipes equinovarus in 4 years and 9 months old boy with DiGeorge syndrome–case report]. Chir Narzadow Ruchu Ortop Pol 2011;76(2):115–7.
20. De Mulder T, Prinsen S, Van Campenhout A. Treatment of non-idiopathic clubfeet with the Ponseti method: a systematic review. J Child Orthop 2018;12(6):575–81.
21. Joseph TN, Myerson MS. Use of talectomy in modern foot and ankle surgery. Foot Ankle Clin 2004;9(4):775–85.
22. Penny JN. The neglegted clubfoot. Tech Orthop 2005;20(2):153–66.
23. Smythe T, Le G, Owen R, et al. The development of a training course for clubfoot treatment in Africa: learning points for course development. BMC Med Educ 2018;18(1):163.
24. Pirani S, Naddumba E, Mathias R, et al. Towards effective Ponseti clubfoot care: the Uganda Sustainable Clubfoot Care Project. Clin Orthop Relat Res 2009; 467(5):1154–63.
25. Asitha J, Zionts LE, Morcuende JA. Management of idiopathic clubfoot after formal training in the Ponseti method: a multi-year, international survey. Iowa Orthop J 2013;33:136–41.
26. Nogueira MP, Pereira JC, Duarte PS, et al. Ponseti Brasil: a national program to eradicate neglected clubfoot - preliminary results. Iowa Orthop J 2011;31:43–8.
27. Lourenço AF, Morcuende JA. Correction of neglected idiopathic club foot by the Ponseti method. J Bone Joint Surg Br 2007;89(3):378–81.
28. de Podestá Haje D. Neglected idiopathic bilateral clubfoot successfully treated with the ponseti method: a case report. JBJS Case Connect 2013;3(1):e9.
29. Ebert N, Ballhause TM, Babin K, et al. Correction of recurrent equinus deformity in surgically treated clubfeet by anterior distal tibial hemiepiphysiodesis. J Pediatr Orthop 2020;40(9):520–5.

30. Malik SS, Knight R, Ahmed U, et al. Role of a tendon transfer as a dynamic check-rein reducing recurrence of equinus following distal tibial dorsiflexion osteotomy. J Pediatr Orthop B 2018;27(5):419–24.
31. Mirzayan R, Early SD, Matthys GA, et al. Single-stage talectomy and tibiocalcaneal arthrodesis as a salvage of severe, rigid equinovarus deformity. Foot Ankle Int 2001;22(3):209–13.
32. Nicomedez FP, Li YH, Leong JC. Tibiocalcaneal fusion after talectomy in arthrogrypotic patients. J Pediatr Orthop 2003;23(5):654–7.
33. Schrantz WF. Arthrogryposis. In: McCarthy JJ, Drennan JC, editors. Drennan's the child's foot and ankle. 2nd edition. Philadelphia: Lippincott Williams & Wilkins; 2009. p. 252–3.
34. Melamed EA, Myerson MS, Schon LC. A review of tendon passing techniques and introduction of a new method using a suction tip. Foot Ankle Int 2000; 21(8):693–6.

The Overcorrected Clubfoot in Children

Johannes Hamel

KEYWORDS

- Clubfoot • Dorsal bunion • Overcorrection • Pedography • Peritalar deformity
- Rigid planovalgus deformity

KEY POINTS

- Clubfoot overcorrection is a serious complication of treatment with major impairment of foot function mainly in late stance phase of gait, observed in all primary correction concepts, but especially after extended surgical release
- Pathomorphology is characterized in most cases by planovalgus deformity with hindfoot valgus, supramalleolar valgus alignment, instability of the medial ray, and dorsal bunion development
- Clinical, radiological, and pedographic examination are useful to specify the different manifestations and degrees of malfunction of overcorrected clubfeet
- Surgical correction includes correction and/or stabilization of the peritalar complex and medial ray as well as realignment of supramalleolar valgus deformity as required in combination with rebalancing of muscular forces in dorsal bunion deformity
- Early surgical correction is recommended in severe cases to prevent further progression

INTRODUCTION AND DEFINITION

Presentation and definition of clubfoot overcorrection in literature is not consistent: whereas Knupp and collegues[1] in 2012 in a study on adult patients confined it mainly to a supramalleolar valgus deformity, others detected it by a footprint that resembles a flatfoot (Hayes and collegues[2] in 2018) or by peak eversion measured with gait analysis (Dussa and collegues[3] in 2020). For this overview a more complex definition seems to be appropriate.

Clubfoot overcorrection on the one hand can be defined in terms of the original deformity components: each single component of clubfoot deformity may be overcorrected. For example, overlengthening of the primary contracted calf muscle-tendon unit leads to calcaneus overcorrection (**Fig. 1**) (O'Brien and collegues[4]), or excessive reduction of the primary cavus component may end up in rocker bottom deformity (**Fig. 2**). **Table 1** shows the most important single components of overcorrection.

Schön Klinik München Harlaching, Harlachinger Straße 51, München D – 81547, Germany
E-mail address: J.Hamel@t-online.de

Foot Ankle Clin N Am 26 (2021) 747–764
https://doi.org/10.1016/j.fcl.2021.07.006
1083-7515/21/

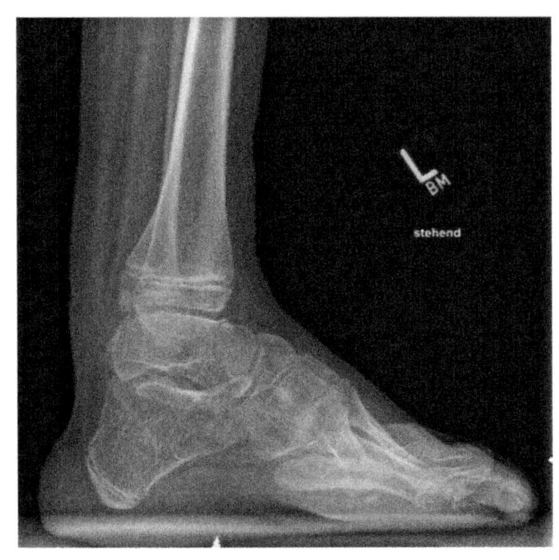

Fig. 1. Calcaneus overcorrection with persisting cavus component after overlengthening of *tendo Achilles.*

Often overcorrection phenomena can be observed in combination with residual clubfoot deformity components (see **Figs. 1** and **2**), signs of iatrogenic spurious malcorrection, complications like talar necrosis with consecutive flat top talus, and compensatory adaptions. Thus a broad spectrum of individual deformities and functional impairment may develop. Clear iatrogenic malcorrection like early rocker bottom deformity as a complication after missed tenotomy of tendo Achilles during primary redression (Koureas and collegues[5]) or surgical dorsal malposition of the navicular in inappropriately executed peritalar release are not in the focus of this overview.

Overcorrection may be defined in a more functional way on the other hand: whereas an undercorrected clubfoot is characterized by strong, overpowering flexors and invertors, absence of a plantigrade weight-bearing position, and a tendency to overload of the forefoot and lateral foot ray, a functionally overcorrected clubfoot often is fairly plantigrade but shows weakness especially in the late stance phase of gait leading to an adynamic way of walking with additional secondary problems. Lau and collegues[6] in 1989 reported unsatisfactory function in 66% of overcorrected clubfeet. Also, overcorrection is associated with a higher probability of foot pain in comparison

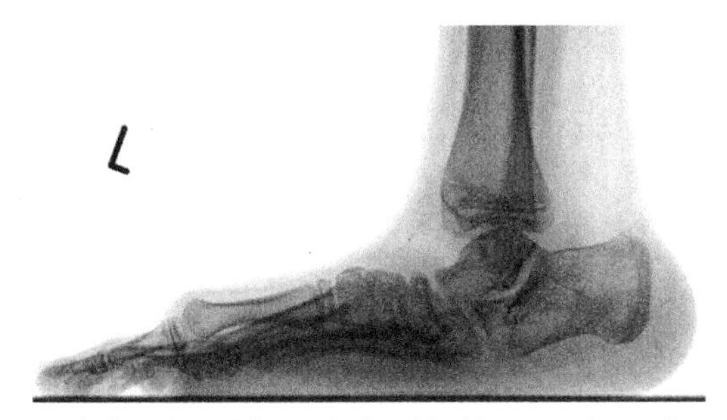

Fig. 2. Rocker bottom deformity with persisting hindfoot equinus after conservative treat*ment with missed lengthening of tendo Achilles.*

Table 1
Original deformity component and corresponding typical overcorrection phenomena

Equinus	*Calcaneus overcorrection* (weak, overlengthened muscle-tendon unit of calf muscles, high calcaneal pitch angle, anterior ankle impingement)
Peritalar inversion with hindfoot varus	*Peritalar eversion* (rotatory and translatory valgus, planovalgus deformity, hindfoot valgus often combined with supramalleolar valgus component, restricted function of posterior tibial muscle, fibulocalcaneal impingement, dislocation of peroneal tendons, weakness of push-off in late stance)
Cavus	*Rocker bottom deformity* (overload of midfoot area, persisting calcaneus equinus, reduction of ankle mobility compensated by hypermobility at Chopart joint line, especially after missed calf muscle lengthening)
Mid-forefoot pronation	*Mid-forefoot supination, dorsal bunion* (instability and reduced weight-bearing capacity of the medial ray, compensatory overactivity of the toe flexors, flexion contracture of the first metatarsophalangeal joint, adduction of the lesser toes)
Mid-forefoot adduction	*Mid-forefoot abduction* (especially located at the naviculocuneiforme joint line in case of incomplete talonavicular correction)

to well corrected clubfeet,[2] although usually pain is neither in undercorrected clubfeet nor in overcorrection the dominating symptom in childhood.

MANIFESTATIONS OF OVERCORRECTION IN DIFFERENT TREATMENT CONCEPTS

Clubfoot overcorrection nearly always is of iatrogenic origin and like clubfoot relapse may be observed in each therapeutic clubfoot concept. However, each treatment concept has its own typical appearance, frequency, and pathogenesis of overcorrection to be expected. Overcorrected clubfeet were observed only rarely in traditional primary treatment including limited posterior release that was popular in the middle of the twentieth century. When relapse occurred and anterior tibial tendon transfer to the lateral side of the foot had to be performed later, this could lead to overcorrection. According to the treatment concept popularized, for example, in Germany by Imhäuser[7] in the 1960s and the 1970s, anterior tibial tendon transfer to the base of the fifth metatarsal led to intended overcorrection until it was rerouted in a second procedure. Lampasi and collegues[8] in 2010 reported 13.2% overcorrections after relapse surgery with anteriortibial tendon transfer to the third or fourth metatarsal ray.

In contrast peritalar release surgery in the first year of life used frequently in the last decades of the twentieth century was prone to end up in progressive overcorrection often arising only after some years (Dobbs and colleagues[9] in 2006, Carroll[10] in 2012). Like in other complications there is a connection to the experience of the treating surgeon; however, the author saw severe cases also from skillful collegues. "Unfortunately, with clubfoot surgery we all have overcorrected clubfeet at one time or another" was stated by Mc Kay[11] in 1994, one of the proposers of this treatment concept. According to Turco[12] in 1970 most of his inferior results after posteromedial release were overcorrected cases. The more radical the release is performed, the more likely overcorrection might happen. Especially section of the deep deltoid ligament fibers or the talocalcaneal interosseus ligaments are considered to result in excessive eversion of the hindfoot complex and planovalgus overcorrection developing gradually over years. After primary surgical release overcorrection is described in 4% to 19.4% of all cases (according to Dussa and collegues[3]).

The rising awareness of this problem was one of the reasons that led to the worldwide radical change in primary clubfoot treatment about 20 years ago. Those who had to deal with clubfoot problems during the last decades, including the author of this overview, were frequently faced with this challenging group of patients who were treated with extended surgical release in infancy. The clinical examples in this overview almost completely come from this group.

Even without any surgery overcorrection might occur (**Fig. 3**). Mainly conservative clubfoot therapy like in the Ponseti primary treatment concept (Ponseti[13] in 1996) may show late overcorrection, but in clearly reduced frequency and severity when compared with extended early surgical release.[14] The main etiologic factor probably is the quality of soft tissue structures, which may vary a lot in different individuals; however, it is recognizable only after infancy.[15] Especially those children with a tendency of hypermobility and loose capsular structures are thought to be prone to develop overcorrection. However, recently this widespread theory could not be supported for the Ponseti treatment concept by Beck and collegues.[16] A recent paper on the outcome of conservative primary treatment found remarkable 12.2% of valgus overcorrection after Ponseti primary treatment documented by clinical examination combined with pedography.[2] Dussa and collegues[3] reported 14 cases of children aged

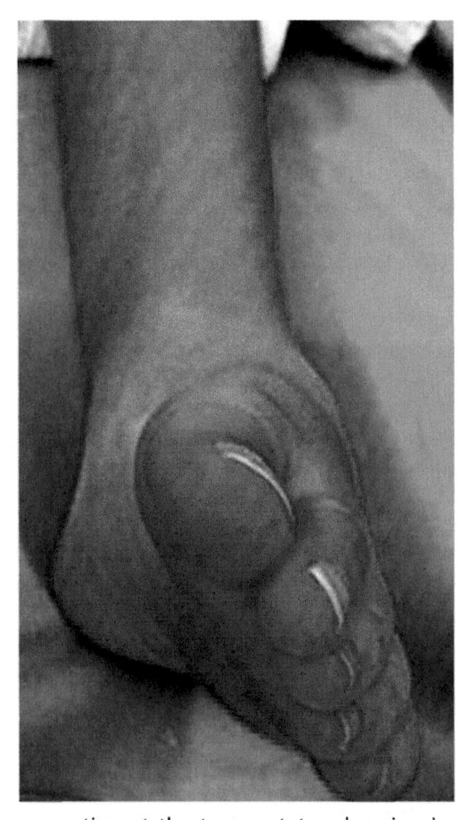

Fig. 3. Supinatory overcorrection at the tarsometatarsal region in a 5-year-old boy after pure conservative clubfoot treatment. The hindfoot alignment in a weight-bearing position was neutral, and the peritalar joints were flexible with complete loss of load distribution at the medial forefoot.

between 7 and 12 years without ligamentous laxity that had been treated by the Ponseti method and developed overcorrection according to their gait analysis criteria. Therefore dealing with clubfoot overcorrection still seems to be of relevance even in the era of mainly conservative primary treatment.

CLINICAL, RADIOLOGICAL, AND FUNCTIONAL EVALUATION OF OVERCORRECTION

Clinical Evaluation

The main clinical features of overcorrection are planovalgus deformity with more or less rigid hindfoot eversion (**Fig. 4**) and instability of the medial ray, weakness of plantarflexion, and dorsal bunion. In severe cases rocker bottom deformity can be observed. The calf muscles in most cases are weak and often still short; the posterior tibial muscle may be functionally inactive. The combination of reduced power of the calf and posterior tibial muscles due to surgical overlengthening or scar formation at the tendon part of these muscle-tendon units and an everted position of the osteoligamentous peritalar complex do not allow the foot to acquire a stable position in late stance phase of walking. The patient more and more will become unable to stand on the forepart of the foot. Further weakening of the long peroneal muscle by tendon instability and dislocation at the distal fibular region may add to the destabilization of the medial ray. Compensatory overactivity of the toe flexors, especially the flexor hallucis longus muscle, in combination with instability of the medial tarsometatarsal ray results in dorsal bunion deformity. Shoe conflict at the elevated first metatarsal bone, restricted motion, and development of arthritis of the first metatarsophalangeal joint may cause problems later.[17,18] Adduction of the lesser toes in a standing position

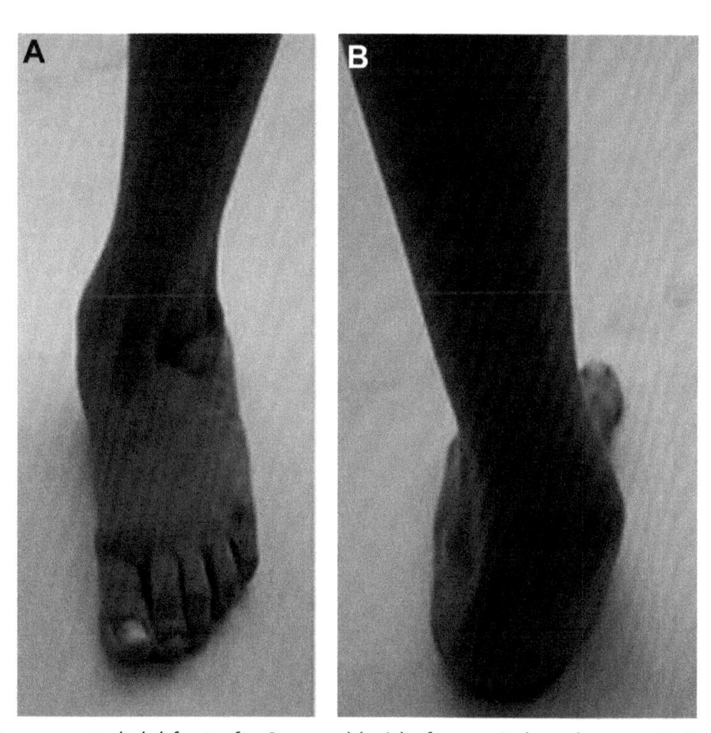

Fig. 4. Overcorrected clubfoot of a 9-year-old girl after peritalar release, anterior (*A*) and posterior (*B*) view.

is another sign of compensatory overactivity of the long toe flexor tendons (See **Fig. 14**).

Radiological Evaluation

The exact location, form, and amount of osteoligamentous peritalar or tarsometatarsal deformity and instability can be assessed by diagnostic radiograph or computed tomography (CT) (digital volume tomography [DVT]) in a weight-bearing position. At the peritalar complex a rotatory valgus can be differentiated from a hinge valgus and a translatory valgus deformity (**Fig. 5**) according to Thompson and Abaza.[19] In a rotatory valgus deformity the ligamentous talocalcaneal connection is mostly preserved, whereas the subtalar joint is completely dislocated in the translatory form. The hypermobility of the medial tarsometatarsal ray can be examined more exactly with a reversed Coleman block test if not apparent in the normal lateral view (**Fig. 6**). The naviculocuneiform joint line and the talonavicular joint are mainly affected, whereas the first tarsometatarsal joint remains stable in most cases. Weight-bearing CT (or DVT) is a very useful tool to display the amount of hindfoot valgus deformity (**Fig. 7**), especially the tibiotalar and talocalcaneal alignment and subtalar or fibulocalcaneal impingement phenomena.

In severe hindfoot valgus conditions always an anteroposterior ankle projection should be added to 3-dimensional examination of the foot to detect an additional supramalleolar valgus component (**Fig. 8**). Fibulocalcaneal impingement can best be examined in the frontal section of a weight-bearing CT. The pathogenesis of

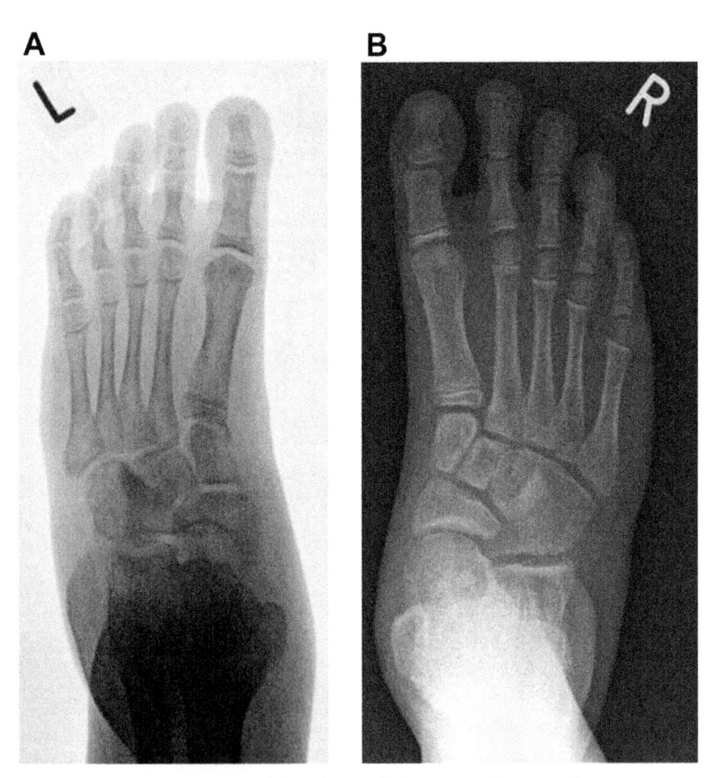

Fig. 5. Translatory (*A*) and rotatory (*B*) valgus of the peritalar complex.

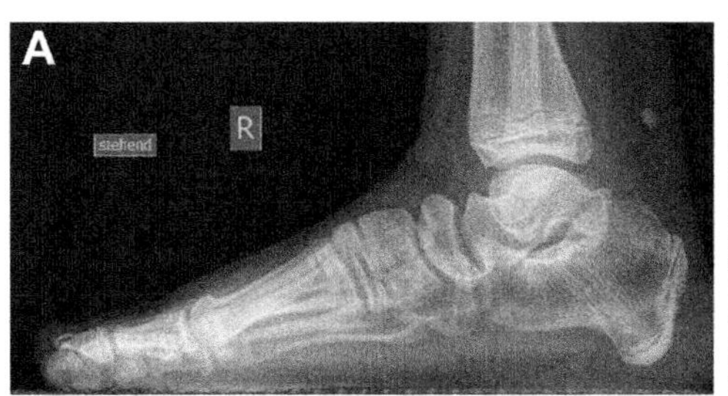

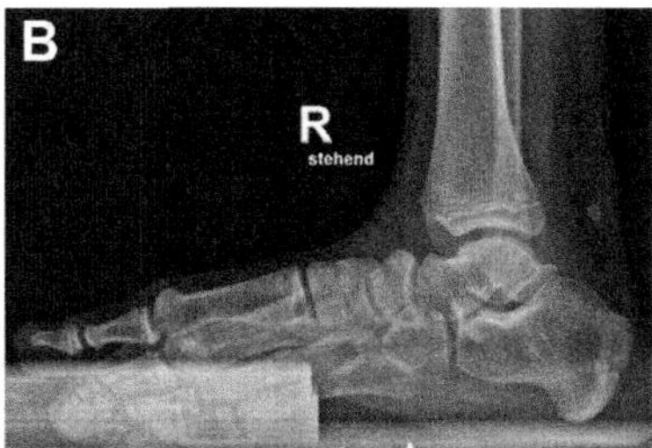

Fig. 6. Overcorrected clubfoot (*A*) with instability of the medial tarsometatarsal ray. The hypermobility of the naviculocuneiform joint line is not apparent in the lateral radiographic projection (*A*) but could be localized by the reversed Coleman block test (*B*).

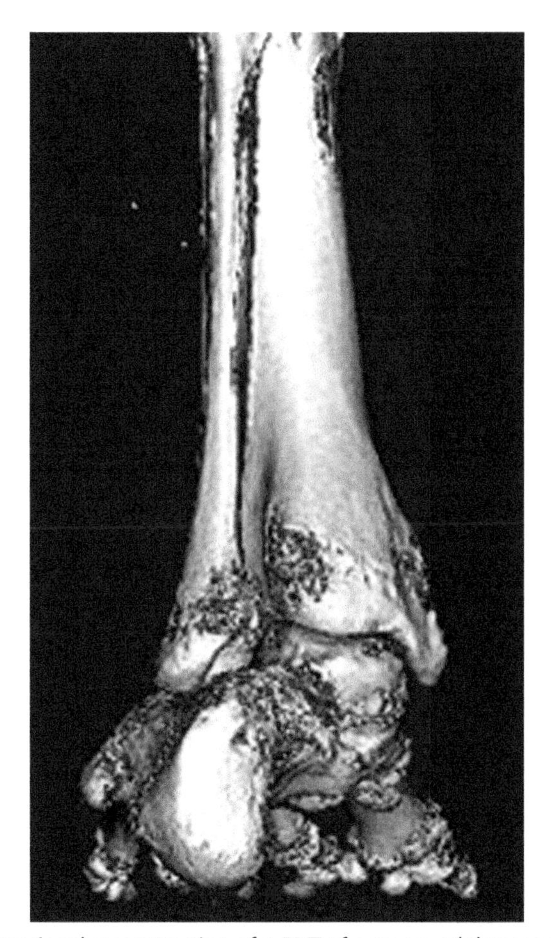

Fig. 7. Three-dimensional reconstruction of a DVT of a severe adolescent clubfoot overcorrection with hindfoot valgus deformity. The amount of malalignment can be quantitatively evaluated by the distance of the load-bearing surface of the calcaneus to the tibial axis.

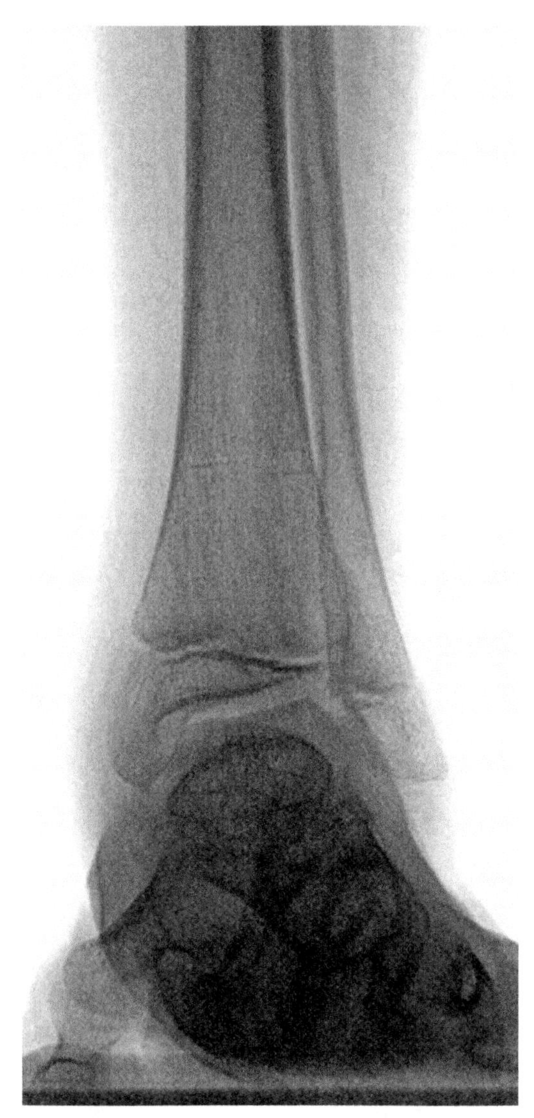

Fig. 8. Severe supramalleolar valgus deformity in a 6-year-old male patient with clubfoot overcorrection and supination of the midforefoot region after conservative treatment (same patient as in **Fig. 3**).

supramalleolar valgus deformity remains unclear. This form of growth disturbance is observed in up to 67% in patients with surgically treated clubfoot[20] but seems to be connected especially to overcorrected cases, where it contributes to overall hindfoot valgus deformity caused additionally by peritalar eversion. Knupp and collegues[1] treated adult patients with clubfoot overcorrection mainly at the supramalleolar region. The author saw the most severe supramalleolar valgus deformities in patients with extreme supination of the midforefoot region and assumes a pathogenetic connection of these 2 phenomena. Supramalleolar valgus deformity is not a phenomenon of

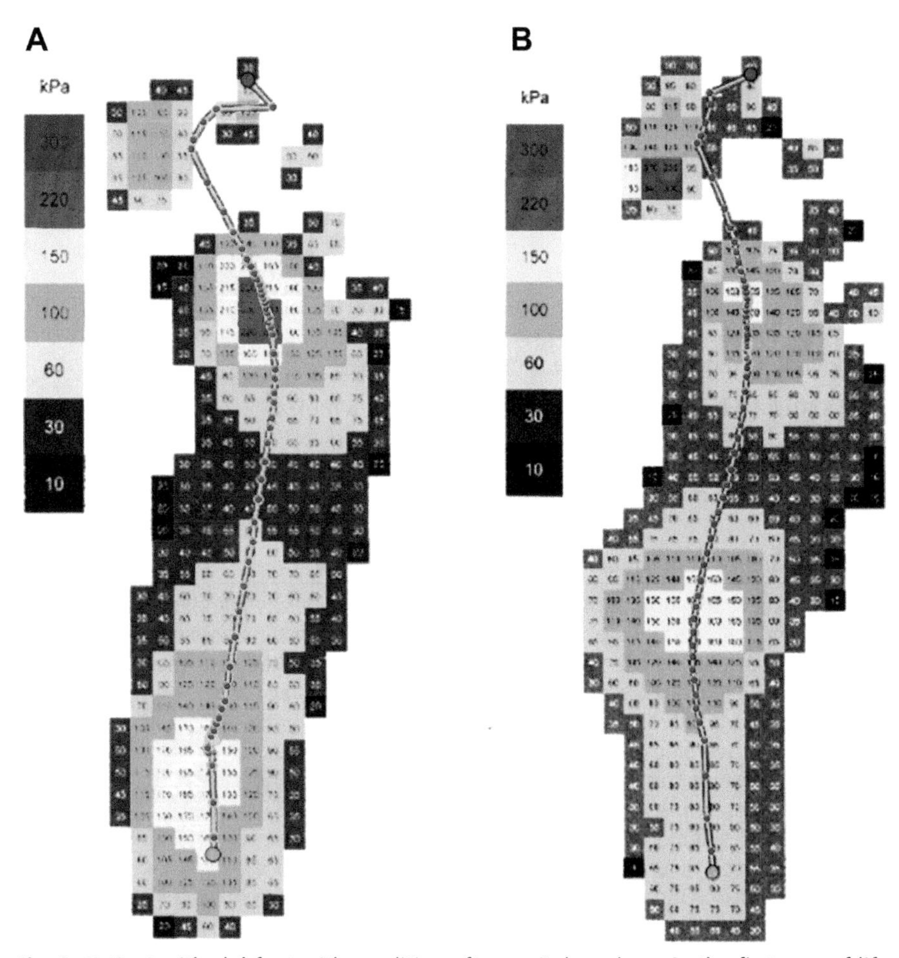

Fig. 9. Patient with clubfoot with condition after peritalar release in the first year of life. The pedographies (peak pressure pictures) at 9 (*A*) and 12 years (*B*) show the serious and progressive increase of the dysfunction with complete loss of load transfer at the medial ray.

overcorrection itself but more a side effect, because supramalleolar varus is never observed in clubfoot.

Functional Evaluation

The functional impairment of overcorrection can be assessed and documented by gait analysis and especially by pedobarographic examination. Typical signs are reduced weight-bearing at the medial metatarsal region and the whole forefoot in late stance, unphysiologic increase of load transfer at the midfoot region, and signs of overactivity of the toe flexors.[21] Repeated examination in most cases reveals deterioration of dysfunction over time (**Fig. 9**). Hayes and collegues[2] defined overcorrection pedographically simply by "the presence of pressure points on the medial side of the midfoot," which according to the author's experience is only one criterion among others and probably not the most important one in severe clubfoot overcorrection. The case in **Fig. 13** shows that it might be missing completely. In contrast the complete deloading of the first metatarsal in severe cases is a specific phenomenon of clubfoot overcorrection and represents a clear difference from a hypermobile pediatric flatfoot.

PRINCIPLES OF SURGICAL TREATMENT

Clubfoot overcorrection in children is a severe complication with a strong tendency to further progression (see **Fig. 9**). Conservative treatment with orthotic devices may be of limited value in early stages especially in younger children. Once any further deterioration is observed, early active intervention should be considered in all cases. It is clearly not advisable to generally postpone surgical treatment until the end of growth. Four therapeutic goals should be pursued individually:

- Correction and/or stabilization of the peritalar complex
- Correction and/or stabilization of the medial ray
- Correction of supramalleolar valgus deformity
- Balancing of muscular forces

Correction and/or Stabilization of the Peritalar Complex

The main feature of clubfoot overcorrection in many cases is weakness and instability in the second half of stance phase. Measures to improve calf muscle power by shortening of Achilles tendon or tendon transfer are clearly limited and merely effective beyond age 6 years.[4] More effect can be expected from stabilization of the tarsometatarsal region and thereby improvement of the efficiency of the given calf muscle power. Excessive eversion of the hindfoot complex can be corrected by calcaneal sliding and/or lengthening osteotomy in minor cases[22] or fusion of single joints of the peritalar complex, for example, by Grice extra-articular fusion (Grice,[23] 1952) (**Fig. 12**); arthroereisis in selected cases; talocalcaneal and/or talonavicular fusion; or triple fusion. Thompson and Abaza[19] in 2010 recommend talocalcaneal extra-articular fusion according to Grice for the age group 4 to 10 years and triple fusion for older children and adolescents. Eberhardt and collegues[24] in 2018 recommend fusion instead of osteotomy especially in cases with translatory valgus deformity of the peritalar complex. If active stabilization of the peritalar complex by the posterior tibial muscle is lost due to prior surgery, this should be taken as an argument for more vigorous bony stabilization. Painful fibulocalcaneal impingement is another clinical situation, where corrective talocalcaneal fusion seems to be inevitable.

Correction and/or Stabilization of the Medial Ray

At the medial ray plantarizing osteotomies of the first metatarsal bone or the medial cuneiform bone are sufficient in minor cases,[17,18,25] whereas fusion of the naviculocuneiform joint line and/or the talonavicular joint (**Fig 14**) are necessary in cases with more severe instability and in later childhood. Supinatory deformity of the whole mid-forefoot requires pronatory correction at the Chopart or naviculocuneiform joint line to restore weight-bearing capacity of the medial metatarsus. Additional rerouting of the flexor hallucis tendon is mandatory in dorsal bunion deformity (see later discussion).

Correction of Supramalleolar Valgus Deformity

In cases with supramalleolar valgus deformity, medial temporary hemiepiphyseodesis[26,27] (**Fig. 10**) and/or supramalleolar osteotomy (**Fig. 13**) should be considered, sometimes with additional correction at the lateral ankle compartment.

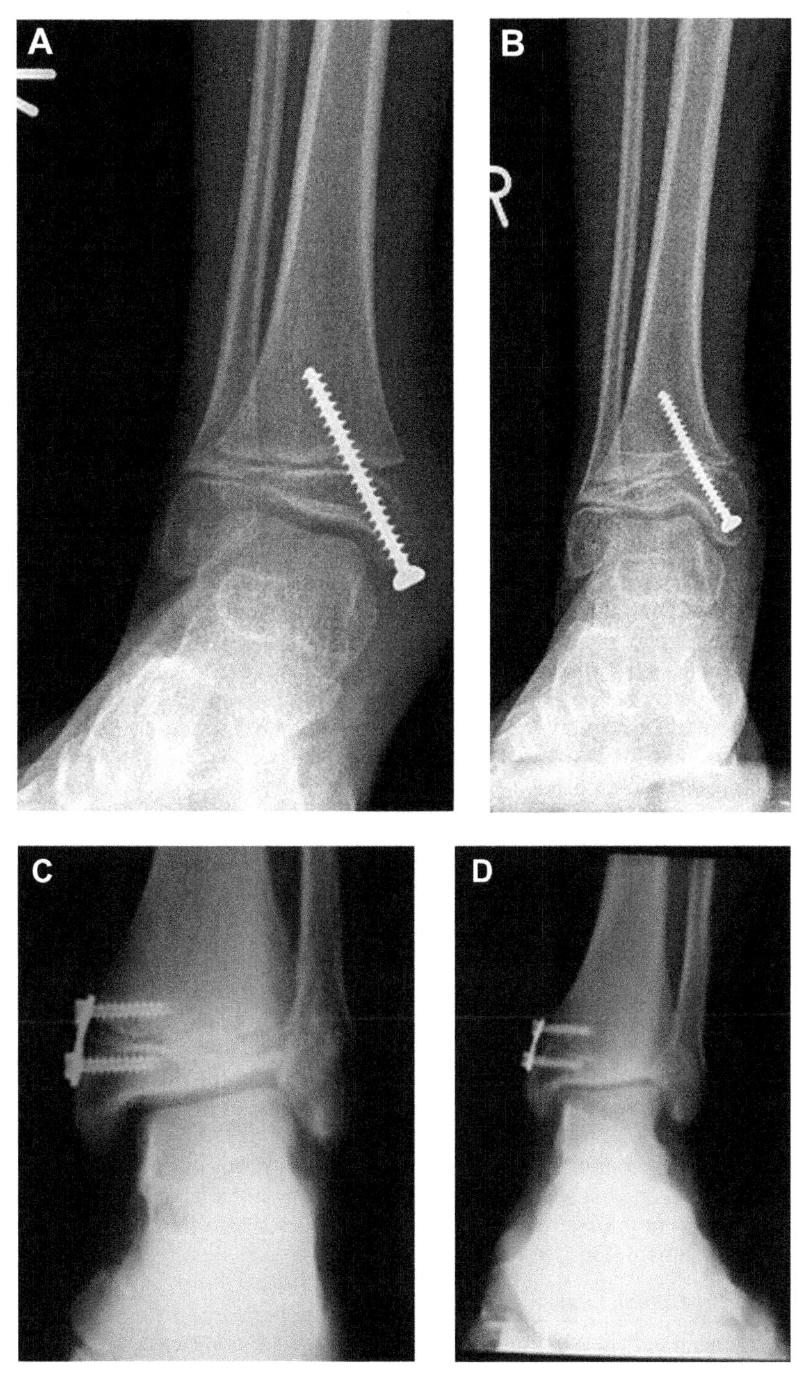

Fig. 10. An 8-year-old girl with multiple clubfoot corrections because of relapse now has supramalleolar valgus malformation (*A*). Temporary hemiepiphyseodesis (*A*) resulted in slight overcorrection within 20 months (*B*). An alternative to the screw technique is the application of an eight plate (*C, D*, these pictures were contributed by Dr M. De Pellegrin).

Balancing of Muscular Forces

As in other complex foot deformities major muscular dysbalance should be corrected by rebalancing of muscular forces, even in combination with fusions. In clubfoot overcorrection especially the dysbalance of the anterior tibial-peroneus longus antagonism on the medial ray and the compensatory overactivity of the M. flexor hallucis longus should be treated by tendon transfer additionally to appropriate bony procedures: transfer of the anterior tibial tendon to the intermediate cuneiform bone and rerouting of the long toe flexor to the first metatarsal bone (reverse Jones procedure) are typical and proven procedures for dorsal bunion deformity and dysfunction.[25] Mc Kay[11] recommended transfer of the flexor hallucis brevis instead. In general, dorsal bunion deformity is an essential part of clubfoot overcorrection in many cases and its correction is as important as hindfoot stabilization.

RESULTS OF SURGICAL TREATMENT

Clinical results of procedures to treat clubfoot overcorrection in childhood are scarce in the literature.

Peritalar Hindfoot Deformity

Eberhardt and collegues[24] in 2018 reported results of 25 cases, most of them in adolescent age. The focus of their study was primarily on hindfoot deformities. This is the only study beyond case reports and expert opinion with a concrete series of patients. The investigators had to converse 32% of those feet to triple arthrodesis, in which they primarily corrected translatory or hinge valgus with calcaneal osteotomy. This approach is in accordance with the experience of the author: only in minor cases of (rotational) hindfoot valgus a calcaneal osteotomy might be sufficient, sometimes in combination with supramalleolar hemiepiphyseodesis or osteotomy. Mosca,[22] however, recommends calcaneal lengthening and/or sliding osteotomy in general for pediatric cases.

Supramalleolar Valgus Deformity

Rupprecht and collegues[26] and Stevens and collegues[27] found about 0.6° correction per month in supramalleolar valgus deformity by temporary hemiepiphyseodesis of the distal tibia. The implant should be removed when slight overcorrection can be observed because of a rebound effect that can be expected afterward. Tibial correction always can be achieved if the procedure is undertaken early enough before closing of the physis (**Fig. 10**); however, one problem may be the still short fibula with lateral ankle compartment malalignment (**Fig. 11**), which can require additional fibula osteotomy at the time of implant removal. Titanium screws should not be used for medial hemiepiphyseodesis because they often cause problems during removal. In older children and adolescents closing wedge osteotomy of the distal tibia with slight lengthening and varus osteotomy of the distal fibula is a safe procedure to achieve complete realignment (**Fig. 13**).

Instability of the Medial Ray and Dorsal Bunion

Yong and collegues[18] in 2007 reported good results with combined osteotomy and tendon transfer in 33 feet, but recurrence in some cases, when osteotomy was omitted. Zide and Myerson[28] in 2013 recommended corrective fusion of the first tarsometatarsal joint in adult patients in combination with anterior tibial tendon transfer without transfer of a flexor tendon. In the author's experience in children plantarizing osteotomy at the medial ray in combination with tendon transfers

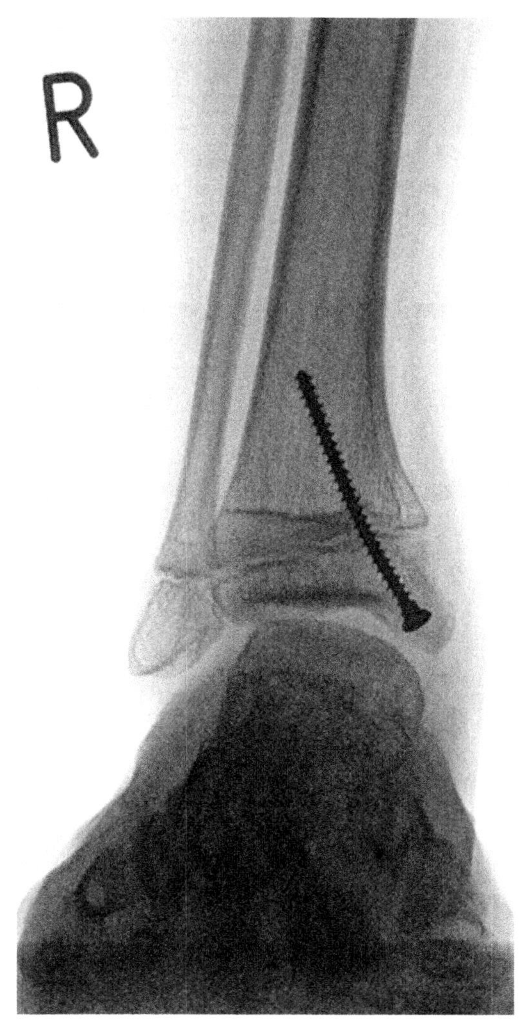

Fig. 11. Successful correction of supramalleolar tibial valgus deformity in a child with clubfoot overcorrection. However, a tibiotalar tilt remains due to medial talar malshaping and missing lateral fibular support. Probably unintentional violation of the deltoid ligament during the primary surgery occurred.

results in a strong effect to overcome dorsal bunion (see **Figs. 12** and **13**). The distal stump of the M. flexor hallucis longus tendon can be sutured to the periosteum of the proximal phalanx to prevent hyperextension of the interphalangeal (IP) joint and later necessity of IP fusion. By pedographic follow-up examination in 10 cases about 70% of the plantarflexion power at the big toe could be saved.[21] In cases of older children with major hypermobility of the talonavicular and/or naviculocuneiform joint fusion seems inevitable. In some of the author's cases a second fusion procedure was necessary, when hypermobility of the neighboring joint was primarily underestimated.

TREATMENT EXAMPLES

Three treatment examples should further illustrate the therapeutic regimen. All 3 children had been treated by peritalar release in the first year of life at another institution. Surgical correction included hindfoot realignment by fusion or osteotomy, stabilization of the medial ray, and dorsal bunion surgery as described earlier. Functional improvement is documented by pedography in the first 2 cases (see **Figs. 12** and **13**). The third, adolescent case required major tarsal fusion to completely correct and stabilize the deformity (**Fig. 14**).

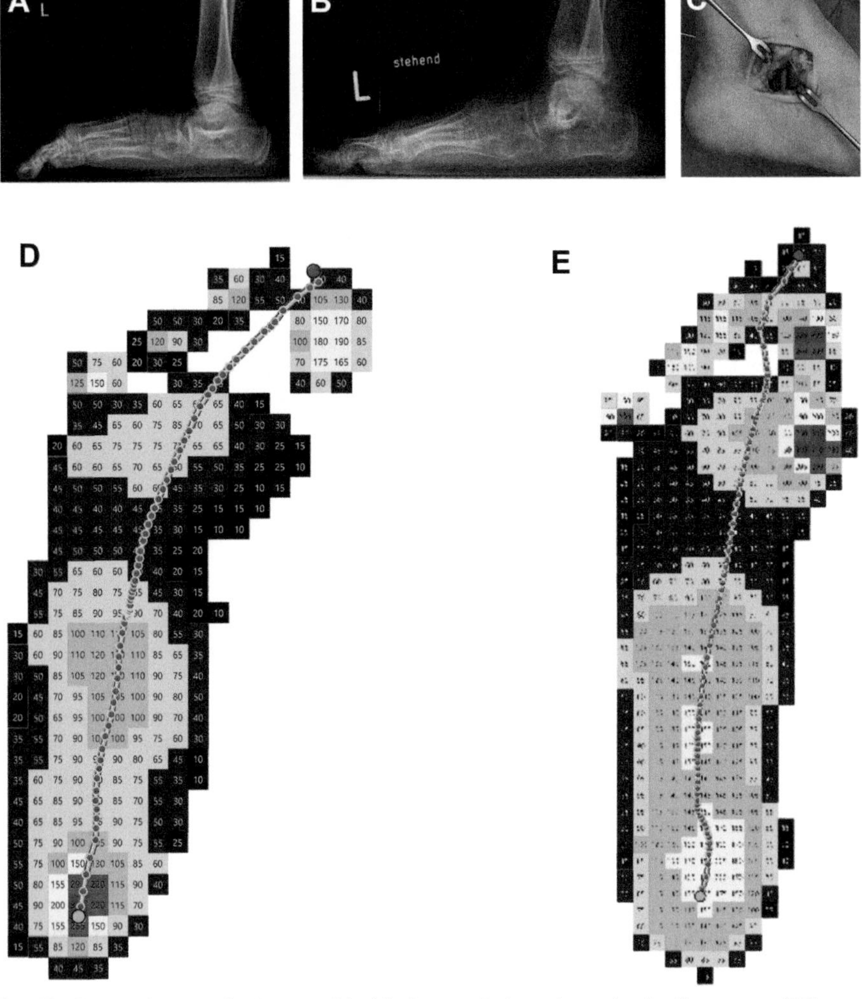

Fig. 12. Case 1. Status of a 9-year-old girl after peritalar release in the first year of life and severe overcorrection with supination of the midforefoot complex and dorsal bunion symptoms (*A*, *D*). Talocalcaneal stabilization with Grice procedure (*C*) and correction of the dorsal bunion with plantarizing cuneiform medial osteotomy, rerouting of the flexor hallucis longus tendon back to the metatarsal I, and transfer of the anterior tibial tendon to the second ray (*B*). Almost 2 years postoperatively (*E*) the load distribution at the forefoot is clearly improved.

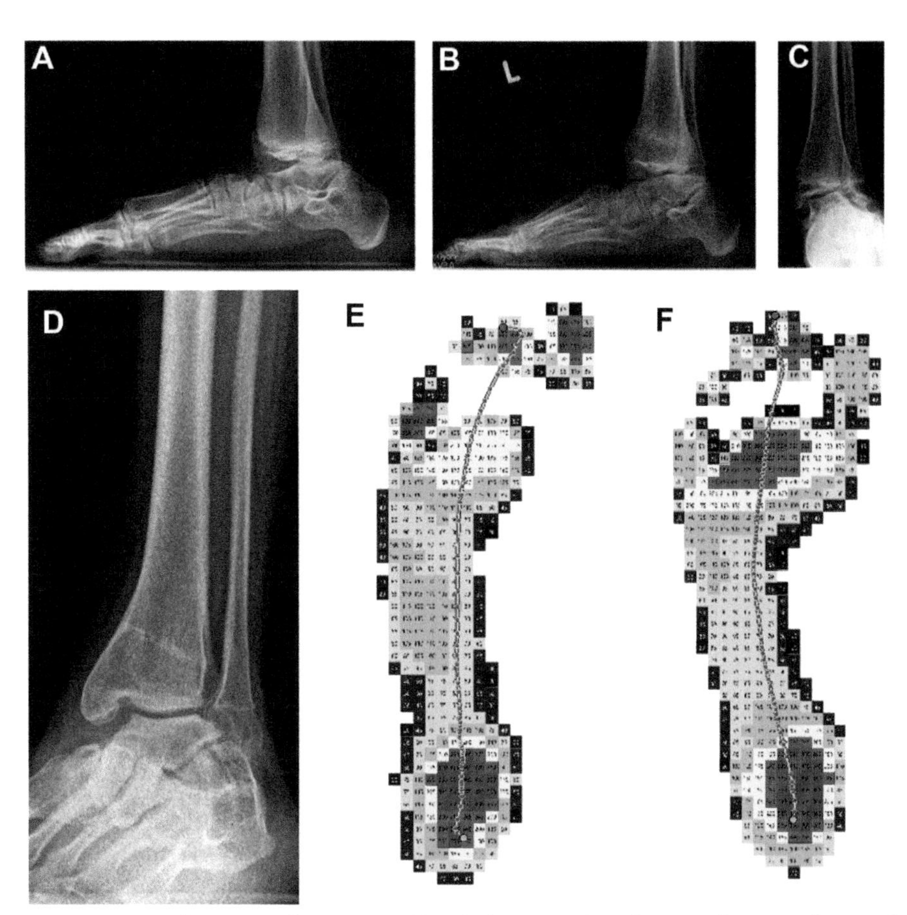

Fig. 13. Case 2. The status of a 12-year-old girl after peritalar release in the second year of life; now there is clinically severe overcorrection problem with clearly reduced load transfer at the forefoot (*E*). Radiologically distinct talar deformity, supramalleolar malformation, and dorsal bunion (*A, C*). After supramalleolar osteotomy with dorsal bunion correction (anterior tibial tendon transfer, metatarsal I base osteotomy, and flexor hallucis longus rerouting (*B, D*), there is significant functional improvement pedographically recognizable by an increased forefoot load (*F*).

TIMINIG OF SURGERY

Overcorrection is rarely observed before school age, and in most cases it becomes obvious not before 8 to 10 years of age. In the series of Eberhard and collegues[24] all the patients requiring planovalgus correction after extensive release surgery in infancy were older than 11 years. Once overcorrection has been diagnosed and provided that there is a promising surgical solution any delay of the intervention is not advisable, because spontaneous improvement cannot be expected. Especially in those cases in which the posterior tibial muscle is without activity, further planovalgus development seems nearly inevitable. In early stages when the situation is not completely clear or the parents do not yet want surgery pedographic examination and control after 1 year is extremely useful to document the functional development.

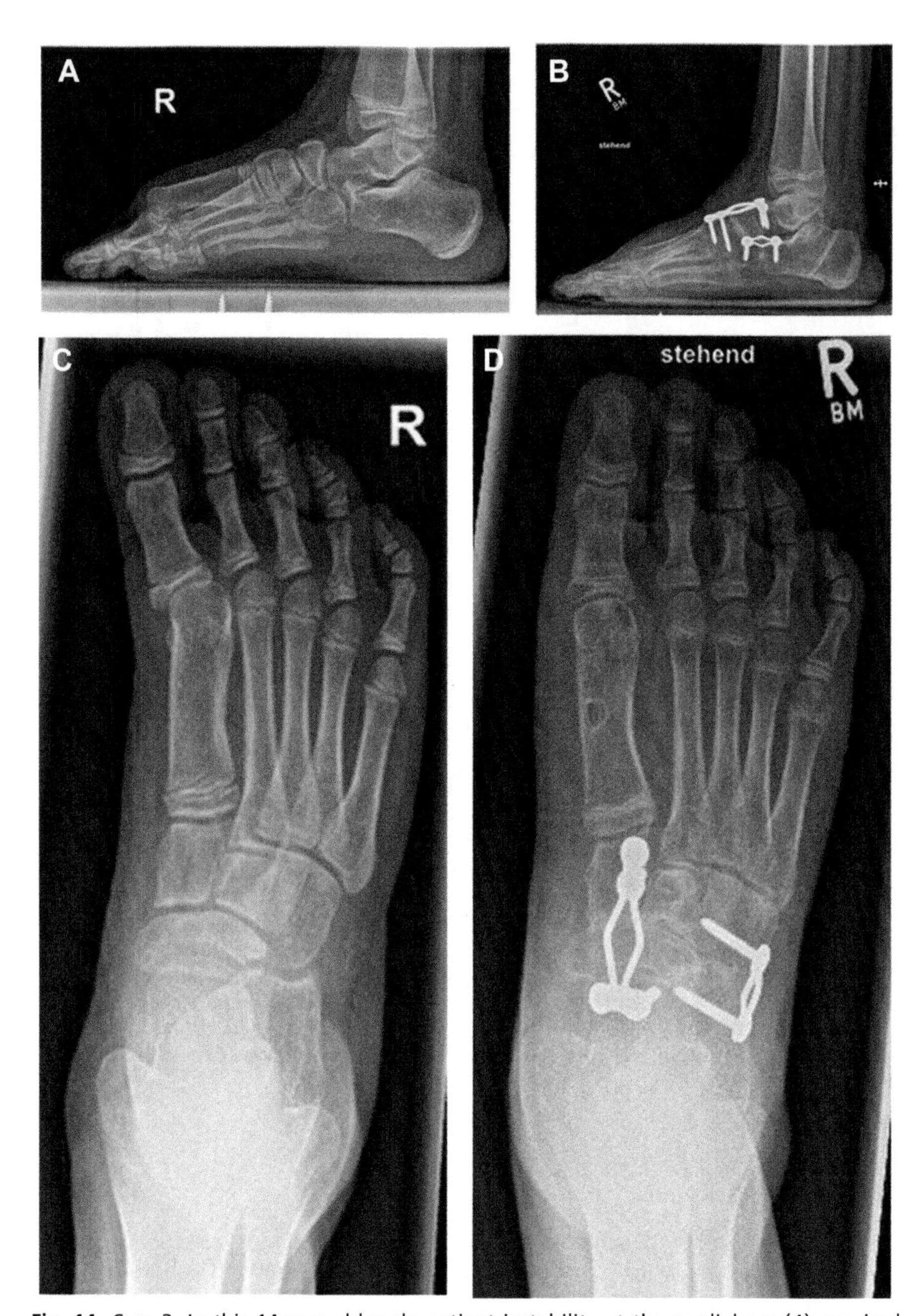

Fig. 14. Case 3. In this 14-year-old male patient instability at the medial ray (*A*) required fusion at the Chopart joint line as well as at the naviculocuneiform joint line (*B*, *D*) in combination with a calcaneal osteotomy. Tendon transfer of the flexor hallucis longus and the anterior tibial tendon was also included in the surgical procedure. Sparing one of these joints in case of severe hypermobility proved not to be sufficiently effective in similar cases. The compensatory adduction of all toes in the metatarsophalangeal region (*C*) disappeared spontaneously (*D*) due to improved stability of the medial ray and better transmission of calf muscle power to the forefoot thereby.

SUMMARY

Clubfoot overcorrection can be observed after any form of primary treatment, but occurred frequently after dorsomedial or peritalar release. The deformity in most cases develops gradually over years and is characterized in school age by hindfoot valgus position due to excessive rigid peritalar eversion, sometimes accompanied by supramalleolar valgus malalignment. In addition, instability and/or elevation of the medial tarsometatarsal ray is observed in all cases together with dorsal bunion deformity. The muscle balance around the foot and ankle shows weakness or malfunction of the calf muscles and the posterior tibial muscle, compensated by overactivity of the long toe flexors. The physiologic antagonism of the anterior tibial muscle and the long peroneal muscle is more or less disturbed. The resulting functional impairment can best be documented by pedography. Surgical treatment is recommended in severe cases and consists of bony realignment at the peritalar complex by osteotomy or fusion, correction of the supramalleolar component in younger children by hemiepiphyseodesis, or osteotomy in adolescents. Correction of the dorsal bunion by stabilization of the medial tarsometatarsal ray and tendon transfer of the anterior tibial and long flexor hallucis muscle is as important as the hindfoot realignment to improve function especially in late stance phase of gait.

CLINICS CARE POINTS

- In follow up examination of clubfoot patients signs of overcorrection like hindfoot valgus, dorsal bunion development and reduced power in tip-toe gait should be evaluated carefully.
- Especially after peritalar release functional overcorrection might develop years after primary surgery.
- Repeated pedobarographic examination is a very useful diagnostic tool in patients at risk for overcorrection.
- Besides X-ray-examination of the foot in at least two planes supramalleolar growth should be monitored by anteroposterior ankle projection.
- If deterioration of overcorrection is detected, early surgical treatment is advisable.

DISCLOSURE

The author has nothing to disclose.

REFERENCES

1. Knupp M, Barg A, Bolliger L, et al. Reconstructive surgery for overcorrected clubfoot in adults. J Bone Joint Surg 2012;94:e1101–7.
2. Hayes CB, Murr KA, Muchow RD, et al. Pain and overcorrection in clubfeet treated by Ponseti method. J Pediatr Orthop 2018;27-B:52–5.
3. Dussa CU, Böhm H, Döderlein L, et al. Does an overcorrected clubfoot caused by surgery or by the Ponseti method behave differently? Gait Posture 2020;77: 308–14.
4. O'Brien SE, Karol LA, Johnston CE. Calcaneus gait following treatment for clubfoot: preliminary results of surgical correction. J Pediatr Orthop 2004;13-B:43–7.
5. Koureas G, Rampal V, Mascard E, et al. The incidence and treatment of rocker bottom deformity as a complication of the conservative treatment of idiopathic congenital clubfoot. J Bone Joint Surg 2008;90-B:57–60.

6. Lau JHK, Meyer LC, Lau HC. The results of surgical treatment of talipes equino-varus congenita. Clin Orthop Relat Res 1989;248:219–26.
7. Imhäuser G. Die Behandlung des idiopathischen Klumpfußes. Germany: Ferdinand Enke Verlag Stuttgart; 1984.
8. Lampasi M, Bettuzzi C, Palmonari M, et al. Transfer of the tendon of tibialis anterior in relapsed congenital clubfoot. J Bone Joint Surg 2010;92-B:277–83.
9. Dobbs MB, Nunley R, Schoenecker PL. Long-term follow-up of patients with club-feet treated with extensive soft-tissue release. J Bone Joint Surg 2006;88:986–96.
10. Carroll NC. Clubfoot in the twentieth century: where we were and where we may be going in the twenty-first century. J Pediatr Orthop 2012;21:1–6.
11. Mc Kay D. Correction of the overcorrected clubfoot. In: Simons GW, editor. The clubfoot – the present and a view of the future. New York: Springer-Verlag; 1994. p. 374–5.
12. Turco VJ. Resistant congenital clubfoot-one-stage posteromedial release with internal fixation: a follow-up report of 15 years experience. J Bone Joint Surg 1979; 61-A:805–14.
13. Ponseti IV. Congenital clubfoot — fundamentals of treatment. Oxford: Oxford University Press; 1996.
14. Smith PA, Kuo KN, Graf AN, et al. Long-term results of comprehensive clubfoot release versus the Ponseti method: which is better? Clin Orthop Relat Res 2014;472:1281–90.
15. Haslam PG, Goddard M, Flowers MJ, et al. Overcorrection and generalized joint laxitiy in surgically treated congenital talipes equino-varus. J Pediatr Orthop B 2006;15:273–7.
16. Beck JJ, Nazif MA, Sangiorgio SN, et al. Does generalized joint hypermobility influence the Ponseti treatment of clubfoot patient? J Pediatr Orthop 2020. https://doi.org/10.1097/BPB.0000000000000747.
17. McKay DW. Dorsal bunions in children. J Bone Joint Surg 1983;65-A:975–80.
18. Yong SM, Smith PA, Kuo KN. Dorsal bunion after clubfoot surgery. J Pediatr Orthop 2007;27:814–20.
19. Thompson GH, Abaza H. Clubfoot: operative treatment. Chapter 6. In: McCarthy JJ, Drennan JC, editors. Drennan's the childs foot and ankle. 2nd edition. Lippincott, Williams & Willkins; 2010.
20. Stevens PM, Otis S. Ankle valgus and clubfeet. J Pediatr Orthop 1999;19:515–8.
21. Hamel J, Nell M. Pedobarographie zur Diagnostik und Therapiekontrolle am Beispiel der Dorsal-Bunion-Deformität. Orthop Technik 2016;8(16):20–3.
22. Mosca VS. Principles and management of pediatric foot and ankle deformities and malformations. Philadelphia: Wolters Kluwer; 2014.
23. Grice DS. An extra-articular arthrodesis of the subastragalar joint for correction of paralytic flat feet in children. J Bone Joint Surg 1952;34-A:927–40.
24. Eberhardt O, Wachowsky M, Wirth T, et al. Limitation of flatfoot surgery in overcorrected clubfeet after extensive surgery. Arch Orthop Trauma Surg 2018;138:1037–43.
25. Kuo KN. "Reverse Jones" procedure for dorsal bunion following clubfoot surgery. In: Simons GW, editor. The clubfoot, the present and a view of the future. New York: Springer-Verlag; 1993. p. 384–6.
26. Rupprecht M, Spiro AS, Breyer S, et al. Growth modulation with a medial malleolar screw for ankle valgus deformity. Acta Orthop 2015;5:1–5.
27. Stevens PM, Kennedy JM, Hung M. Guided growth for ankle valgus. J Pediatr Orthop 2011;31:878–83.
28. Zide JR, Myerson M. The overcorrected clubfoot in the adult: evaluation and management – topical review. Foot Ankle Int 2013;34:1312–8.

Subtalar Arthroereisis for Surgical Treatment of Flexible Flatfoot

Maurizio De Pellegrin, MD[a], Désirée Moharamzadeh, MD[b,*]

KEYWORDS

- Flatfoot • Arthroereisis • Children • Flexible • Flexible flatfoot • Pes planus
- Subtalar arthroereisis • Calcaneo-stop

KEY POINTS

- The persistent forefoot abduction might lead to poor quality of propulsion, instability and necessitate kinematic adaptations at the foot; individuals with pronated feet may have implications on the underlying mechanisms of overuse injuries.
- Publications about flatfoot treatment with subtalar arthroereisis procedures in children and the number of surgical treatments have been increased in the last 10 years.
- According to the different biomechanical effect, the subtalar arthroereisis with endorthesis into tarsal canal (SAE) must be distinguished from the subtalar arthroereisis with calcaneo-stop procedures (SAC-stop).
- Data collected in a review of the last 10-year period (2010–2020) show that among the 691 feet undergoing SAE, average age at surgery was 11.40 years and in the 1856 feet that underwent SAC-stop 11.69 years, while the complications rate was 9.00% and 6.38%, respectively. These data confirm that SAC-stop may have an advantage over SAE as the screw is not placed across the subtalar joint but instead into the calcaneus.

 **Video content accompanies this article at http://www.foot.theclinics.com.**

INTRODUCTION

Flatfoot (FF) deformities include valgus position of calcaneus,[1] medial-plantar tilt of the talus, and reduction (absence) of the longitudinal arch.[2] Clinical evaluation is well described in recent publications.[1,3–5] According to Banwell and colleagues,[5] no universally accepted criteria for diagnosing flexible flatfoot (FFF) were found in a systematic review including 27 studies. The outcome of this review indicates that only the Staheli arch index (>1.07),[6] the Chippaux-Smirak index (>62.7%), and the Foot Posture Index-Six item version (FPI-6) (>+6) are reliable and age-specific.

[a] Pediatric Orthopedic and Traumatology Unit, San Raffaele Hospital, Via Olgettina 60, Milan 20132, Italy; [b] Orthopedic and Traumatology Unit, San Raffaele Hospital, Via Olgettina 60, Milan 20132, Italy
* Corresponding author.
E-mail address: depellegrin.maurizio@hsr.it

Foot Ankle Clin N Am 26 (2021) 765–805
https://doi.org/10.1016/j.fcl.2021.07.007
foot.theclinics.com

Distinction between rigid and flexible FF is very important. Rigid forms are usually symptomatic and associated with coalitions, neurologic or neuromuscular conditions, whereas flexible forms are asymptomatic with patient able to restore the medial arch when standing on tiptoes (**Fig. 1**) or performing Jack's test.

Within the first years of life, a flat shape of the foot has to be considered physiologic, often spontaneously correcting by the age of 10 years.[4,7]

Despite this, an abnormal foot shape may become a reason for concern for parents and triggers subsequent medical referral. Children are usually able to walk without symptoms, but sometimes feel pain located over the medial aspect of the foot, the sinus tarsi, and the distal fibula. Surgery goals are to reduce pain, deformity, and foot instability.

Treatment of FFF is extremely variable. Conservative treatment efficacy with foot orthoses lacks good-quality evidence.[4,8–10]

Various surgical techniques have been applied with a range of results.[11–20] Procedures including tendon transfers,[14,17] osteotomies,[19,21] and arthrodesis[22] are possible.

Cohen-Sobel and colleagues[23] reported 12 severe symptomatic FF treated with combined surgical techniques such as Evans calcaneal osteotomy, Young tenosuspension, and Achilles tendon lengthening (ATL) in children younger than 10 years

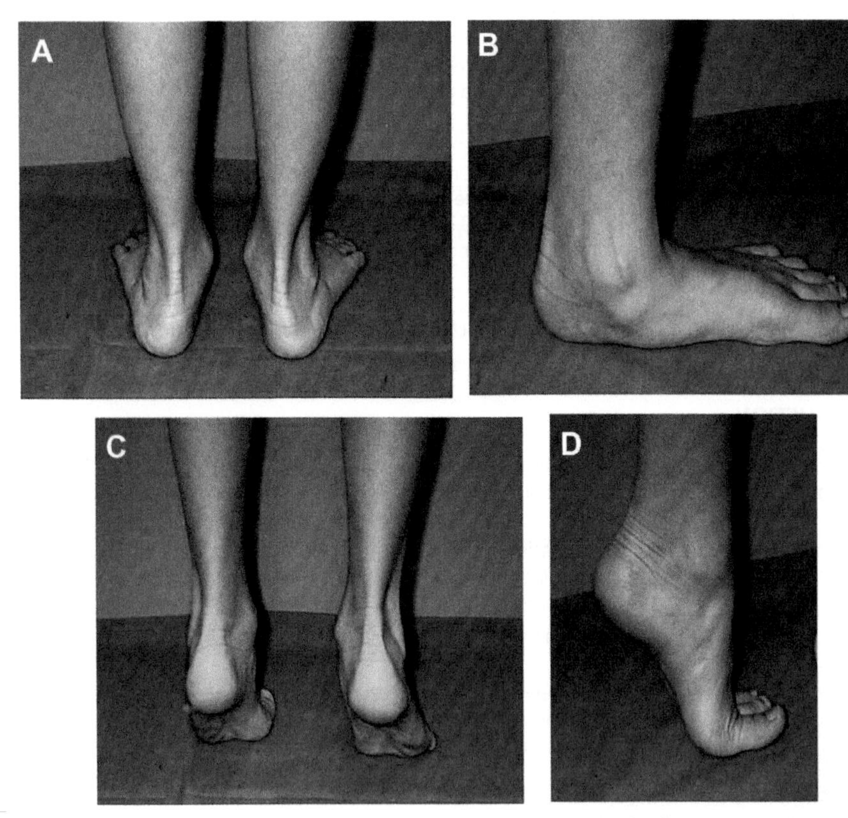

Fig. 1. An 11-year-old boy with severe asymptomatic flexible flatfoot. In weight-bearing hindfoot valgus with "too many toes sign" (*A*) and collapse of the medial longitudinal arch with talus protrusion (*B*). Restoring of the hindfoot valgus (*C*) and of the medial arch (*D*) when standing on tiptoes.

and modified Young tenosuspension, talonavicular desmoplasty, and subtalar arthroereisis (SA) in children older than 10 years.

Jacobs[17] reported for correction of FFF, without specific indications for children, following techniques: Cobb procedure (tibialis posterior tendon reinforcement and tibialis anterior tendon splitting), Young's tenosuspension, Durham plasty, and Kidner procedure (spring ligament reconstruction and tibialis posterior tendon reconstruction). Mosca modified Evans osteotomy, reporting good results in 93.5% of the 25 cases,[24] whereas Su and colleagues 2019 reported a success rate between 69% and 89% after lateral column lengthening (LCL).[25] Rathjen and Mubarak developed triple C osteotomy (sliding and medial closing wedge osteotomy of the posterior calcaneus, plantar-based closing wedge osteotomy of the cuneiform and opening wedge osteotomy of the cuboid) for pediatric valgus foot deformity.[26]

Kwon and Myerson[19] reported in a focus of FFF management in children the medial calcaneal translational osteotomy, the LCL (Evans procedure), and the medial cuneiform osteotomy (open wedge osteotomy).

Vora and colleagues 2006[27] suggested that less severe FFF might be appropriately treated with a combination of medialized calcaneal osteotomy and flexor digitorum longus transfer together with SA.

Among these surgical options, subtalar "arthroereisis" (Greek: arthro- "joint," -ereisis "sustaining, supporting, pushing against something") limits, without blocking, excessive subtalar joint movement.

From 1946, after the first description of a surgical technique for FFF correction,[28] many authors described and studied the concept of arthroereisis for pathologic pronation of the foot. In 1970, LeLièvre introduced the term "lateral arthroereisis" to describe the process of decreasing motion of the hindfoot without eliminating it.[29] In the following years, the devices implanted inside the sinus tarsi were many (STA peg, threaded polyethylene plug, silicone implants, metallic).[2,11,13,15,16,18,30]

In the 1980s, Pisani[31] introduced in Italy the technique suggested in Spain by Recaredo Alvarez in 1970, subsequently published by Burutaran in 1979.[32] This technique, also known as "calcaneo-stop" or "subtalar extra-articular arthroereisis," is performed outside the bony sinus tarsi. This technique is common in Italy and Europe[33–40] but not in North America.[10] Many different variations have been introduced in the technique throughout years.[34,35,37,39]

Chong and colleagues[41] compared LCL and SA and found no differences between the outcomes of both groups, concluding that SA is a valid less-invasive alternative to LCL. Suh and colleagues compared systematic review outcomes of LCL and SA and conclude that LCL achieved more radiographic corrections and more improvements in the American Orthopedic Foot and Ankle Score (AOFAS), but with more complications. Reoperation rates were similar between LCL and SA.[25]

In a recent article by Bauer,[42] the authors answer to the question "What's new in Pediatric Flatfoot?": among the surgical techniques subtalar extra-articular screw arthroereisis (Calcaneo-stop procedure) is reported.

Also, Vulcano and colleagues[43] described SA as the first choice in the surgical management of pediatric FF.

The numbers of reports of pediatric FF treatment with arthroereisis have been increasing in the last 10 years.[36,38,40,41,44–67] Evaluation of outcomes became more accurate and sophisticated as well. SA effectiveness is analyzed through pedobarography,[54,65] gait analysis,[60] Kinematics,[68,69] and 2D gait analysis.[62] Cadaver studies were conducted to analyze the biomechanical effects of surgical procedures.[47,70,71]

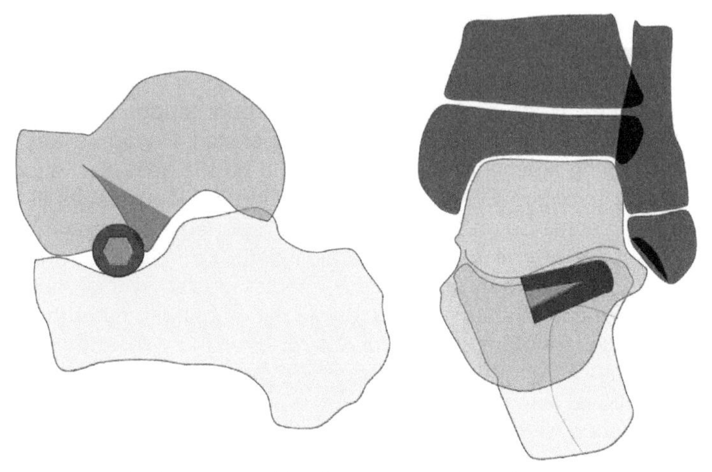

Fig. 2. SAE showing the implant position into the tarsal canal.

The SA with endorthesis (SAE; arthroereisis into tarsal canal; **Fig. 2**) and the SA with Calcaneo-stop procedures (SAC-stop; **Fig. 3**) will be treated separately in this article, according to their different biomechanical effect.

SUBTALAR ARTHROEREISIS

Indications

According to Zaret and Myerson, the indication for SA procedure is a symptomatic patient who failed all conservative treatment options.[72] Evans and Rome[73] concluded in a review that surgery is rarely indicated for pediatric FF and only after failure of prolonged nonsurgical attempt to relieve pain under the medial midfoot and/or in the sinus tarsi interfering with normal activities.

Although indications for surgical correction of symptomatic FFF are clear, its symptomatology is less clear. So what does it mean "symptomatic"? Some authors report as symptom calluses, fatigue, as well as failure of nonsurgical treatment such as

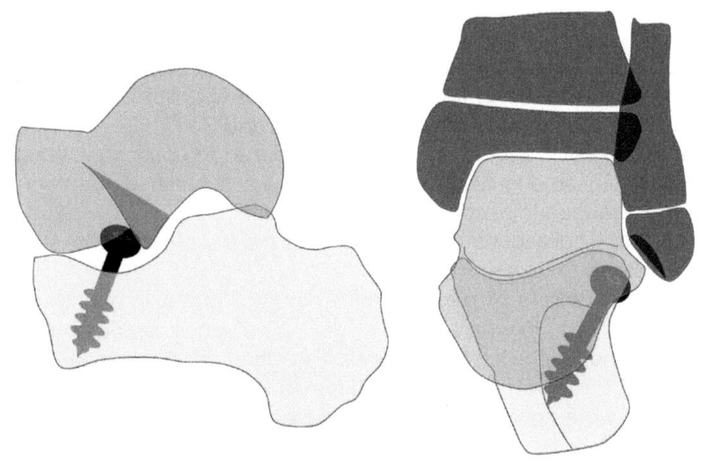

Fig. 3. SAC-stop procedure showing the screw into the calcaneus.

orthosis and physiotherapy. The high percentage of complications reported in literature conditioned surgical treatment in the past, especially referring to SAE into tarsal canal. Many authors reported complications mainly for this type of SA.[1,3,20,74]

Pain symptoms are more common in FFF with a short Achilles tendon.[1] The Silverskiöld test is still commonly used for identifying a contracture of gastrocnemius-soleus complex.[4]

However, as literature showed good and excellent results with less invasive surgical techniques, SA became a topic and the number of surgical treatments has increased.

Evidences are not strong enough to define indications for SA.[1,3] However, a painful FFF causing abnormal gait in an 8 to 14 years old after conservative treatment failure is an indication according to Aranjio and colleagues.[71]

According to Martinelli and colleagues,[47] SA was indicated when the deformity induced pain during and/or after exercise, postural fatigue, or cramping sensation in the foot or medial arch. Surgical indication was also established when parents noticed abnormal gait or a decrease in activity in their child.[75]

Kerr and colleagues demonstrated in a recent study how in young patients with symptomatic flatfeet the persistent forefoot abduction might lead to poor quality of propulsion, instability and necessitate kinematic adaptations at the foot.[76] In untreated symptomatic flatfeet, Zhang and colleagues showed differences in foot muscles morphology with respect to asymptomatic patients, in a physically active adult population. Results of this study may have implications on the underlying mechanisms of overuse injuries in individuals with pronated feet.[69]

Sharer and colleagues[46] reported in 39 patients (mean age 12 years; 68 feet) SA that all patients who underwent surgical treatment did not respond to nonsurgical care such as functional foot orthoses, bracing, and immobilization.

Arbab[63] indications are symptomatic FFF and/or progressive deformity in a clinical and radiographical follow-up.

De Pellegrin and colleagues[59] indications for surgery were at a median age at surgery of 11.5 years: painful FFF, FFF with Achilles tendon shortening (positive Silverskiöld test), Staheli arch index greater than 1, and pathologic values of 2 of 3 weight-bearing x-ray angles (Calcanel Pitch, Costa-Bartani angle, Talar inclination angle).

Radiological Evaluation

A multitude of radiographic measurements has been described for the evaluation of FFF.[77] The most common angles used preoperatively and postoperatively for FFF evaluation are as follows: Calcaneal pitch (CP), Meary's angle in both views, Talar inclination angle, Costa-Bartani angle, and TMT-I angle[34,51,58,59] (**Fig. 4**).

Contraindications

Contraindications for SA is a rigid FF.

An exception represents the tarsal coalitions after their removal when the foot becomes mobile in the subtalar joint and a severe valgus deformity remains.[78] A SAC-stop can follow the coalition resection as a one-step procedure.[79]

Bilateral SA in One Step?

Roth and colleagues[37] 2007 reported SA bilaterally at the same time in 46 of 48 patients, whereas Indino and colleagues[56] in a sample of 56 patients (mean age of 15.5 years). Caravaggi and colleagues[49] reported a 13 patients series with 26 feet operated at the same time using 2 types of implants (on the right foot a bioreabsorbable Calcaneus screw and on the left foot a bioreabsorbable expanding endorthesis).

Instead, Richter and Zech reported one foot at a time and the contralateral 3 months later.[58] De Pellegrin and colleagues[59] reported that among 732 cases, 247 had FFF bilaterally and 238 monolaterally. In the bilateral cases, surgery was performed on one foot—the second foot operated on an average of 6 months after the first (if the indication was still present). In syndromic patients, the Calcaneo-stop procedure as minimally invasive approach to FFF can be bilaterally performed in one step without postoperative immobilization and weight-bearing restriction.[80]

Outcomes Overview

Many authors reported good results and patients satisfaction—among the 20 patients in the report of Cao and colleagues,[48] 12 rated the result as excellent, 6 as good, and 2 as fair; among the 44 patients, Giannini and colleagues[61] reported 33 excellent clinical outcomes, 9 good outcomes, and 2 poor outcomes; Arbab patients[63] reported 95% excellent and good results; among 19 of 25 patients in the report of Kellermann and colleagues,[57] 5 rated the result as good and 1 as poor; De Pellegrin and colleagues[59] reported 95.4% (2005) in 152 patients and 93.7% in 485 patients in a 22-year observation period (2014) of good clinical results and radiographic improvement. Interestingly, only 1 patient[48] reported SAE results, whereas the others reported SAC-stop outcomes.

Comparing the 2 techniques (SAE and SAC-STOP), data have been collected in the last 10-year period (2010–2020). Among the 691 feet undergoing SAE, the average

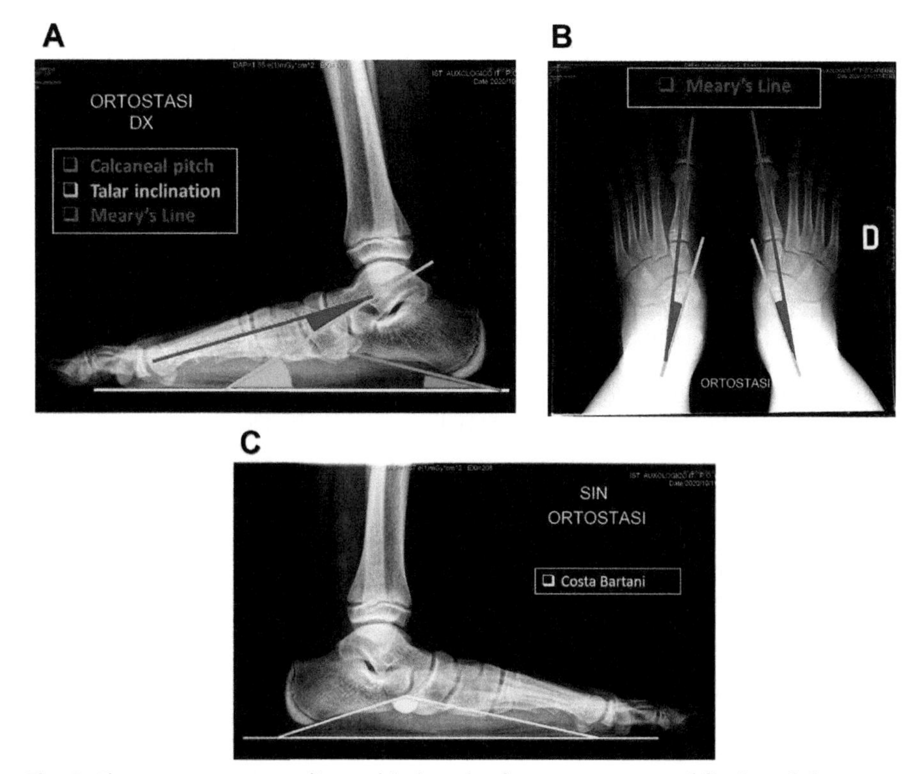

Fig. 4. The most common radiographical angles for measurement of flatfoot deformity in children. Calcaneal pitch, talar inclination angle and Meary's line (*A*), Costa Bartani angle (*B*), Meary's line with TMT-I angle in anteroposterior view (*C*).

Table 1
Subtalar arthroereisis with endorthesis (SAE)

Author	Patients	Feet	Mean Age at Surgery (y)	Complications (%)
Scharer et al,[46] 2010	39	68	12	14.71
Chong et al,[41] 2015	7	13	12.8	15.38
Martinelli et al,[47] 2017	49	98	10.7	8.16
Cao et al,[48] 2017	20	27	12.1	3.70
Caravaggi et al,[49] 2018	13	13	11.3	Not specified
Memeo et al,[50] 2019	200	200	12.8	12.50
de Bot et al,[51] 2019	16	26	12.5	23.08
Ruiz-Picazo et al,[52] 2019	16	32	9	12.50
Megremis et al,[53] 2019	14	28	10.7	0.00
Papamerkouriou et al,[54] 2019	6	12	11.05	0.00
Bernasconi et al,[55] 2020	31	62	10.5	Not specified
Indino et al,[56] 2020	56	112	Not specified	0.00
	Tot. 467	*Tot. 691*	*Mean 11.40*	*Mean 9.00*

Literature data of a review of the period 2010-2020 regarding the total number of patients and feet operated, the average age at surgery and the complications rate (%)

age at surgery was 11.40 years and in the 1856 feet that underwent SAC-stop 11.69 years, while the complications rate was 9.00% and 6.38%, respectively (**Tables 1** and **2**).

These data confirm what Kwon and Myerson suggested[19]: SAC-stop may have an advantage over SAE as the screw is not placed across the subtalar joint but into the

Table 2
Subtalar arthroereisis with calcaneo-stop procedure (SAC-stop)

Author	Patients	Feet	Mean Age at Surgery (y)	Complications (%)
Kellermann et al,[57] 2011	25	43	10	0.00
Pavone et al,[36] 2013	242	410	11	5.12
Richter et al,[58] 2013	18	31	10.6	0.00
De Pellegrin et al,[59] 2014	485	732	11.5	[a]6.28
Das et al,[60] 2017	15	25	12.5	4.00
Giannini et al,[61] 2017	44	88	11.7	2.27
Caravaggi et al,[49] 2018	13	13	11.3	Not specified
Arbab et al,[63] 2018	41	71	11.7	14.08
Hagen et al,[62] 2019	14	27	12.38	3.70
Franz et al,[65] 2020	39	78	11.3	Not specified
Memeo et al,[50] 2019	202	202	13.6	15.84
Pavone et al,[66] 2018	68	136	12.7	12.50
	Tot. 1206	*Tot. 1856*	*Mean 11.69*	*Mean 6.38*

Literature data of a review of the period 2010-2020 regarding the total number of patients and feet operated, the average age at surgery and the complications rate (%)

[a] Complication rate is recorded from 2004 for a total of 398 feet.

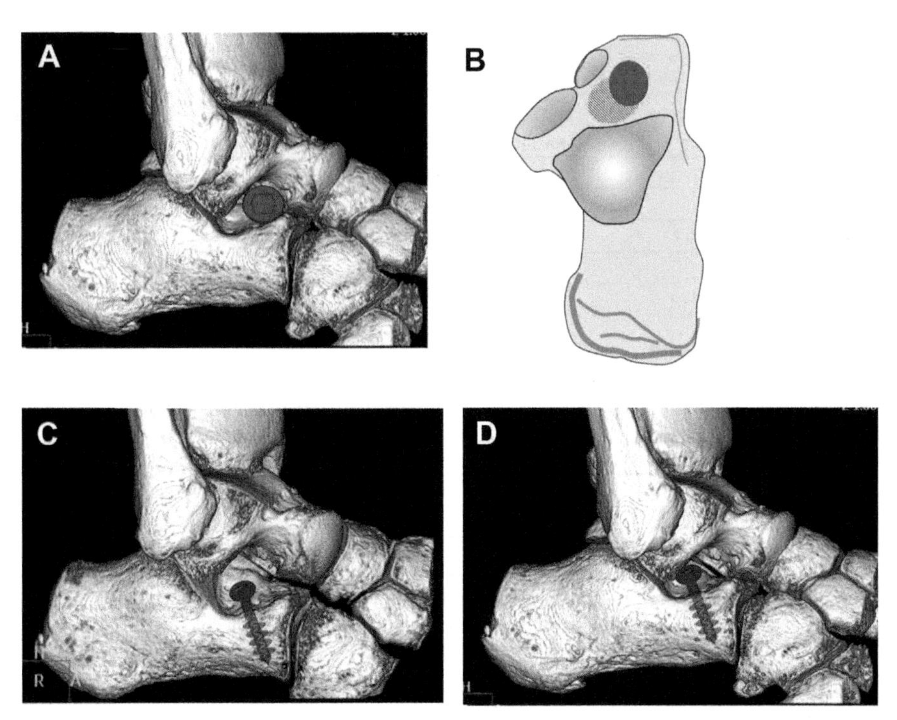

Fig. 5. The working mechanism of the 2 types of subtalar arthroereisis. SAE into tarsal canal decreasing the motion of the hindfoot (*A, B*), SAC-stop procedure with foot in supination (*C*) and stopping the calcaneus eversion against the plantar surface of the talus lateral process in pronation (*D*).

calcaneus (**Fig. 5**). Rein and colleagues[81] showed that the inlet of the sinus tarsi was richly innervated with free nerve endings; therefore, we assumed that pain of the sinus tarsi syndrome mainly originates at the inlet of this structure, giving explanation to these data.

SAE (ARTHROEREISIS INTO THE TARSAL CANAL)

Surgical Technique

With patient in supine position (prone position is also described[67]), 1 to 2 cm skin incision over the sinus tarsi avoiding the sometime crossing branch of Nervus suralis (**Fig. 6**, Video 1). A blunt probe or a closed small scissor is inserted into the subtalar joint along the sinus tarsi floor to determine the correct angle for insertion of the implant anteriorly to the posterior facet. In Maxwell-Brancheau arthroereisis (MBA) technique, a guide-pin is inserted from anteromedial to posterolateral into the tarsal canal, which is shaped as an oblique cone and should reach (exit) medially just inferior to the posterior tibialis tendon.[72] A trial sizer (cannulate) beginning with the smallest sizer is inserted in neutral position of the rearfoot. A fluoroscopy check can be useful to verify the proper position of the implant. The implant is well-positioned if in anteroposterior view is located 1 cm deeper in relation to the lateral calcaneus border and occupying less than half of the width of the talus (**Fig.7**). On the lateral view, it must be positioned exactly above the floor of the sinus tarsi. The appropriate sizer should limit abnormal subtalar joint eversion (few degrees of eversion should remain). The definitive implant will substitute the trial. The foot has to be evaluated clinically to

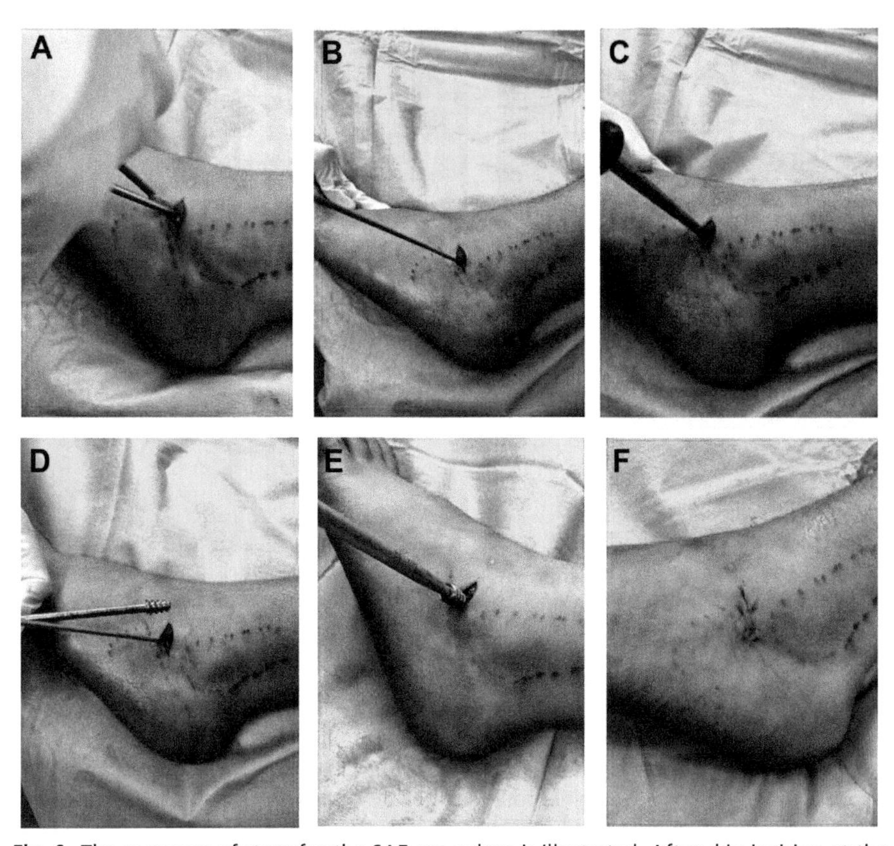

Fig. 6. The sequence of steps for the SAE procedure is illustrated. After skin incision at the level of sinus tarsi, gently spreading of the subcutaneous tissue (*A*), the guide pin is inserted from anterolateral to posteromedial into the tarsal canal (*B*), tissue spreading with dilator (*C*), trial sizers and spacer are inserted beginning with the smallest sizer (*D*), after clinical (subtalar joint range of motion) and radiological (position of the implant in lateral and anteroposterior view) assessment, the trial implant will be replaced by the endorthesis (*E*), suture in layers and skin suture (*F*).

choose the correct size of the implant. Choosing a too small implant will result in an undercorrected foot with residual valgus deformity and will increase the risk of implant extrusion. On the contrary, a too large implant could cause a varus deformity of the rearfoot and a reduced subtalar motion.

Choosing the right size of the implant, which means the appropriate diameter size, is a challenge. According to Ruiz-Picazo and colleagues,[52] the trial implants (with increasing diameters) were inserted until the appropriate implant size was determined. The authors chose the smallest implant that corrected the deformity and remained stable in the sinus tarsi while moving the subtalar joint. According to Chong and colleagues,[41] care must be taken to avoid overcorrection of the hindfoot into varus. According to Bernasconi and colleagues,[55] the right size is appropriate if the expandable device (with effective opening of the fins) leads to "self-stabilization." According to Cao and colleagues[48] and de Bot and colleagues,[51] trial implants were introduced with increasing diameters in the sinus tarsi to achieve an optimal filling of the cavity. Then, the definitive implant with the corresponding trial size was screwed and fixed with a frangible screw.[48]

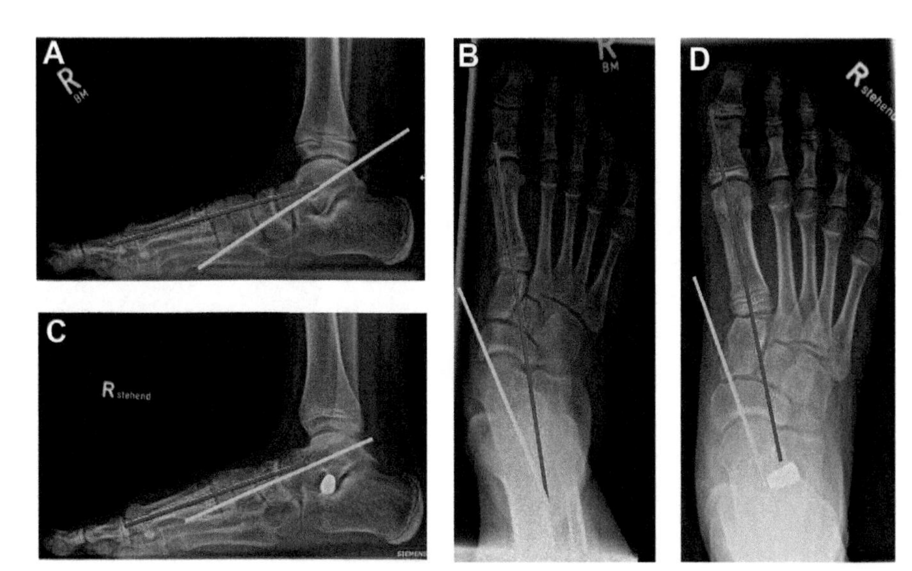

Fig. 7. Preoperative (*A, B*) and postoperative radiographs (*C, D*) of FFF of a 12-year-old boy after SAE showing correction of the deformity with decreased Meary's angle in both views and correct position of the implant (Tornier size 9). (Case from M. Poschmann, Munich, Germany.)

There are many different implants developed.[41,45–49,51,52,54–56,82] An expanding endorthotic implant was presented by Giannini and colleagues.[83] Gutierrez and Lara reported outcomes of a Giannini prosthesis for FF[84] with complications in 10.7% of the cases. Scharer and colleagues[46] and Megremis and Megremis[53] reported treatment with MBA implant, while the second authors group reported an average size of diameters of 10 mm in 71.42% and 8 mm in 28.57% of the cases. Martinelli and colleagues[47] used a standardized conic subtalar implant ranging from 8 to 9 mm as well as Indino and colleagues[56] in 35.7% of the case. In the remaining patients, a BRM Subtalar screw was implanted. Ruiz-Picazo and colleagues[52] used a cannulated titanium device in 32 feet, whereas Chong and colleagues cannulated Vilex titanium conical screw in 24 feet. Bernasconi and colleagues[55] implanted a composed steel screw with peripheral threaded Teflon and the sizes reported were between 8 and 10 mm of diameters. Papamerkouriou and colleagues[54] implanted an expandable device (Kalix2/Viladot) in 12 feet as well de Bot and colleagues[51] in 26 feet and Cao and colleagues[48] in 27 feet. Caravaggi and colleagues[49] reported a series of 13 patients (bilaterally operated in one step) using a PLLA subtalar bioabsorbable expanding implant (expanding screw comprised in an internally threaded cylinder) on the left foot and a bioabsorbable calcaneo-stop screw on the right foot reporting in a 1-year follow-up similar results of both implants in restoring foot alignment but better effectiveness of frontal plane mobility of the endorthotic implant. Memeo and colleagues[50] reported also a comparison between subtalar bioabsorbable expandable implant (Poly-L-lactic acyd) in 200 feet and Calcaneo-stop with steel screw in 202 feet with no statistical differences between the 2 techniques even though 12.5% of feet had complications (with 10.0% of inflammatory processes and 2.5% of failure due to technical errors) in the bioabsorbable endorthesis patients.

According to a biomechanical analysis of MBA, choosing the right size for the implant is important for range of movement (ROM) which decreases progressively

Table 3
Literature review of flatfoot treatment in children with subtalar arthroereisis with endorthesis (SAE)

Authors	Title	Journal	Patients (y) (Feet)	Mean age at surgery (y) (Range)	Period of Surgery	Indications	Preoperative Evaluation	Surgery ± Concomitant Procedures	Complications	Mean FU (Range) + Postoperative Evaluation + Results
Giannini et al,[45] 2001 Italy	Surgical treatment of flexible flatfoot in children	J Bone Joint Surg	21 (21)	(8–15)	Not reported	FFF	Clinical x-rays Gait analysis	SAE (Bioabsorbable implant) = 21 Achilles tendon lengthening = 6 Accessory navicular excision = 12	Device fragments impingements = 2	Mean FU 4 y X-rays: Improvement of all measures considered Gait analysis: improvement No significative clinical improvement: • Plantar flexion • Supination • Pronation Clinical improvement: • Ankle dorsiflexion • Discomfort • Resting heel valgus • Jack's test • Footprint grading

(continued on next page)

Table 3
(continued)

Authors	Title	Journal	Patients (y) (Feet)	Mean age at surgery (y) (Range)	Period of Surgery	Indications	Preoperative Evaluation	Surgery ± Concomitant Procedures	Complications	Mean FU (Range) + Postoperative Evaluation + Results
Scharer et al,[46] 2010 USA	Treatment of painful pediatric flatfoot with Maxwell-Brancheau Subtalar Arthroereisis implant a retrospective x-rays review	Foot and Ankle Spec	39 (68) (R 34, L 34)	12 (6–16)	Jul 2000-Nov 2006	FFF Failed nonsurgical care	X-rays: • Lateral talocalcaneal angle • Talocalcaneal angle • Talonavicular coverage	SAE (MBA) = 68 Gastrocnemius Recession = 12 Achilles' tendon lengthening = 6 Kidner procedure = 4	Migration, undercorrection, overcorrection = 9 Persistent pain (implant removal) = 1	X-rays: Improvement of all measures considered
Chong et al,[41] 2015 USA	Prospective comparison of subtalar arthroereisis with lateral column lengthening for painful flatfeet	J Pediatr Orthop Part B	7 (13) (6 bil)	12.8 (8–17)	2010–2011	FFF Failed nonsurgical care	Kinematic motion analysis Pedobarometry X-rays Oxford Ankle-Foot Questionnaire for Children	SAE (Vilex) = 7	Persistent pain (implant removal) = 2	Mean FU 12.75 mo Improvement of all measures considered: • Kinematic motion analysis • Pedobarometry • X-rays
Martinelli et al,[47] 2017 Italy, Denmark	Return to sport activities after subtalar arthroereisis for correction of pediatric	J Pediatr Orthop Part B	49 (98) (R 49, L 49)	10.7 (7–14)	Jan 2008 - Dec 2011	Deformity induced pain Postural fatigue Cramping sensation in the foot	X-rays CHQ in the child and parent form	SAE	Residual pain = 3 Residual deformity = 1 Sport limitations = 1 Persistent	Mean FU 4.9 y (2–5.8 y) Asymptomatic: no x-rays in FU CHQ: Improvement of:

	flexible flatfoot					or medial arch Abnormal gait Decrease in activity			pain (implant removal) = 3	• School and play (parent) • Emotional (child) • Footwear (child + parent) • Successful return to sport activities Bilateral gastrocnemius recession = 6
Cao et al,[48] 2017 China	Therapeutic outcomes of kalix II in treating juvenile flexible flatfoot	Orthop Surg	20 (27) (R 11, L 16)	12.1 (7–16)	Jan 2008-Sept 2012	Flexible flatfoot Failed nonsurgical care	VAS AOFAS X-rays: • Meary's angle • Calcaneal pitch angle • Talar declination angle	SAE (Kalix II) Reconstruction of the end point of the posterior tibialis tendon after dissection of the accessory scaphoid = 11	Displaced device due to a fall i n inversion position = 1	Mean FU 28.1 mo (range, 23–60 mo) Improvement of scores and measures considered: • VAS • AOFAS • X-rays
Caravaggi et al,[49] 2018 Italy	Functional evaluation of bilateral subtalar arthroereisis for the correction of flexible flatfoot in children: 1-y follow-up.	Gait Posture	13 (26) (R 13, L 13)	11.3	Not reported	FFF (8–14 y)	VAS X-rays: • Meary's line • Talocalcaneal angle Kinematic	SAE (Bioabsorbable implant) = 13 SAC-Stop (Bioabsorbable implant) = 13	Not reported	Mean FU 12.5 mo Improvement of scores and measurement considered in both implants: • VAS • X-rays • Kinematic

(*continued on next page*)

Table 3
(*continued*)

Authors	Title	Journal	Patients (y) (Feet)	Mean age at surgery (y) (Range)	Period of Surgery	Indications	Preoperative Evaluation	Surgery ± Concomitant Procedures	Complications	Mean FU (Range) + Postoperative Evaluation + Results
Memeo et al,[50] 2019 Italy	Flexible Juvenile Flat foot surgical correction: a comparison between 2 techniques after 10 y experience	J Foot Ankle Surg	(402)	13.4 (8–16)	Not reported	Positive clinical evaluation Pain	Clinical: • medial longitudinal arch collapse • Achilles tendonitis • plantar fasciitis • juvenile hallux valgus X-rays: • Costa-bertani angle • Heel inclination angle • Talar declination angle • Kite angle	SAE (Bioabsorbable implant) = 202 + Percutaneous lengthening of the Achilles tendon = 185 SAC-Stop (metallic screw) = 200 + Percutaneous lengthening of the Achilles Tendon = 142	SAE: Soft tissue inflammation, device reimplant for technical error = 25 SAC-Stop: Incomplete correction, device breakage = 32	Mean FU 130 mo (range, 35–150 mo) Clinical improvement of all feet in both groups No statistical differences between the 2 groups X-rays: Standardization of the angles considered: • SAE 94.5% • SAC-Stop 84.2%
de Bot et al,[51] 2019 Netherlands	Clinical and radiological outcomes of subtalar Kalix II arthroereisis	Foot Ankle Spec	16 (26) (R 12, L 14)	12.5 (10–15)	2009–2014	FFF Failed nonsurgical care Pain	X-rays: • Calcaneal pitch • Meary's angle	SAE (Kalix II) Spring ligament reconstruction = 14 Achilles tendon	Revision surgery = 6	Mean FU 47 mo (range, 19–79 mo) X-rays improvement

	for a symptomatic pediatric flexible flatfoot					Walking problems No previous foot surgical procedures		lengthening = 20		Dutch PROM tool adapted for flatfeet Symptoms improvement = 68.75%
Ruiz-Picazo et al,[52] 2019 Spain	X-rays and functional results following subtalar arthroereisisin pediatric flexible flatfoot	Adv Orthop	16 (32)	9 (7–11)	2008–2015	Not precise because it is a retrospective study mostly focused on radiological aspects	X-rays: • Moreau-Costa-Bartani angle • talocalcaneal angle (dorsoplantar and lateral) • talonavicular coverage • naviculo-cuboid overlap OxAFQ-C	SAE	Overcorrection, expulsion of the implant due to erroneous measurements = 4	FU not reported Improvement of: • X-rays angles • OxAFQ-C (School and play, Emotional, Footwear)
Megremis and Megremis,[53] 2019 Greece	Arthroereisis for symptomatic flexible flatfoot deformity in young children: radiological assessment and short-term follow-up	Foot Ankle Surg	14 (28)	10.7 (8–14)	Not reported	FFF Pain Decreased endurance in sports activities and long walks Failed nonsurgical care	X-rays: • Meary's angle • Calcaneal pitch angle • Talocalcaneal angle (Kite's angle) • Talar declination angle • Talonavicular joint subluxation AOFAS rating scale	SAE + percutaneous triple-hemisection Achilles tendon lengthening	None	Mean FU 35. 14 mo (range, 19–60 mo) Improvement of AOFAS Radiological angles improvement except for a slight improvement of calcaneal inclination
Papamer-kouriou et al,[54] 2019	Prospective early clinical, radiological, and kinematic pedobarigraphic	Cureus	6 (12)	11.05 (6.2–15.5)	Not reported	FFF Failed nonsurgical care	Clinical evaluation X-rays: • Meary's angle • Calcaneal pitch Pedobarographic	SAE (Kalix II)	None	Improvement of measures considered: • Clinical • X-rays:

(continued on next page)

Table 3 (*continued*)

Authors	Title	Journal	Patients (y) (Feet)	Mean age at *surgery* (y) (Range)	Period of Surgery	Indications	Preoperative Evaluation	*Surgery* ± Concomitant Procedures	Complications	Mean FU (Range) + Postoperative Evaluation + Results
Greece, UK	analysis following subtalar arthroereisis for pediatric pes planovalgus						MOXFQ score			• Pedobarographic • MOXFQ score
Bernasconi et al,[55] 2020 Italy	Midterm assessment of subtalar arthroereisis for correction of flexible flatfeet in children	Orthop Traumatol Surg Res	31 (62)	10.5 (8–15)	2012–2015	FFF Failed nonsurgical care	Clinical X-rays: • Talonavicular coverage angle • Talocalcaneal divergence angle • Calcaneo-fifth metatarsal angle on dorsoplantar view • Dijan-Annonier angle • Meary's angle • Calcaneal pitch • Talocalcaneal divergence angle on lateral view VAS-FA score	SAE	Not reported	Mean FU 62 mo Clinical improvement Radiological angles improvement except for: • talonavicular coverage angle (dorsoplantar view) • calcaneo-fifth metatarsal angle (dorsoplantar view) VAS-FA score: • higher pain at rest and during activity • felt limited when standing on one and running

Indino C et al, 2020 Italy	Effectiveness of subtalar arthroereisis with endorthesis for pediatric flexible flatfoot: a retrospective cross-sectional study with final follow-up at skeletal maturity	Foot Ankle Surg	56 (112)	(9–14)	Jan 2011 - Mar 2015	FFF Pain Failed nonsurgical care	Clinical and functional scores X-rays: • Meary's angle • Lateral talocalcaneal angle • Talonaviculat coverage • Calcaneal Pitch angle • Talonavicular uncoverage percentage	SAE	None	Mean FU 40.1 mo Improvement of: • Clinical and functional scores • X-rays measurement

Abbreviations: CHQ, Child health questionnaire; MOXFQ, Manchester Oxford Foot Questionnaire; PROM, patient-reported outcome measurement; OxAFQ-C, The Oxford Ankle Foot Questionnaire for Children; VAS, visual analog scale; VAS-FA, visual analog scale foot and ankle.

Mean age is referred at the time of surgery.

with respect to the diameter of the implant. Changing the foot from a pronated to a supinated position leads to a tension of the Achilles tendon.[85]

Postoperative Care

Cao and colleagues[48] suggested early postoperative rehabilitative training and protective strategy avoiding extreme inversion within 3 months after surgery.

Bernasconi and colleagues[55] reported no cast immobilization and weight-bearing allowed after 2 days and sport activities after 3 months.

Indino and colleagues[56] reported plaster cast immobilization for 2 weeks and weight-bearing to tolerance.

Martinelli and colleagues[47] reported in 49 patients a cast immobilization for 2 weeks and weight-bearing allowed with crutches; jumping and running were not permitted for additional 12 weeks but swimming and riding bicycle was recommended 3 weeks after surgery. Memeo and colleagues[50] reported in 200 patients a cast immobilization for 2 weeks and weight-bearing allowed with crutches after the cast removal for 1 week. After ATL, 1 week more immobilization. No sport activities for 3 months.

Megremis and Megremis[53] reporting 14 children (28 feet) who underwent SAE in association with percutaneous triple-hemisection ATL recommended scotch cast for 4 weeks and a brace for another 3 months time.

For SAE associated with Kidner procedure, an immobilization for 6 weeks in a cast; a 6-week period of protected weight-bearing and following physical therapy was suggested by Garras and colleagues[86]

Literature review of FF treatment in children with SAE is reported in **Table 3**.

SAC-STOP PROCEDURES

The technique was first described by Alvarez and later published by Burutaran[32] (**Fig. 8**, Videos 2 and 3). Original technique contemplates the manual reduction of the talocalcaneal derotation, which is then kept in the correct position by means of a cortical screw inserted from out-to-in, from lateral to medial, from posterior to anterior, into the calcaneus, at the level of the floor of sinus tarsi. A variation that had already been suggested by Pisani[31] consists in substituting the cortical screw with a cancellous screw.[34,59] The screw is positioned under the talus lateral process and it maintains the correction of the calcaneus valgus, in a mechanical and proprioceptive manner, therefore, forcing the hindfoot in the correct position.

The skin incision, at the sinus tarsi level, is approximately 1.0 cm. Attention must be paid to the sensitive branch of the sural nerve, which may cross the incision. Bluntly, the calcaneus and the floor of the sinus tarsi, are reached. The foot is kept by the assistant in maximum supination, with a neutral tibiotarsal position. Different variables are possible from now on: (1) a K-wire with a diameter of 2.0 mm is inserted craniocaudally, from posterior to anterior with an angle of approximately 20°, from lateral to medial, with the anatomic barrier of the lateral malleolus (which does not allow a perfectly sagittal introduction of the K-wire). The correct position of the K-wire is controlled with fluoroscopy. The K-wire is then removed and a 3.2 mm reamer is inserted in the same position. The screw used is a partially threaded cancellous screw[34] between 2.5 and 3.5 cm long, and with a diameter of 4.5/6.5 mm. The screw length mostly used is 3.0 cm. The screw is inserted until it reaches a position under the talus lateral process; the thread disappears completely in the calcaneus (**Fig. 9**). (2) A self-threaded screw is introduced directly with respect to the above-explained principles (see Video 2).[59] (3) A cannulated screw is introduced with respect to the above-explained principles (see Video 3).[59] (4) A

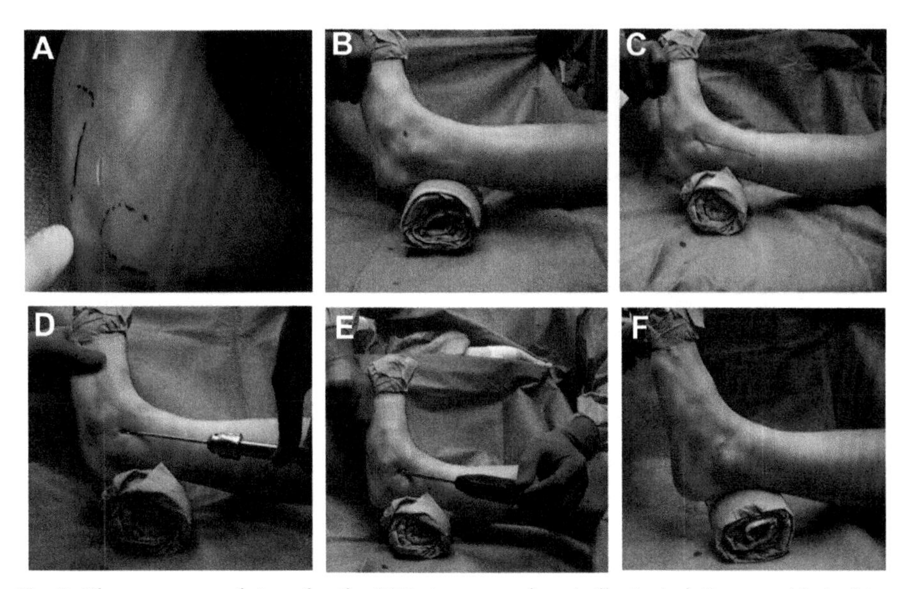

Fig. 8. The sequence of steps for the SAC-stop procedure is illustrated. One cm skin incision at the level of sinus tarsi (*A*), the foot is in neutral position and maximal supination (avoid equinus position). (*B*) Introduction of a K-wire in the calcaneus with an angle of approximately 20° from posterior to anterior and from lateral to medial (*C*), the K-wire is then removed and a 3.2 mm reamer is inserted in the same position (*D*), the screw is inserted until it reaches a position under the talus lateral process. Effectiveness of the procedure is tested using the plantar malleoli view sign (Videos) (*E*), suture in layers and skin suture (*F*).

bioabsorbable screw.[61] (5) A special screw with a plastic/metallic cup.[34] (6) A special conical screw. (7) A titanium screw. (8) Other screws with different shapes. Firstly, the correction is verified by observing the position of the hindfoot with respect to the longitudinal axis of the leg and the effectiveness of the stop of the calcaneus against the talus, more anatomic precisely against the plantar surface of the talus lateral process. The position against the lateral aspect of the talus and minimal variations of the screw direction are tolerated. The postoperative correction can also be controlled using the "Plantar Malleoli View Sign." If a foot is properly corrected, both malleoli will be seen from a plantar view. If undercorrected, the medial malleolus is seen and the screw has to be pulled out a few threads from the calcaneus so that it protrudes more; vice-versa, if overcorrected only the lateral malleolus is seen and the screw has to be inserted more into the calcaneus.[59]

The deep tissues (fibrous-fatty flap) are sutured above the head of the screw; then, the subcutaneous tissues and skin are sutured. An elastic bandage is positioned.

Other variables of calcaneo-stop procedures are as follows: (1) retrograde talus screw introducing a cancellous[37] or a conical screw[35] into the talus starting from sinus tarsi. The unthreaded portion of the screw conflicts with calcaneus lateral border. (2) Retrograde calcaneus special screw introduced from plantar into the calcaneus perforating the sinus floor and producing an impingement against the talus.[39] Screw malpositioning and screw breakage are reported in 12% of the cases with these techniques.[37]

Postoperative Care

Kellermann and colleagues[57] and Roth and colleagues[37] suggested nonimmobilization, postoperative foot exercises, and full weight-bearing as soon as possible. If

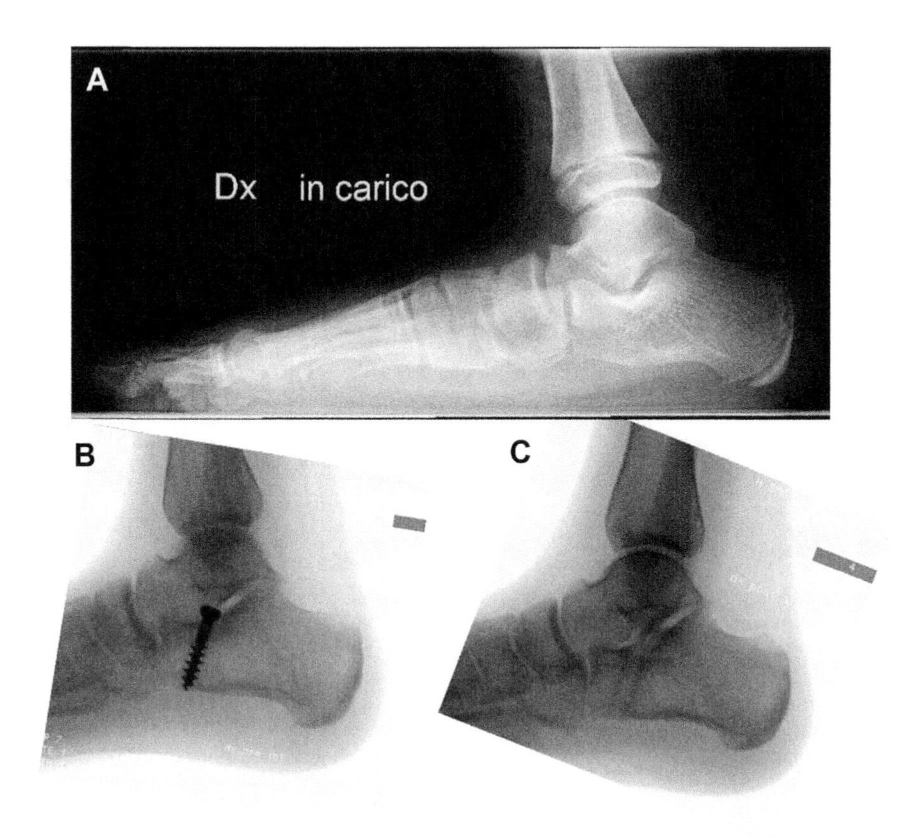

Fig. 9. An 11-year-old girl with symptomatic FFF. Preoperative radiograph. Note the anterodorsal bony "nose" on the talar head with impingement of the talonavicular joint (*A*). At 3 years follow-up before removal of the screw (*B*), after removal of the screw (*C*) maintaining the correct anatomic talocalcaneal relationship and still avoiding impingement.

pain persisted, gradual weight-bearing was suggested by Roth and colleagues.[37] Sports were allowed when perioperative pain ended.

The patient is instructed to actively perform flexion-extension exercises of the ankle in the postoperative period. At day 5 postoperative, the patient is allowed a partial weight-bearing, which becomes complete by day 11 postoperative, when the stitches are removed. Sport activities are forbidden for 1 month. No cast is required.[59]

Pavone and colleagues[36] stated full weight-bearing within 3 days and 3 weeks cast if ATL was associated.

Richter and Zech allowed 15 kg partial weight-bearing for 6 weeks.[58] Arbab and colleagues[63] reported full weight-bearing achieved after an average of 8.1 days (range, 2–21 days), whereas Kubo and colleagues[64] allowed immediately postoperative as tolerated.

Memeo and colleagues[50] reported in 202 patients a cast immobilization for 2 weeks and weight-bearing allowed with crutches after the cast removal for 1 week. After ATL, 1 week more immobilization. No sport activities for 3 months.

Jerosch and colleagues[38] allowed full weight-bearing as soon as possible and in case of gastrocnemius recession (GR), walker in neutral position for 2 to 4 weeks was prescribed. A supporting insole was recommended for 2 to 3 months as well as exercises for tibialis post muscle.

Literature review of FF treatment in children with SAC-stop is reported in **Table 4**.

Additional Procedures

The most common associated procedures are GR, ATL, and accessory navicular excision. Data reported in the literature varied from 0% to 91.5% additional procedures. According to Zaret and Myerson,[72] approximately 60% of the feet required additional correction including ATL and GR. Many authors reported nonconcomitant procedures,[41,52,54,56,57,59] whereas other authors did not mention if performed any concomitant procedure.[49,55,59,62,63]

De Pellegrin and colleagues reported in a previous study[34,87] a tight AT after SAC-stop in a third of 226 feet, which was postoperatively successfully treated with a stretching program.

Cohen–Sobel and colleagues[23] reported 12 severe symptomatic FF treated with a combined surgical technique such as a modified Young tenosuspension, talonavicular desmoplasty, and SA in children older than 10 years.

Memeo and colleagues[50] reported percutaneous ATL in 142 feet associated with 202 SAE and 185 associated with 202 SAC-stop. Richter and Zech[58] stated that GR was necessary in 25 of 31 patients, Pavone and colleagues[36] in 18 of 410 patients, Martinelli and colleagues[47] in 12 of 98 patients (49 patients bilaterally), Das and colleagues[60] in 7 of 25 patients, de Bot and colleagues[51] in 20 of 26 patients, Kubo and colleagues[64] in 35 of 95 patients, and Franz and colleagues[65] in 11 of 78 patients.

Giannini and colleagues[45] reported in a sample of 21 treated with SAE 6 ATL and 12 accessory navicular excision in 21 feet. Gutierrez and Lara[84] reported ATL in 38 of 65 feet (58.5%), 7 of the Z-type and 31 of the Hoke type, whereas Sharer and colleagues[46] in 68 SAE, 6 ATL, 12 GR, and 4 Kidner procedures (accessory navicular excision).

Cao and colleagues[48] reported that in 27 FFF with surgery at an average age of 12.1 years, a reconstruction of the end point of posterior tibialis tendon was performed after dissection of the accessory scaphoid in 11 feet.

de Bot and colleagues[51] reported spring ligament reconstruction as an additional procedure in 14 of 26 feet and a percutaneous ATL in 20 of 26 feet treated with SAE (Kalix II).

Highlander and colleagues[75] reported in a review that GR and ATL are the most common adjunctive procedures followed by Kidner procedure and medial column reconstruction.

Garras and colleagues[86] reported the modified Kidner procedure combined with a SA resulted in significant pain and functional improvement (no data available).

Megremis and Megremis[53] reported 14 children (28 feet) who underwent SAE in association with percutaneous triple-hemisection ATL reporting improvement of AOFASs and Meary's angles.

Cicchinelli and colleagues[88] reported 3 groups of patients who underwent: (1) SAE (n = 9); (2) SAE and distal GR (n = 9); (3) SAE, distal GR, and medial column stabilization (n = 10). The last group showed poorer results.

According to Zaret and Myerson,[72] SA has been performed together with additional hindfoot procedures (eg, calcaneal osteotomy, flexor digitorum longus tendon transfer, tarsometatatarsal arthrodesis, and ATL; **Fig. 10**).

Another association with SAC-stop is described in symptomatic rigid flatfeet affected by coalitions; Calcaneonavicular and Talocalcaneal coalitions can be treated after resection, creating a mobile subtalar joint in association with SA for correction of

Table 4
Literature review of flatfoot treatment in children with subtalar arthroereisis with calcaneo-stop procedure (SAC-stop)

Authors	Title	Journal	Patients (feet)	Mean Age at Surgery (y) (Range)	Period of Surgery	Indications	Preoperative Evaluation	Surgery ± Concomitant Procedures	Complications	Mean FU (Range) + Postoperative Evaluation + Results
Jerosch et al,[38] 2009 Germany	The stop-screw technique—A simple and reliable method in treating flexible flatfoot children	Foot Ankle Surg	18 (21)	11.9 (8–14)	1999–2007	FFF	Clinical X-rays: • Meary's line	SAC-Stop Gastrocnemius lengthening = 5	Limitations of daily activities (no objective reason) = 2	Mean FU 2.7 y (range, 6 mo-7 y) Clinical improvement: • Heel valgus angle • Dorsiflexion • Podographic grad. Improvement of x-rays measurements Device removal
Kellermann et al,[57] 2011 Hungary	Calcaneo-stop procedure for pediatric flexible flatfoot	Arch Ortho Trauma Surg	25 (43)	10 (7–14)	Aug 2008-Jan 2010	FFF Failed nonsurgical care Meary's angle <170° on lateral view Age limit 7–14 y	Clinical X-rays: • Meary's angle Dynamic Pedography	SAC-Stop	None	Mean FU 9.7 y (range, 3–19 mo) Clinical Patients satisfaction (standard visual analog scale): • 33 feet (77%) of 19 children had excellent

										• 8 feet (19%) of 5 children had good • 1 child's 2 feet (4%) gained poor outcome (highest BMI [29.9]) Improvement of radiological angles Improvement of podographic grading
Pavone et al,[36] 2013 Italy	Calcaneo-stop procedure in the treatment of the juvenile symptomatic flatfoot	J Foot Ankle Surg	242 (410) (168 bil, 33 R, 41 L)	11 (7–14)	Jan 1999-Mar 2010	FFF Failed nonsurgical care Pain	Clinical Podoscopic X-rays: • Kite angle • Costa-Bartani angle • Talar declination • Calcaneal inclination	SAC-Stop Achilles tendon lengthening (if not dorsiflexion min 5°–10° when C-stop performed) = 14	Screw l oosening = 2 Pain in the surgical scar = 9 Local symptoms at incision = 10 Contractures of peroneal muscles = 3 Superficial infection = 7	Mean FU 88 y (range, 14–157 mo) Satisfactory outcome: 397 feet (96.83%) Evident Heel valgus: 12 feet (2.92%) Normalized footprint: 328 feet (80%) Improvement of radiological angles Device removal

(continued on next page)

Table 4
(continued)

Authors	Title	Journal	Patients (feet)	Mean Age at Surgery (y) (Range)	Period of Surgery	Indications	Preoperative Evaluation	Surgery ± Concomitant Procedures	Complications	Mean FU (Range) + Postoperative Evaluation + Results
2013 Germany	corrects Talo-1st Metatarsal -Index (TMT-Index)						Pedography Visual Analogue Scale Foot and Ankle (VAS-FA)			• Clinical • X-rays: • Pedography • VAS-FA Device removal
De Pellegrin et al,[59] 2014 Italy	SESA for the treatment of flexible flatfoot in children	J Child Orthop	485 (732) (247 bil)	11.5 (5–17.9)	1990–2012	Clinical Pain Fatigue If bilateral, second foot after 6 mo if indications still present	Clinical X-rays: • Costa-Bartani • Calcaneal pitch • Talar inclination Pedography	SAC-Stop	25 (6.3%): • Ankle joint effusion hemarthrosis = 8 • Contracture of the peroneal muscles due to an antalgic position in pronation = 14 • Stress fractures of the fourth metatarsal bones due to abnormal gait with excessive weight-bearing on the fourth to fifth rays = 3	Mean FU 4.5 y Evaluation of " Plantar Malleoli view sign" during surgery 93.7% improvement of all parameters considered Device removal
Das et al,[60]	Effectiveness of surgically	J Taibah Univ	15 (25)	12.5	Jan 2007-Oct 2010	FFF Failed	Clinical ROM	SAC-Stop Achilles tendon	Screw loosening = 1 Local symptoms	Mean FU 4.5 y (range, 2 y 8 mo

2017 India	treated symptomatic plano-valgus deformity by the calcaneo stop procedure according to radiological, functional and gait parameters	Med Sci				nonsurgical care	VAS-FA AOFAS OxAFQ-C X-rays: • Costa-Bartani • Kite • Calcaneal inclination • Talar declination • Meary's angle Kinematic and kinetic analysis	lengthening (if not dorsiflexion min 5°–10° when C-Stop performed) = 7	and peroneal muscles contracture = 3	to 6 y 3 mo) Improvement of all parameters considered
Giannini et al,[61] 2017 Italy	Bioabsorbable calcaneo-stop implant for the treatment of flexible flatfoot: a retrospective cohort study at a minimum follow-up of 4 y	J Foot Ankle Surg	44 (88)	11.7 (8–14)	Sept 2010-Jan 2012	Idiopathic, flexible, symptomatic flatfeet in pts aged 8–14 y	Clinical X-rays: • Meary's angle • Talocalcaneal angle Viladot classification	SAC-Stop Achilles tendon lengthening = 24 (12 pts)	Pain (screw breakage) = 2	FU not reported Clinical Outcome: • 33 (75%) excellent • 9 (20.5%) good • 2 (4.5%) poor Improvement of X-rays angles Improvement of foot print rate (Viladot classification)
Arbab et al,[63]	Die subtalare Schraubenar-	Z Orthop Unfall	41 (71)	11.8 (9–14)	Not reported	FFF Pain	Clinical X-rays:	SAC-Stop	Contracture peroneal	Mean FU 30.6 y (12–80 mo)

(continued on next page)

Table 4
(continued)

Authors	Title	Journal	Patients (feet)	Mean Age at Surgery (y) (Range)	Period of Surgery	Indications	Preoperative Evaluation	Surgery ± Concomitant Procedures	Complications	Mean FU (Range) + Postoperative Evaluation + Results
2018 Germany	throrise zur Behandlung des symptomatischen, flexiblen Pes planovalgus – Ergebnisse und eine aktuelle Literaturübersicht					Failure nonsurgical care	• calcaneal pitch angle • talus inclination • Meary's angle • Costa-bartani angle • talo-metatarsal base 1 angle		muscle = 2 Wound inflammation (removal of the screw) = 1 Reduction of sport activities = 3 Sporadic pain without reduction of daily activities = 4	Clinical improvement Improvement of x-rays angles
Hagen et al,[62] 2019 Germany	Are there benefits of a 2D gait analysis in the evaluation of the subtalar extra-articular screw arthroereisis? Short-term investigation in children	Clin Biomech	14 (27)	12.38	Oct 2016-Mar2017	FFF Pain Fatigue Failed nonsurgical care	2-D gait analysis Clinical	SAC-Stop	3.7% rate = 1	Functional improvement: • 2-D gait analysis • Clinical
Kubo et al,[64] 2020 Germany	Outcome after subtalar screw arthroereisis in children with flexible flatfoot	J Orthop Sci	50 (95)	11.3	Aug 2007-Ded 2015	FFF Pain X-rays: • Calcaneal pitch	Clinical Muscle and achilles tendo length Bony maturation X-rays	SAC-Stop Achilles tendon lengthening = 35	None	Mean FU 35.8 y (range, 13–79 mo) X-rays:

	depends on time of treatment: midterm results of 95 cases					• Lateral talocalcaneal angle • Talocalcaneal angle • Navicular cuboid index • Meary's angle				Improvement of all angles considered When surgery is performed at: • 9–12 y of age: best results • 5–8 y of age: inferior results with poorer long-term success with only an improvement in the a.p. TCA • 13–15 y of age: mixed results. While CP and NCI improved, the lat. TCA deteriorated in FU
Franz et al,[65] 2020 Germany	Pedobarographic outcome after subtalar screw arthroereisis in flexible juvenile flatfoot	Foot Ankle Surg	39 (78)	11.3	Not reported	FFF	Clinical Pedography	SAC-Stop Gastrocnemius soleus recession (Vulpius) = 11	Not reported	FU not reported Improvement of all parameters considered

(continued on next page)

Table 4
(continued)

Authors	Title	Journal	Patients (feet)	Mean Age at Surgery (y) (Range)	Period of Surgery	Indications	Preoperative Evaluation	Surgery ± Concomitant Procedures	Complications	Mean FU (*Range*) + Postoperative Evaluation + Results
	after 10 years' experience						• plantar fasciitis • juvenile hallux valgus X-rays: • Costa-bertani angle • Heel inclination angle • Talar declination angle • Kite angle	of the Achilles Tendon = 142 SAE (Bioabsorbable implant) = 202 + Percutaneous lengthening of the Achilles tendon = 185	Soft tissue inflammation, device reimplant for technical error = 25	No statistical differences between the 2 groups X-rays: Standardization of the angles considered: • SAE. 94.5% • SAC-Stop 84.2%
Pavone et al,[66] 2018 Italy	Outcomes of the calcaneo-stop procedure for the treatment of juvenile flatfoot in young athletes	J of Child Orthop	68 (136)	12.7 (9–15)	2008–2016	FFF Pain Failed nonsurgical care	Clinical X-rays: Talar declination Cosa-bertani Calcaneal pitch	SAC-Stop	17: • Pain at surgical scar = 5 • Local symptoms = 4 • Screw loosening = 3 • Superficial infections = 4 • Screw breakage = 1	Mean FU 57.6 mo Improvement of all parameters considered Device removal

Caravaggi et al,[49] 2018 Italy	Functional evaluation of bilateral subtalar arthroereisis for the correction of flexible flatfoot in children: 1-y follow-up.	Gait Posture	13 (26) (R 13, L 13)	11.3 y	Not reported	FFF (8–14 y)	VAS X-rays: • Meary's line • Talocalcaneal angle Kinematic	SAE (Bioabsorbable implant) = 13 SAC-Stop (Bioabsorbable implant) = 13	Not reported	Mean FU 12.5 mo Improvement of scores and measurement considered in both implants: • VAS • X-rays • Kinematic

Abbreviations: OxAFQ-C, the Oxford Ankle Foot Questionnaire for Children; SESA, subtalar extra-articular screw arthroereisis; VAS-FA, visual analog scale foot and ankle.

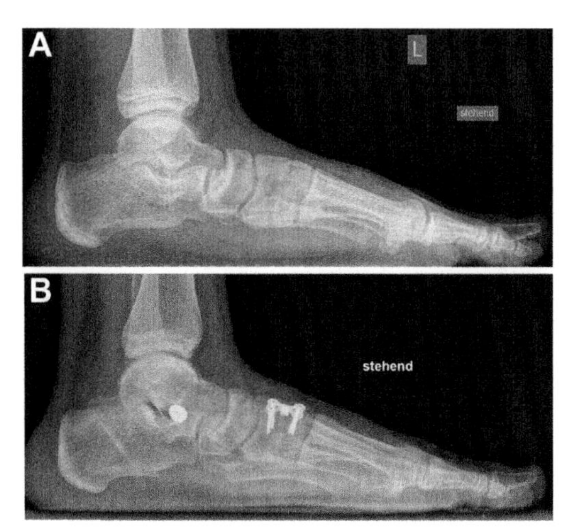

Fig. 10. A 13-year-old boy (*A*) pre-operatively (*B*) after SAE and additional bony procedures (Calcaneal osteotomy and medial cuneiform osteotomy) (Case from J. Hamel, Munich, Germany.)

the most frequent valgus-hind foot deformity in one step and achieve good to excellent results in 95.2% of patients.[79]

Complications

Preoperative complications (or rather "risk factors") are rigid flatfeet with unrecognized coalitions; intraoperative complications include technical errors with malpositioning of the implant, undercorrection and overcorrection. The most common postoperative complication is pain. Bernasconi and colleagues[55] reported sinus tarsi pain, peroneal spasm, soft tissue entrapment, and biomaterial failure.[72] Yen-Douangmala and colleagues[44] attributed pain directly to the implant.

Implant-specific complications are related to specific properties of the implant (material, geometry, fixation) and how it is designed to function (biomechanical explanation). Wear products, foreign body reaction, implant degradation, and implant fracture are implant-specific complications. Case reports describe also intraosseous ganglion cysts and avascular necrosis of talus, peroneal muscle spasm, and fractures of either the talus or the calcaneus. Giannini and colleagues[45] described implant degradation (4.8%), whereas Gutierrez and Lara reported 10.7% complications with postoperative pain the most frequently.[84] Mosca V. reported in the past literature complications rates of 3.5% to 30% for synthetic implants, whereas in a more recent review, a rate range of 3.5% to 11%.[1] Soomekh and Baravarian[89] reported improper application, sinus tarsi pain, implant malpositioning, or failure. Bouchard and Mosca[3] referred the same complications rate (30%) due to implant resorption, inflammatory reactions, persistent pain, undercorrection; data are presumably referred to SAE. Kumar and Clough[90] reported talar neck fracture. Tompkins and colleagues[91] reported a rate of 7.3% (n = 3) complications of STA-peg procedures: SA (n = 2); talar fracture (n = 1).[30] de Bot and colleagues[51] reported implant migration (SAE) and the need for revision surgery in 6 of 26 feet. Oloff and colleagues[92] referred implant deformation in SAE.

Rockett and colleagues[93] described in case-report intraosseous talar cyst formation after STA-peg implant. Smith and Millar[30] reported 2 complications (3.8%) in 53

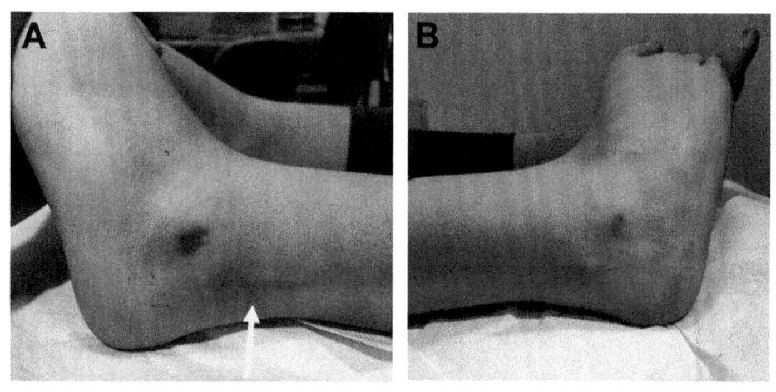

Fig. 11. A 13-year-old girl with peroneal spasm (*yellow arrow*) and painful limitation of the supination persisting 3 months after SAC-stop (*A*). Normal supination without spasm on the contralateral foot (*B*).

feet at an FU of 3 years: one child developed a reactive synovitis and the second sustained a calcaneus fracture and peroneal spasm.

Pavone and colleagues[66] reported in a large number of treated feet with SAC-stop a complications rate of 12.5% including local incision symptoms, painful surgical scar, screw loosening or breakage, superficial infections.

Needleman RL[74] reported complications after an analysis of 3 different devices: (1) free-floating device (MBA), (2) axis altering device (STA-peg), and (3) impact blocking device or direct impact implants (Sgarlato implant) which is fixed on the floor of the sinus tarsi by making a hole in the bone. The author divided complications into general and implant specific. General are as follows: implant malpositioning, undercorrection, overcorrection, loss of position wrong implant size, persistent tarsal sinus pain, and tenderness. Implant-specific complications are as follows: foreign body reactions, arthritis, synovitis, implant fracture, intraosseous ganglion cyst, and osteonecrosis of the talus. Trieb and colleagues described a case with loosening of the screw after trampolining.[94]

The review of Metcalfe and colleagues[20] summarizing the outcomes of 5 different SAE devices (nonbespoke silicone, bespoke silicone, seated within calcaneus [STA-peg and Koning], free-floating bioresorbable [Giannini], and free-floating nonbioresorbable [MBA, Kalix]) referred sinus tarsi pain, device extrusion, synovitis, superficial and deep infection, overcorrection and undercorrection, peroneal spasm in a range of 4.8% to 19%; transient symptoms (peroneal tendonitis, leg cramps, heel pain, and gait abnormalities) were excluded.

Despite the majority of these findings are related to the SAE technique, often the complications are grouped together for SAE and SAC-stop. Bernasconi and colleagues[55] in a recent study divided complications into 4 main categories (inappropriate indications, technical errors, adaptation/irritation, and biomaterial failure) still not differentiating between the 2 different arthroereisis procedures. To date, there are no studies where calcaneo-stop complications have been exclusively analyzed and described. De Pellegrin and colleagues focused only on this technique's postoperative complications and reported 6.3% of complications in 398 treated feet with SAC-stop.[59]

In literature, reported complications rates range from 4% to 46%,[3,20,59,66,72,74,89–93,95] with unplanned removal rates between 7% and 39%.

Contracture/spasm of the peroneal muscles starting from the immediate postoperative period is a reaction to pain and to stimulation of the sinus tarsi receptors (**Fig. 11**).

Rein and colleagues[81] showed that the inlet of the sinus tarsi was richly innervated with free-nerve endings, assuming that pain of the sinus tarsi syndrome mainly originates at its inlet, suggesting a proprioceptive role of the sensory nerve endings at the sinus tarsi in regulating the activities of gamma-motor neurons of the peroneal muscles. The interruption of this mechanism by local injection of methylprednisolone acetate probably confirms involvement of free-nerve endings at the entrance of sinus tarsi as also suggested by Zaret and Myerson, and Needleman[72,74] suggested if pain persisted after SA.

Removal of the Implants

Removal of the implant is not frequently described in the literature. Although some authors describe implant removal as the consequence of a complication,[20,46,47,51,55,56,86] others considered removal not only for complications but also as the last surgical step.[36–38,50,58,59,66]

Memeo and colleagues reported[50] that implants removal may represent a problem indicating in the own experience that the older the patients, the less well they tolerate the devices and will need to remove them in adulthood.

Ruiz-Picazo and colleagues 2019[52] reported that the implants were not removed because patients had not yet achieved bone maturity, whereas Megremis and Megramis[53] with a short-term follow-up did not mention removal.

The surgical correction of deformity is maintained even if the arthroereisis plug was removed.[86]

SAE

Removal of the implant is reported mainly for complication.

Metcalfe and colleagues[20] rates for nonscheduled removal of implants was 7.1% to 19.3%.

In 26 feet (16 patients) treated with SAE, according to de Bot and colleagues,[51] a removal after 34 ± 12 months was necessary in 15 of 17 feet evaluated at follow-up; 7 of 15 patients experienced sinus tarsi pain, which completely disappeared after removal.

Bernasconi and colleagues[55] reported routine removal was not planned but was performed for persistent pain in the sinus tarsi in 14 of 62 after 7.2 ± 3.3 months. No loss of correction was found after removal of the implant.

Indino and colleagues[56] reported removal for complications after 38 and 28 months in 2 cases.

Garras and colleagues[86] reported 3 patients of 20 requiring removal of plug because of impingement pain laterally.

Papamerkouriou and colleagues[54] reported screw removal between 15 and 18 months postinsertion and no complications in all cases (n = 12).

SAC-Stop

Removal of the implant is considered as the last surgical step at the end of growth and an established correction.

According to Kellermann and colleagues,[57] screws are scheduled for removal. De Pellegrin and colleagues[59] reported removal of the screw in 138 patients (227 feet) on average 2.9 years after SAC-stop at median age of 14 years maintaining the clinical and radiographical results after removal (**Figs. 12–15**). Roth and colleagues[37] left the screw in place for approximately 30 months and developed a formula for removal timing.

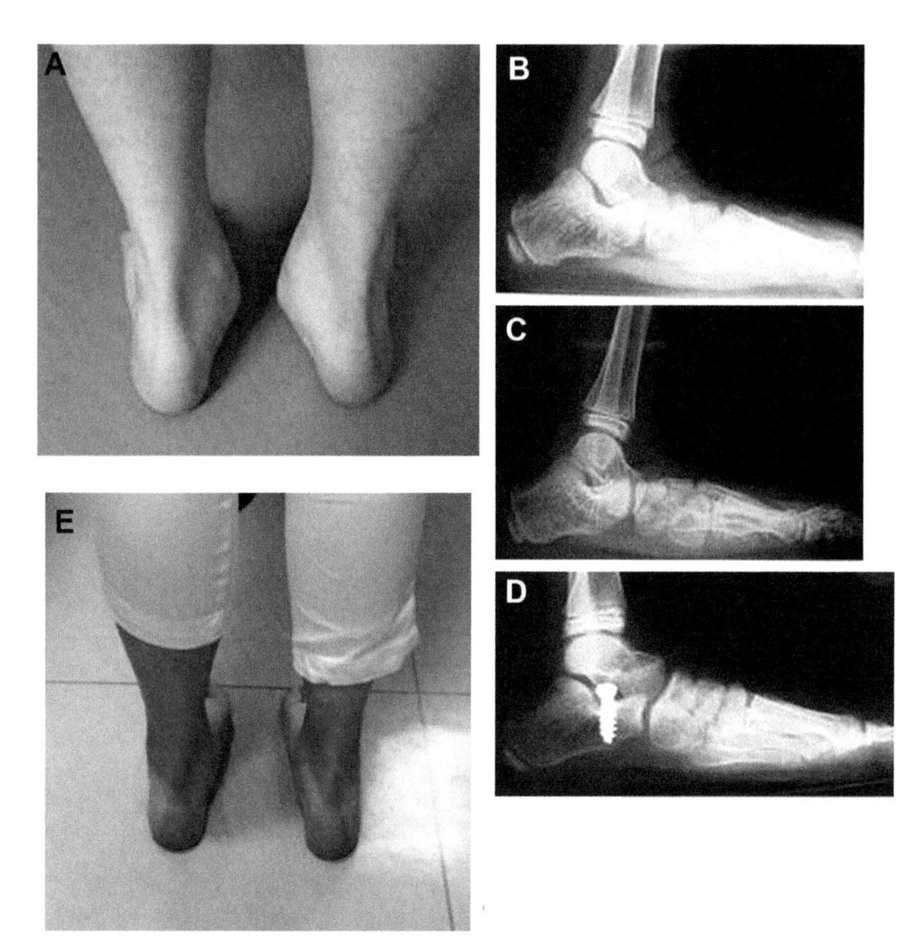

Fig. 12. A 9-year-old girl affected by autism with severe FFF bilaterally (*A*). Preoperative radiographic evaluation of both feet (*B, C*), postoperative result after SAC-stop of the right foot (*D*), clinical evaluation at 9 years follow-up (*E*).

Jerosch and colleagues[38] performed removal of the screw 2 to 3 years after implantation, but not before growth arrest of the foot (approximately 12 years of age in female patients and 14 years of age in male patients). There were no complications encountered in this series.

Richter and Zech[58] reported that the screws were removed after a 2-year follow-up and that all relevant parameters (stage of posterior tibialis insufficiency, TMT dorsoplantar/lateral/Index, pedographic midfoot contact area and force, VAS-FA scores) improved after arthroereisis with calcaneo-stop screw (before and after screw removal). Also, Pavone and colleagues[36] stated that removal of the screw was performed 3 years after arthroereisis with no complications encountered, whereas in a later publication,[66] a rate of 12.5% of minor complications has been reported.

Arbab and colleagues[63] described 2 early removals (one for pain and one for skin infection) out of 73 feet operated.

Giannini and colleagues[61] reported there was no need for removal because of biodegradability.

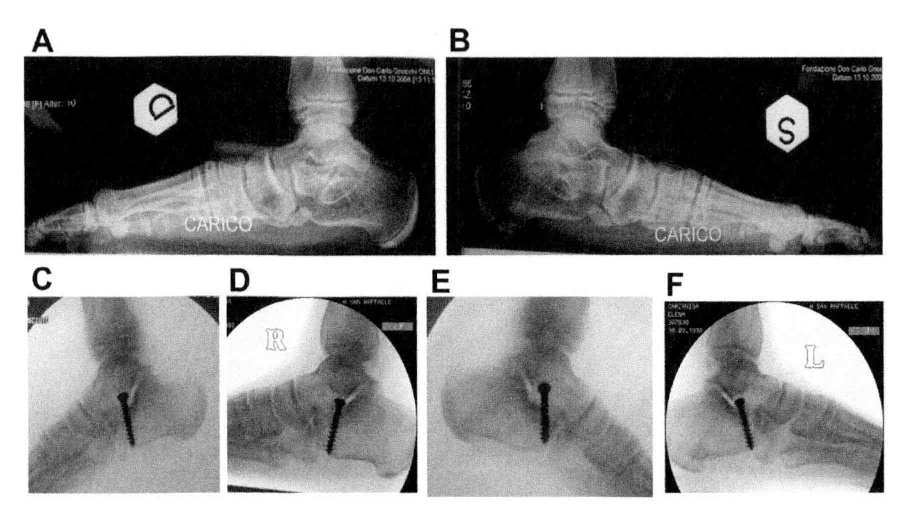

Fig. 13. A 10-year-old girl affected by Trisomie 20 with symptomatic FFF bilaterally. Preoperative (*A*, *B*) and immediate postoperative (*C*, *D*) radiographic evaluation of both feet. Radiological 4-year follow-up before removal of the screws (*E*, *F*).

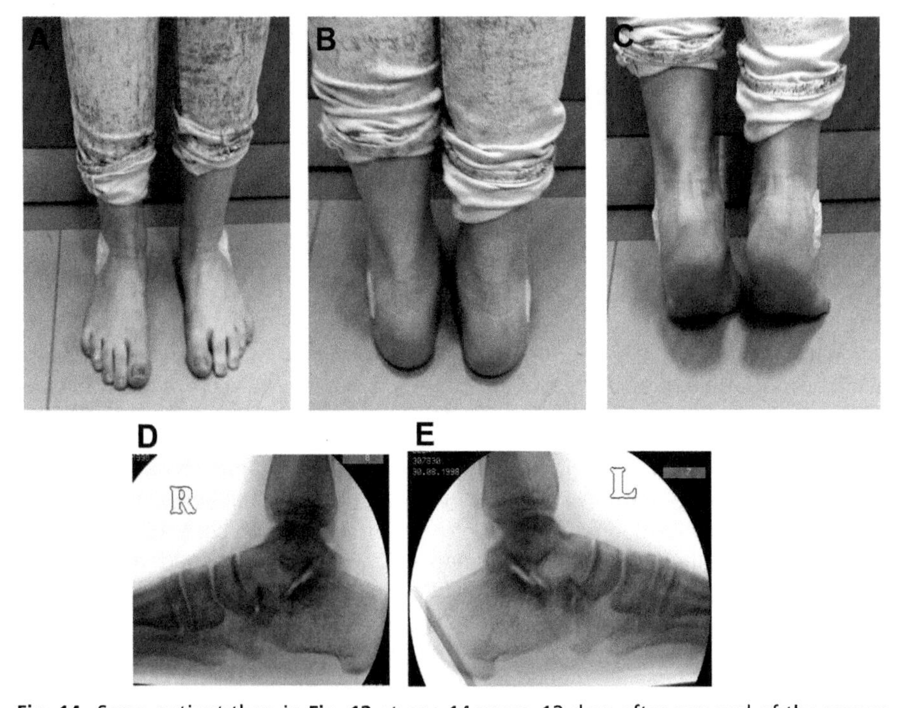

Fig. 14. Same patient than in **Fig. 12** at age 14 years, 12 days after removal of the screws. Clinical aspect with full weight-bearing, normal hindfoot alignment and free subtalar motion in tiptoes standing (*A–C*). Radiographic evaluation after removal of the screws (*D*, *E*).

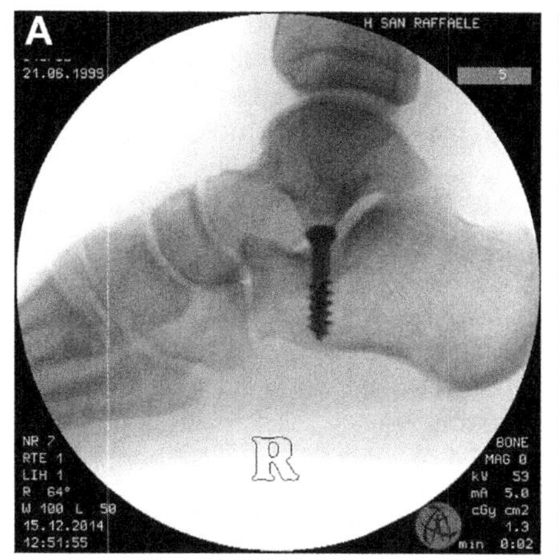

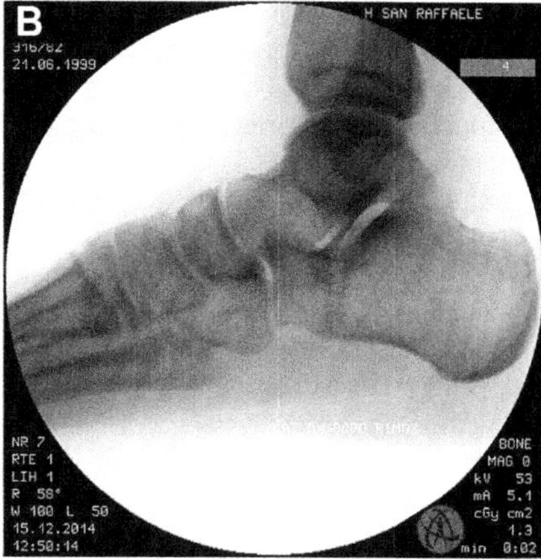

Fig. 15. A 15-year-old boy at screw removal 3 years after SAC-stop. Preoperative (*A*) and postoperative (*B*) radiographic evaluation showing unaltered angles between them.

How Do the Implants Work?

The correction is mechanically maintained first and proprioceptively later.[2,19,37,40,59] SA maintains the physiologic alignment between talus-calcaneus-scaphoid during growth; bone remodeling while correcting the deformity before it becomes rigid.[67]

Christensen and colleagues[70] studied the effect of SA in the adult cadaver model of a normal foot and concluded that SA did not alter the normal closed kinetic chain mechanics. Otherwise, we know it has a mechanical effect because the result is immediate after surgery; in younger children, the correction decreases with growth; and in 8 cases, a protrusion of the screw head into the talus, where there is the greatest contact, has been reported.[59] It is known that joint stability is constituted by static and dynamic elements, where the first one depends on the anatomic congruity of joint surfaces and on ligamentous restraints that limit joint translations. Instead, the dynamic joint stability implies a proprioceptive control of the compressive and directional muscular forces acting on the joint.[96] Subtalar joint plays a proprioceptive key role in adapting the foot to the ground, thus increasing stability.[97] Harris underlines the influences of proprioception in maintaining and correcting supination and pronation. The role of proprioception after SA has been suggested previously.[35] De Pellegrin and colleagues[59] performed SA in patients with osteogenesis imperfecta,[34] with a lower bone resistance. In these patients, there was no screw protrusion or osteolysis. Another aspect we considered is that the screw becomes shorter during foot growth, as seen at removal surgery, but correction is persistent in most of the cases, implying another correction other than the mechanical one. Furthermore, a painful peroneal contracture has been described in 14 patients without a real verifiable complication.

According to Akiyama and colleagues,[98] there were abundant free-nerve endings and 3 types of mechanoreceptors (Pacini-, Ruffini-, and Golgi-corpuscles). Particularly, the free-nerve ending appeared to predominate, indicating that sinus tarsi is relatively sensitive to pain.

In a study, Rein and colleagues[99] analyzed the pattern and types of mechanoreceptors (Ruffini endings, Pacini corpuscles, Golgi-like endings, free-nerve endings, and unclassifiable corpuscles) in the different anatomic complexes of ankle ligaments using designated immunohistochemical markers. The free-nerve endings were the predominant mechanoreceptor type, followed by Ruffini endings, indicating that nociception and joint position have enormous importance in ankle proprioception. Patients with functional ankle instability and pain near the sinus tarsi have a prolonged peroneal reaction time (PRT).[100] This suggests a proprioceptive role of the sensory nerve endings at the sinus tarsi in regulating the activities of gamma-motor neurons of the peroneal muscles, which in turn may cause the symptoms of functional ankle instability and prolonged PRT. The aforementioned studies allowed us to explain how the screw works at the level of the lateral subtalar joint, below the talar lateral process. As a matter of fact, there is an explanation of the proprioceptive effect of the screw on one hand, and on the other hand, it may elucidate those cases of peroneal muscle contracture without identifiable failure of the surgical technique.

Arangio and colleagues[71] studied the effect of SA on adult FFF after SA performing a biomechanical model. SA moved the calcaneus into relative varus and prevented eversion of the subtalar joint. In the normal foot, the 2 medial metatarsals support 15% of total load, whereas in FF, the percentage increases to 31%; after SA, the percentage reduced to normal values (13%).

Martinelli and colleagues[47] reported in a cadaveric FF model the effect of SA performed with canalis tarsi implant demonstrating a lateral shift of the medial pressure.

Papamerkoriuo and colleagues[54] and Franz and colleagues[65] confirmed these data performing a perdobarographic analysis.

Hagen and colleagues reported 4 weeks after calcaneo-stop procedure (subtalar extra-articular screw arthroereisis) with 2D gait analysis a functional improvement of all 14 patients examined.[62] Das reported significant improvement for all radiographic parameters, functional measures, and ROM after calcaneo-stop procedure in all patients.[60]

Kerr and colleagues in a recent study demonstrated kinematic differences between neutral and flatfeet underlying indirectly the need of correction of symptomatic flatfeet to improve quality of propulsion and stability.[76]

The action of the screw in calcaneo-stop is not only mechanical; as seen in a few cases of bilateral involvement, we observed a spontaneous correction of the nonoperated foot before surgery on the contralateral.[59] The mechanism underlying this correction is the proprioceptive one. This is supported by a recent description of the mirror cortical neuron as well as the rich concentration of receptors in the subtalar joint.[67] This hypothesis might explain why a correction persists after implant removal. Proprioception has a critical role in ankle joint stability; in particular, the subtalar joint plays a key role in adapting the foot to the ground.[81,99]

CLINICS CARE POINT

- Many procedures for treatment of FFF have been described; subtalar arthroereisis with calcaneo-stop may have an advantage compared to other techniques as the screw is inserted in the calcaneus and not placed across the subtalar joint.
- An unanimous indication for SA procedure is a painful flatfoot.
- Complications differ between SAC and SAE procedures.

DISCLOSURE

The authors have nothing to disclose.

SUPPLEMENTARY DATA

Supplementary data to this article can be found online at https://doi.org/10.1016/j.fcl.2021.07.007.

REFERENCES

1. Mosca VS. Flexible flatfoot in children and adolescents. J Child Orthop 2010;4:107–21.
2. Viladot A. Surgical treatment of the child's flatfoot. Clin Orthop Relat Res 1992;34–8.
3. Bouchard M, Mosca VS. Flatfoot deformity in children and adolescents: surgical indications and management. J Am Acad Orthop Surg 2014;22:623–32.
4. Ueki Y, Sakuma E, Wada I. Pathology and management of flexible flat foot in children. J Orthop Sci 2019;24:9–13.
5. Banwell HA, Paris ME, Mackintosh S, et al. Paediatric flexible flat foot: how are we measuring it and are we getting it right? A systematic review. J Foot Ankle Res 2018;11:21.
6. Staheli LT, Chew DE, Corbett M. The longitudinal arch. A survey of eight hundred and eighty-two feet in normal children and adults. J Bone Joint Surg Am 1987;69:426–8.
7. Gould N, Moreland M, Alvarez R, et al. Development of the child's arch. Foot Ankle 1989;9:241–5.
8. Wenger DR, Leach J. Foot deformities in infants and children. Pediatr Clin North Am 1986;33:1411–27.
9. Jane MacKenzie A, Rome K, Evans AM. The efficacy of nonsurgical interventions for pediatric flexible flat foot: a critical review. J Pediatr Orthop 2012;32:830–4.
10. Dare DM, Dodwell ER. Pediatric flatfoot: cause, epidemiology, assessment, and treatment. Curr Opin Pediatr 2014;26:93–100.
11. Addante JB, Chin MW, Loomis JC, et al. Subtalar joint arthroereisis with SILASTIC silicone sphere: a retrospective study. J Foot Surg 1992;31:47–51.
12. Adelman VR, Szczepanski JA, Adelman RP. Radiographic evaluation of endoscopic gastrocnemius recession, subtalar joint arthroereisis, and flexor tendon transfer for surgical correction of stage II posterior tibial tendon dysfunction: a pilot study. J Foot Ankle Surg 2008;47:400–8.
13. Brancheau SP, Walker KM, Northcutt DR. An analysis of outcomes after use of the maxwell-brancheau arthroereisis implant. J Foot Ankle Surg 2012;51:3–8.
14. Dragonetti L, Ingraffia C, Stellari F. The young tenosuspension in the treatment of abnormal pronation of the foot. J Foot Ankle Surg 1997;36:409–13.
15. Forg P, Feldman K, Flake E, et al. Flake-Austin modification of the STA-Peg arthroereisis: a retrospective study. J Am Podiatr Med Assoc 2001;91:394–405.
16. Giorgini R, Schiraldi F, Hernandez P. Subtalar arthroereisis: a combined technique. J Foot Surg 1988;27:157–61.
17. Jacobs AM. Soft tissue procedures for the stabilization of medial arch pathology in the management of flexible flatfoot deformity. Clin Podiatr Med Surg 2007;24:657–65, vii–viii.
18. Koning PM, Heesterbeek PJ, de Visser E. Subtalar arthroereisis for pediatric flexible pes planovalgus: fifteen years experience with the cone-shaped implant. J Am Podiatr Med Assoc 2009;99.
19. Kwon JY, Myerson MS. Management of the flexible flat foot in the child: a focus on the use of osteotomies for correction. Foot Ankle Clin 2010;15:309–22.

20. Metcalfe SA, Bowling FL, Reeves ND. Subtalar joint arthroereisis in the management of pediatric flexible flatfoot: a critical review of the literature. Foot Ankle Int 2011;32:1127–39.
21. Koutsogiannis E. Treatment of mobile flat foot by displacement osteotomy of the calcaneus. J Bone Joint Surg Br 1971;53:96–100.
22. Carr JB 2nd, Yang S, Lather LA. Pediatric pes planus: a state-of-the-art review. Pediatrics 2016;137:e20151230.
23. Cohen-Sobel E, Giorgini R, Velez Z. Combined technique for surgical correction of pediatric severe flexible flatfoot. J Foot Ankle Surg 1995;34:183–94.
24. Mosca VS. Calcaneal lengthening for valgus deformity of the hindfoot. Results in children who had severe, symptomatic flatfoot and skewfoot. J Bone Joint Surg Am 1995;77:500–12.
25. Suh DH, Park JH, Lee SH, et al. Lateral column lengthening versus subtalar arthroereisis for paediatric flatfeet: a systematic review. Int Orthop 2019;43: 1179–92.
26. Rathjen KE, Mubarak SJ. Calcaneal-cuboid-cuneiform osteotomy for the correction of valgus foot deformities in children. J Pediatr Orthop 1998;18:775–82.
27. Vora AM, Tien TR, Parks BG, et al. Correction of moderate and severe acquired flexible flatfoot with medializing calcaneal osteotomy and flexor digitorum longus transfer. J Bone Joint Surg Am 2006;88:1726–34.
28. Chambers EFS. An operation for the correction of flexible flat feet of adolescents. West J Surg Obstet Gynecol 1946;54:77–86.
29. LeLièvre J. Current concepts and correction in the valgus foot. Clin Orthop Relat Res 1970;70:43–55.
30. Smith S, Millar E. Arthrorisis by means of a subtalar polyethylene peg implant for correction of hindfoot pronation in children. Clin Orthop Relat Res 1983;181: 15–23.
31. Pisani G. Piede calcaneo-valgo. In: Trattato di chirurgia del piede. II Edizione. Edizioni Minerva Medica Torino; 1993. p. 243–50.
32. Burutaran JM. El calcaneo-stop para el tratiamento del valgo de talon infantile. Chir Del Piede 1979;3:319–22.
33. Milano L, Scala A. La risi extrarticolare della sottoastragalica con endortesi calcaneale nel trattamento chirurgico delle deformità in valgo del calcagno. Chir Del Piede 1985;9:303–9.
34. De Pellegrin M. Subtalar screw-arthroereisis for correction of flat foot in children. Orthopade 2005;34:941–53, quiz 954.
35. Castaman E. L'intervento di calcaneo-stop nel piede piatto valgo. Chir Del Piede 1985;9:319–29.
36. Pavone V, Costarella L, Testa G, et al. Calcaneo-stop procedure in the treatment of the juvenile symptomatic flatfoot. J Foot Ankle Surg 2013;52:444–7.
37. Roth S, Sestan B, Tudor A, et al. Minimally invasive calcaneo-stop method for idiopathic, flexible pes planovalgus in children. Foot Ankle Int 2007;28:991–5.
38. Jerosch J, Schunck J, Abdel-Aziz H. The stop screw technique–a simple and reliable method in treating flexible flatfoot in children. Foot Ankle Surg 2009; 15:174–8.
39. Nogarin L, Brigantini A, Magnan B, et al. Calcaneo-stop: modifiche all'endortesi e alla via chirurgica. Chir Piede 1987;11:57–60.
40. Usuelli FG, Montrasio UA. The calcaneo-stop procedure. Foot Ankle Clin 2012; 17:183–94.

41. Chong DY, Macwilliams BA, Hennessey TA, et al. Prospective comparison of subtalar arthroereisis with lateral column lengthening for painful flatfeet. J Pediatr Orthop B 2015;24:345–53.
42. Bauer K, Mosca VS, Zionts LE. What's new in pediatric flatfoot? J Pediatr Orthop 2016;36:865–9.
43. Vulcano E, Maccario C, Myerson MS. How to approach the pediatric flatfoot. World J Orthop 2016;7:1–7.
44. Yen-Douangmala D, Vartivarian M, Choung JD. Subtalar arthroereisis and its role in pediatric and adult population. Clin Podiatr Med Surg 2012;29:383–90.
45. Giannini BS, Ceccarelli F, Benedetti MG, et al. Surgical treatment of flexible flatfoot in children a four-year follow-up study. J Bone Joint Surg Am 2001;83-A Suppl 2 Pt 2:73–9.
46. Scharer BM, Black BE, Sockrider N. Treatment of painful pediatric flatfoot with Maxwell-Brancheau subtalar arthroereisis implant a retrospective radiographic review. Foot Ankle Spec 2010;3:67–72.
47. Martinelli N, Bianchi A, Martinkevich P, et al. Return to sport activities after subtalar arthroereisis for correction of pediatric flexible flatfoot. J Pediatr Orthop B 2017;27:82–7.
48. Cao L, Miao X-D, Wu Y-P, et al. Therapeutic outcomes of kalix ii in treating juvenile flexible flatfoot. Orthop Surg 2017;9:20–7.
49. Caravaggi P, Lullini G, Berti L, et al. Functional evaluation of bilateral subtalar arthroereisis for the correction of flexible flatfoot in children: 1-year follow-up. Gait Posture 2018;64:152–8.
50. Memeo A, Verdoni F, Rossi L, et al. Flexible juvenile flat foot surgical correction: a comparison between two techniques after ten years' experience. J Foot Ankle Surg 2019;58:203–7.
51. de Bot RTAL, Stevens J, Hermus JPS, et al. Clinical and radiological outcomes of subtalar kalix ii arthroereisis for a symptomatic pediatric flexible flatfoot. Foot Ankle Spec 2019;14(1):9–18.
52. Ruiz-Picazo D, Jiménez-Ortega P, Doñate-Pérez F, et al. Radiographic and functional results following subtalar arthroereisis in pediatric flexible flatfoot. Adv Orthop 2019;2019:5061934.
53. Megremis P, Megremis O. Arthroereisis for symptomatic flexible flatfoot deformity in young children: radiological assessment and short-term follow-up. J Foot Ankle Surg 2019;58:904–15.
54. Papamerkouriou Y-M, Rajan R, Chaudhry S, et al. Prospective early clinical, radiological, and kinematic pedobarographic analysis following subtalar arthroereises for paediatric pes planovalgus. Cureus 2019;11:e6309.
55. Bernasconi A, Iervolino C, D'Alterio R, et al. Midterm assessment of subtalar arthroereisis for correction of flexible flatfeet in children. Orthop Traumatol Surg Res 2020;106:185–91.
56. Indino C, Villafañe JH, D'Ambrosi R, et al. Effectiveness of subtalar arthroereisis with endorthesis for pediatric flexible flat foot: a retrospective cross-sectional study with final follow up at skeletal maturity. Foot Ankle Surg 2018;26:98–104.
57. Kellermann P, Roth S, Gion K, et al. Calcaneo-stop procedure for paediatric flexible flatfoot. Arch Orthop Trauma Surg 2011;131:1363–7.
58. Richter M, Zech S. Arthrorisis with calcaneostop screw in children corrects Talo-1st Metatarsal-Index (TMT-Index). Foot Ankle Surg 2013;19:91–5.
59. De Pellegrin M, Moharamzadeh D, Strobl WM, et al. Subtalar extra-articular screw arthroereisis (SESA) for the treatment of flexible flatfoot in children. J Child Orthop 2014;8:479–87.

60. Das SP, Das PB, Ganesh S, et al. Effectiveness of surgically treated symptomatic plano-valgus deformity by the calcaneo stop procedure according to radiological, functional and gait parameters. J Taibah Univ Med Sci 2017;12:102–9.
61. Giannini S, Cadossi M, Mazzotti A, et al. Bioabsorbable calcaneo-stop implant for the treatment of flexible flatfoot: a retrospective cohort study at a minimum follow-up of 4 years. J Foot Ankle Surg 2017;56:776–82.
62. Hagen L, Kostakev M, Pape JP, et al. Are there benefits of a 2D gait analysis in the evaluation of the subtalar extra-articular screw arthroereisis? Short-term investigation in children. Clin Biomech (Bristol, Avon) 2019;63:73–8.
63. Arbab D, Frank D, Bouillon B, et al. [Subtalare screw arthroereisis for the treatment of symptomatic, flexible pes planovalgus]. Z Orthop Unfall 2018;156:93–9.
64. Kubo H, Lipp C, Hufeland M, et al. Outcome after subtalar screw arthroereisis in children with flexible flatfoot depends on time of treatment: Midterm results of 95 cases. J Orthop Sci 2020;25:497–502.
65. Franz A, Herz D, Raabe J, et al. Pedobarographic outcome after subtalar screw arthroereisis in flexible juvenile flatfoot. Foot Ankle Surg 2020;27(4):389–94.
66. Pavone V, Vescio A, Di Silvestri CA, et al. Outcomes of the calcaneo-stop procedure for the treatment of juvenile flatfoot in young athletes. J Child Orthop 2018;12:582–9.
67. Ortiz CA, Wagner E, Wagner P. Arthroereisis: what have we learned? Foot Ankle Clin 2018;23:415–34.
68. Hsieh C-H, Lee C-C, Tseng T-H, et al. Body weight effects on extra-osseous subtalar arthroereisis. J Clin Med 2019;8.
69. Zhang X, Pauel R, Deschamps K, et al. Differences in foot muscle morphology and foot kinematics between symptomatic and asymptomatic pronated feet. Scand J Med Sci Sports 2019;29:1766–73.
70. Christensen JC, Campbell N, DiNucci K. Closed kinetic chain tarsal mechanics of subtalar joint arthroereisis. J Am Podiatr Med Assoc 1996;86:467–73.
71. Arangio GA, Reinert KL, Salathe EP. A biomechanical model of the effect of subtalar arthroereisis on the adult flexible flat foot. Clin Biomech (Bristol, Avon) 2004;19:847–52.
72. Zaret DI, Myerson MS. Arthroerisis of the subtalar joint. Foot Ankle Clin 2003;8: 605–17.
73. Evans AM, Rome K. A Cochrane review of the evidence for non-surgical interventions for flexible pediatric flat feet. Eur J Phys Rehabil Med 2011;47:69–89.
74. Needleman RL. Current topic review: subtalar arthroereisis for the correction of flexible flatfoot. Foot Ankle Int 2005;26:336–46.
75. Highlander P, Sung W, Weil LJ. Subtalar arthroereisis. Clin Podiatr Med Surg 2011;28:745–54.
76. Kerr CM, Zavatsky AB, Theologis T, et al. Kinematic differences between neutral and flat feet with and without symptoms as measured by the Oxford foot model. Gait Posture 2019;67:213–8.
77. Lamm BM, Stasko PA, Gesheff MG, et al. Normal foot and ankle radiographic angles, measurements, and reference points. J Foot Ankle Surg 2016;55:991–8.
78. Giannini S, Ceccarelli F, Vannini F, et al. Operative treatment of flatfoot with talocalcaneal coalition. Clin Orthop Relat Res 2003;178–87.
79. Fracassetti D, Moharamzadeh D, De Pellegrin M. Resection of tarsal coalition and surgical correction of the hindfoot deformity in one step. J Child Orthop 2017;10:S159–60.
80. De Pellegrin M, Moharamzadeh D. Severe flat foot in syndromic patients. a minimally invasive surgical option. J Child Orthop 2012;6:s25.

81. Rein S, Hanisch U, Zwipp H, et al. Comparative analysis of inter-and intraligamentous distribution of sensory nerve endings in ankle ligaments: a cadaver study. Foot Ankle Int 2013;34:1017–24.
82. Faldini C, Mazzotti A, Panciera A, et al. Bioabsorbable implants for subtalar arthroereisis in pediatric flatfoot. Musculoskelet Surg 2018;102:11–9.
83. Giannini S, Girolami M, Ceccarelli F. The surgical treatment of infantile flat foot. A new expanding endo-orthotic implant. Ital J Orthop Traumatol 1985;11:315–22.
84. Gutiérrez PR, Lara MH. Giannini prosthesis for flatfoot. Foot Ankle Int 2005;26: 918–26.
85. Husain ZS, Fallat LM. Biomechanical analysis of Maxwell-Brancheau arthroereisis implants. J Foot Ankle Surg 2002;41:352–8.
86. Garras DN, Hansen PL, Miller AG, et al. Outcome of modified Kidner procedure with subtalar arthroereisis for painful accessory navicular associated with planovalgus deformity. Foot Ankle Int 2012;33:934–9.
87. De Pellegrin M. Subtalar screw arthroereisis for correction of flat foot in children-15 years experience. Fuss Und Sprunggelenk 2007;5:12.
88. Cicchinelli LD, Huerta JP, Carmona FJG, et al. Analysis of gastrocnemius recession and medial column procedures as adjuncts in arthroereisis for the correction of pediatric pes planovalgus: a radiographic retrospective study. J Foot Ankle Surg 2008;47:385–91.
89. Soomekh DJ, Baravarian B. Pediatric and adult flatfoot reconstruction: subtalar arthroereisis versus realignment osteotomy surgical options. Clin Podiatr Med Surg 2006;23:695–708, v.
90. Kumar V, Clough TM. Talar neck fracture-a rare but important complication following subtalar arthroereisis. Foot (Edinb) 2014;24:169–71.
91. Tompkins MH, Nigro JS, Mendicino S. The smith STA-peg: a 7-year retrospective study. J Foot Ankle Surg 1993;32:27–33.
92. Oloff LM, Naylor BL, Jacobs AM. Complications of subtalar arthroereisis. J Foot Surg 1987;26:136–40.
93. Rockett AK, Mangum G, Mendicino SS. Bilateral intraosseous cystic formation in the talus: a complication of subtalar arthroeresis. J Foot Ankle Surg 1998;37: 421–5.
94. Trieb K, Fingernagel T, Petershofer A, et al. Loosening of a calcaneo-stop screw after trampolining. Sportverletz Sportschaden 2015;29:122–3.
95. Corpuz M, Shofler D, Labovitz J, et al. Fracture of the talus as a complication of subtalar arthroereisis. J Foot Ankle Surg 2012;51:91–4.
96. Frank CB. Ligament structure, physiology and function. J Musculoskelet Neuronal Interact 2004;4:199–201.
97. Stagni R, Leardini A, O'Connor JJ, et al. Role of passive structures in the mobility and stability of the human subtalar joint: a literature review. Foot Ankle Int 2003; 24:402–9.
98. Akiyama K, Takakura Y, Tomita Y, et al. Neurohistology of the sinus tarsi and sinus tarsi syndrome. J Orthop Sci 1999;4:299–303.
99. Rein S, Hagert E, Hanisch U, et al. Immunohistochemical analysis of sensory nerve endings in ankle ligaments: a cadaver study. Cells Tissues Organs 2013;197:64–76.
100. Khin-Myo-Hla, Ishii T, Sakane M, et al. Effect of anesthesia of the sinus tarsi on peroneal reaction time in patients with functional instability of the ankle. Foot Ankle Int 1999;20:554–9.

Juvenile Hallux Valgus

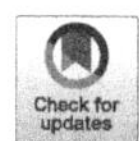

Susan T. Mahan, MD, MPH[a,*], Emily O. Cidambi, MD[b]

KEYWORDS

- Juvenile hallux valgus • Hallux valgus • Adolescent bunion
- Adolescent foot deformity • Juvenile bunion • Foot pain

KEY POINTS

- Etiology and treatment of hallux valgus is different for juvenile hallux valgus (JHV) than in adult-onset hallux valgus.
- Conservative treatment should be exhausted prior to procedural intervention for JHV and treatment should be for pain and not just deformity
- Radiographically, the "typical" JHV deformity includes elevated distal metatarsal articular angle (DMAA), elevated intermetatarsal angle (IMA), higher metatarsal cuneiform angle (MCA) and an oblique medial cuneiform; variability from foot to foot is common. Incongruent metatarsophalangeal joint (MTPJ) is more common with increased severity of JHV.
- Surgical treatment is highly variable, and many options exist with generally inconsistent results. Recurrence is likely. Lateral release should be considered when MTPJ incongruity is present.
- Minimally invasive surgical options are tempting but unproven.
- Treatment algorithm for JHV is presented.

INTRODUCTION

In the 19th century, hallux valgus was thought to be purely an enlargement of the first toe metatarsophalangeal joint[1] (MTPJ); however, this was before the availability of radiographic assessment. The definition is now accepted to be a lateral deviation of the proximal phalanx relative to the first metatarsal, which creates a symptomatic medial prominence at the MTPJ.[2] These days, the diagnosis of hallux valgus is made radiographically, when the hallux valgus angle (HVA) is 15° or more.[3] Most hallux valgus occurs in adults, typically in women in their fourth to sixth decade of life; this is often a result of poor fitting shoewear.[3] However, the onset of hallux valgus in childhood has been noticed to occur and has some unique features; it is not associated with poor fitting shoewear.[4] To qualify as juvenile hallux valgus (JHV), the onset of the deformity must occur in the preteen or teenage years, regardless of when

[a] Department of Orthopaedics and Sports Medicine, Boston Children's Hospital, Harvard Medical School, 300 Longwood Avenue, Boston, MA 02115, USA; [b] Department of Orthopaedics, Rady Children's Hospital, UC San Diego Medical School, 3020 Children's Way, MC 5062, San Diego, CA 92123, USA
* Corresponding author.
E-mail address: susan.mahan@childrens.harvard.edu

Foot Ankle Clin N Am 26 (2021) 807–828
https://doi.org/10.1016/j.fcl.2021.07.008

treatment is initiated. It is estimated that 40% to 50% of adult bunions actually had onset in childhood.[5] The etiology of the juvenile onset hallux valgus is not known, but it is felt that genetics plays a role.[4]

EPIDEMIOLOGY

Though the overall prevalence of hallux valgus is highest in the elderly population (older than 65 years), the deformity may frequently start in the adolescent, or even juvenile age in many cases.[4,6] A female predominance for the deformity is reported across all age groups and has been reported to be as high as 88% of JHV patients. One meta-analysis reported the prevalence in pediatric patients (younger than 18 years) as 7.8%, and a relative prevalence of 15% for women and 5.7% for men.[6] This is compared to a prevalence of 23% in adults aged 18 to 65 years, and 35.7% in those aged 65+ years. Women were affected at more than 2 times the rate of men across age groups. When examining juvenile patients alone, 40% of the patients already had some hallux valgus deformity by age 10 years or less,[4] indicating that a JHV population exists as its own entity, beyond early adult pathology.

INHERITANCE

The inheritance pattern is not well-defined in the setting of JHV and is likely multifactorial. A maternal family history is the most commonly reported, 73% in a cohort including all ages and 77% in JHV patients.[4,7] Overall patients with hallux valgus reported some form of family history in 84% of patients, 27% of which was a multigenerational history. In addition, there is an increased association between the presence of bilateral hallux valgus in patients younger than 30 years and a family history of bunions.[7] One study found as high as 90% of JHV patients with a history of at least one family member affected, and some with family members affected across 3 generations, with female family members more commonly affected.[8] This is thought to suggest an inheritance pattern compatible with autosomal dominant with incomplete penetrance. There was no relationship found between the severity of the HVA and family history of deformity.[7,8]

ETIOLOGY

The true etiology of hallux valgus deformity seems to be multifactorial. It includes a combination of both intrinsic and extrinsic factors that contribute to onset and progression of the deformity, as well as a general progression of changes that occur with worsening deformity.[9] The underlying pathology is thought to be primus varus, both in the adult and pediatric population.[5]

Although adult and juvenile bunions share many similar characteristics regarding the appearance and progression of deformity, there are a few key factors that are unique to JHV[4,5,10]:

1. Some authors have proposed that the etiology of the JHV deformity is metatarsus primus varus, which can present as an increased angle between the first and second metatarsals, or as metatarsus adductus.[11] However, more recent data suggest that the etiology may lay with the deformity in the MTPJ itself, which causes an elevated distal metatarsal articular angle (DMAA).[4] Some propose that it is the elevated DMAA and not the metatarsus primus varus that may be driving the JHV deformity.[4,10] Coughlin[4] found that early-onset hallux valgus (before age 10 years) was associated with a much higher DMAA.

2. There may be an oblique (medially angulated) first metatarsal-medial cuneiform joint which is contributory to the medial angulation of the metatarsal as well as the increased intermetatarsal angle (IMA).[10,12]
3. The first MTP joint may have irregular morphology (flat or conical)
4. Increased length of the first metatarsal which is associated with increased DMAA and hypermobility of the first ray.

The general progression of adult hallux valgus has been well-described[2,9,13,14]; however, there are clinical factors that differentiate an adult-onset hallux valgus (AHV) from JHV. In children, the MTP joint is laterally deviated (increased DMAA), whereas the first metatarsal migrates medially. The medial metatarsal shift may be augmented by laxity at the tarsometatarsal (TMT) joint of the first ray.[9] This creates a prominence of the MTPJ, which can be painful when placed into narrow-based shoes. As the deformity worsens, the sesamoids migrate laterally due to the pull of the short flexors and adductors, and the great toe pronates. The proximal phalanx follows the pull of the sesamoids, deep transverse ligament, and adductor hallucis which tether it laterally.[9] The lateral sesamoid moves to rest in the intermetatarsal space between the first and second rays.[13] Lateral subluxation of the sesamoid complex results in *pronation* of the metatarsal due to pulling of the soft tissues. One study demonstrated an average metatarsal diaphyseal pronation of 12.7° in patients with hallux valgus compared with neutral, to slight supination in unaffected feet.[15] The medial soft tissues become stretched and the pronation causes the abductor hallucis to migrate in a plantar direction, such that it no longer counterbalances the adductor.[5] Medial eminence bursal thickening is much less prominent in JHV than in AHV. Degenerative arthritis of the first MTP is rarely seen in JHV, rather MTP congruity is thought to be a significant factor.[4]

There are extrinsic factors that may play a role in the development of deformity. Unlike AHV, shoe wear in JHV is felt to be an aggravating factor rather than causative.[4] Certainly, in a patient with JHV who is having symptoms from their shoes, alteration of footwear and the recommendation for wider shoes precedes surgical intervention. Excessive loading has also been proposed as a mechanism for deformity progression but has poor support in young patients. Although weight distribution changes in the foot after deformity is present, there is no proven support for an overload or impact etiology to the evolution of hallux valgus based on occupation or body weight.[9]

Generalized ligamentous laxity, which is common in women with hallux valgus, may also play a significant role in deformity. Female patients with symptomatic hallux valgus (aged 20–40 years) had a higher rating of ligamentous laxity when compared with normal female controls.[16] In conditions associated with increased ligamentous laxity such as Marfan syndrome and Ehlers-Danlos, hallux valgus is common and more difficult to treat.[17] The rate of deformity recurrence is higher in the setting of ligamentous laxity and therefore requires thoughtful assessment with regards to surgical treatment,[18,19] particularly in patients with known pathologic ligamentous laxity (eg, Trisomy 21, cerebral palsy).[20–22]

CLINICAL PRESENTATION

The primary presenting symptom related to JHV is pain over the medial eminence at the MTPJ.[3] In patients who present with JHV, more than 80% are girls[5] and half present before age 10 years.[5] Pain from shoe wear is the most common complaint, but pain can persist out of shoes as well. In addition, skin changes over the medial MTPJ can also be present including callous and bursal swelling, or even skin breakdown.

The foot should be examined both in the seated and standing positions. When seated, the examiner may assess motion and flexibility of the metatarsophalangeal (MTP) and interphalangeal joints, as well as the passive reducibility of the MTP joint to neutral alignment.[3] It is also important for the examiner to assess the stability of the first tarsometatarsal joint. Pedobarograph examination has demonstrated an association between increased dorsiflexion excursion of the first ray and increased pressure on central to lateral forefoot, contributing to transfer metatarsalgia.[23] Presence of callosities at sites other than the medial eminence may suggest transfer metatarsalgia and possible TMT instability.[5] The examiner should assess patients for signs of general ligamentous laxity and hypermobility, as this plays an important role in surgical decision-making.[16]

In stance, the foot can be examined for pes planovalgus (PPV) deformity, Achilles contracture, and pronation deformity of the first metatarsal with weight-bearing.[3] The true deformity may not be fully appreciated on a sitting or supine examination. Tightness of the gastrocnemius muscle places tension on the plantar aponeurosis, which can accentuate the valgus deformity of a pre-existing hallux valgus,[24] especially during gait at the end of stance phase. Furthermore, this can contribute to limited extension of the MTPJ in dorsiflexion when the MTPJ is held in neutral, which is sometimes seen in JHV. One can also assess for the presence of concomitant deformities such as hallux valgus interphalangeus and metatarsus adductus in the standing position.[5]

There has been some debate about the relationship between JHV and PPV in children. Some studies have not shown a relationship between JHV and PPV,[10,25–27] whereas others report or claim that a relationship exists.[28] When a painful bunion is found in the setting of PPV, use of an accommodative/low-profile orthotic can be helpful in reducing pain symptoms[5]; however, the patient should be advised that orthotics will not provide deformity correction. One study demonstrated that the use of an arch support was unsuccessful at preventing the progression of the HVA, and in fact, some patients developed hallux valgus on the previously unaffected side.[29] Another group examined the efficacy of a thermoplastic night splint for the MTP joint used for at least 2 years, combined with stretches in 25 patients with an average age of 10 years, finding that approximately 50% of patients had an improvement in either the IMA or HVA, and there was no recurrence in those who had improvement.[30] Despite the possible efficacy of night splinting, and temporary pain relief with orthotics, cooperation with bracing and splinting is generally poor, especially in adolescent females who are generally resistant to shoes that can accommodate an orthotic insert.[5]

Conservative care should be used first before any invasive procedures. Significant deformity can occur without any pain, and invasive treatment should not be initiated for deformity alone, except in the instance of severe deformity causing skin compromise (more common in developmentally delayed or neuromuscular patients who may not be able to express discomfort). Shoe and activity modifications are usually the first line of treatment. Night splints, bunion pads, and other commercial devices can be used to help relieve symptoms. Surgical treatment should be reserved for bunions that are persistently painful despite failure of conservative measures, typically in a patient who has reached skeletal maturity.[5]

RADIOGRAPHIC PRESENTATION

When assessing hallux valgus, it is imperative to obtain standing anterior-posterior (AP) and standing lateral views of the feet. The diagnosis of JHV is made radiographically when the HVA is 15° or more. Mild to moderate (**Fig. 1**) hallux valgus is generally considered an HVA of 15° to 35°, whereas severe (**Fig. 2**) hallux valgus is greater than 35°. The DMAA measures the angle of the distal metatarsal articular surface relative to the perpendicular to the metatarsal axis (**Fig. 3**); in normal feet, these are parallel but in most cases of JHV, this is significantly elevated.[4,10] One study found that the DMAA was independently associated with JHV and its severity.[10] The IMA is the angle between the axis of the first and the axis of the second metatarsal (**Fig. 4**); in normal feet, this is under 10°; however, this is often elevated in JHV. MTPJ congruity is a dichotomous measure of the reduction versus subluxation of this joint; in AHV, this joint is often incongruent (ie, subluxated); however, this is more commonly congruent (reduced) in JHV (**Fig. 5**). With the increasing severity of JHV, increased incongruity is generally noted.[10]

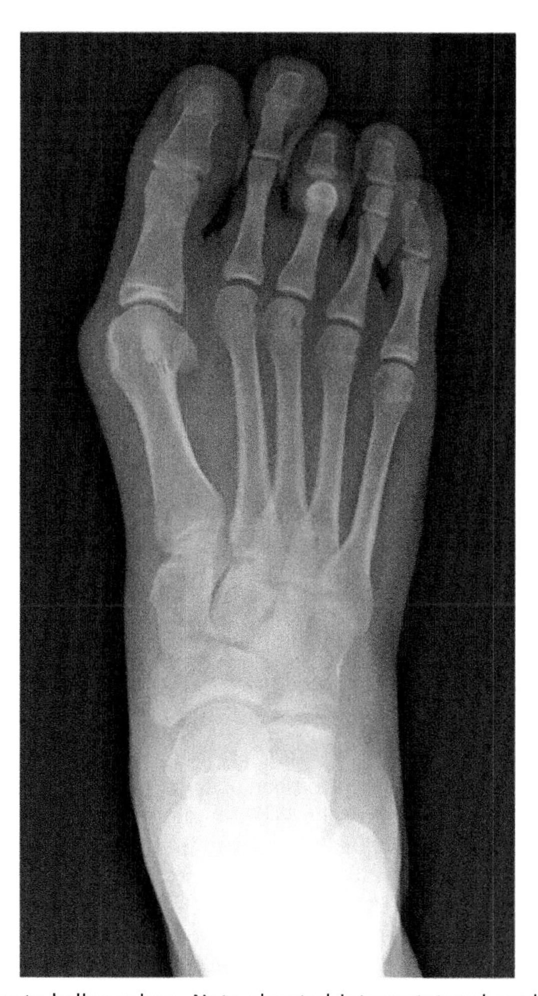

Fig. 1. Mild-moderate hallux valgus. Note elevated intermetatarsal angle, elevated distal metatarsal articular angle, prominent medial metatarsal head, and congruent metatarsophalangeal joint. The lateral sesamoid is just starting to slip out from underneath the metatarsal head.

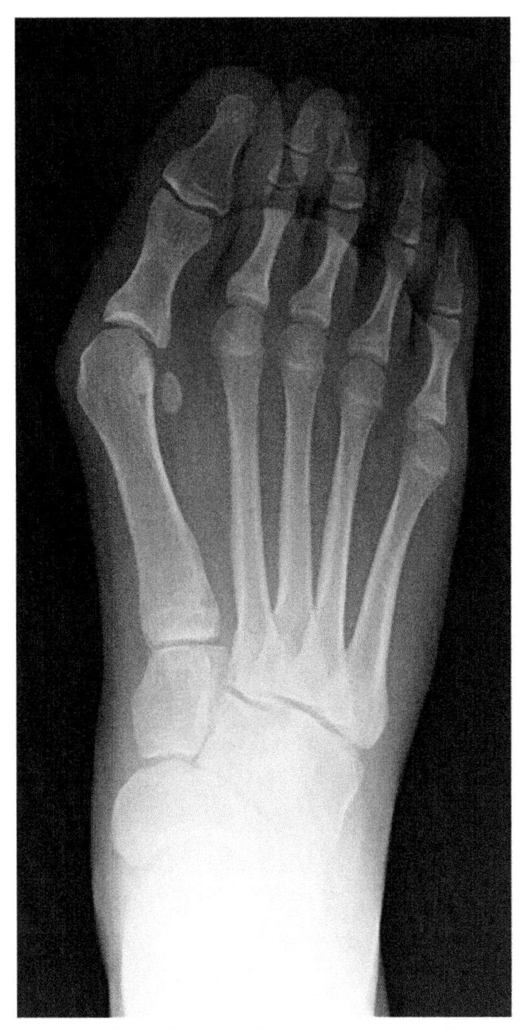

Fig. 2. Severe hallux valgus. Note elevated distal metatarsal articular angle and incongruency of the metatarsophalangeal joint. His lateral sesamoid is now completed uncovered by the metatarsal head.

Other radiographic parameters have been used to help determine the severity and potential etiology of JHV. Metatarsal cuneiform angle (MCA) was first described by Vyas and colleagues[12] and describes the angle between the long axis of the first metatarsal and the medial cuneiform articular surface (**Fig. 6**); they found this to be higher in JHV, which was supported by a subsequent study.[10] The obliquity of the medial cuneiform has also been noted, which was described as the angle between the proximal and distal articular surfaces of the medial cuneiform. It has been noted by several authors that the hallux valgus deformity appears to originate from the medial cuneiform.[10,12] A long first metatarsal has also been noted by some authors[31] and hypermobility of the first ray has also been thought to contribute to the deformity[5] (see **Fig. 4**).

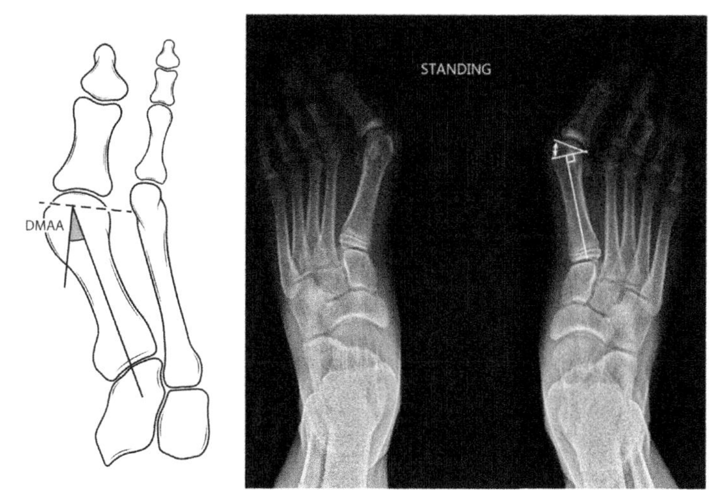

Fig. 3. Two techniques for measuring the DMAA.

The "typical" pattern of deformity in JHV includes an elevated DMAA, an elevated IMA, a higher MCA, and an oblique medial cuneiform.[10] As the severity of the JHV increases, the greater the likelihood that the MTPJ is incongruous (see **Fig. 2**). In addition, with increasing severity, the sesamoids are less likely to be underneath the MTPJ and instead subluxate laterally, signifying the increased pull of the soft tissues to worsen the deformity (see **Figs. 1** and **2**).

In growing children (younger than 15 years) with radiographic evidence of JHV, the HVA has been shown to increase about 0.8° per year.[25] The DMAA increases in children younger than 10 years at 1.5° per year, but does not increase significantly in the older child. This demonstrates that the development of JHV originates at a young age with the increased DMAA, and the HVA increases afterward. This suggests that the DMAA may be the driver of the deformity, which is further supported by the study showing DMAA to be independently associated with JHV and its severity.[10] However, others have considered the metatarsus primus varus (from increased IMA) to be the etiologic deformity.[5]

SURGICAL TREATMENT

It is worth emphasizing again that surgical treatment should be reserved for symptomatic hallux valgus that has been recalcitrant to conservative means, typically in a skeletally mature patient. One exception may be the use of guided growth, as discussed later. Once the decision to pursue acute corrective surgery of the hallux valgus is made, then comes the unenviable decision as to which procedure(s) to use.

There have been algorithms produced for the treatment of AHV; however, these algorithms typically do not cover the constellation that is JHV. Several authors have emphasized that treatment of JHV has a different set of considerations than AHV.[5,10,32]

When choosing an operative plan for JHV, an important initial consideration is determining if the MTPJ is congruent or incongruent. Although this comes as a dichotomous option, this is not always a clear choice. If the joint is congruent, then the surgical technique must respect the congruent joint or an incongruent joint may result; this typically involves bony procedures to reorient the bone rather than soft tissue

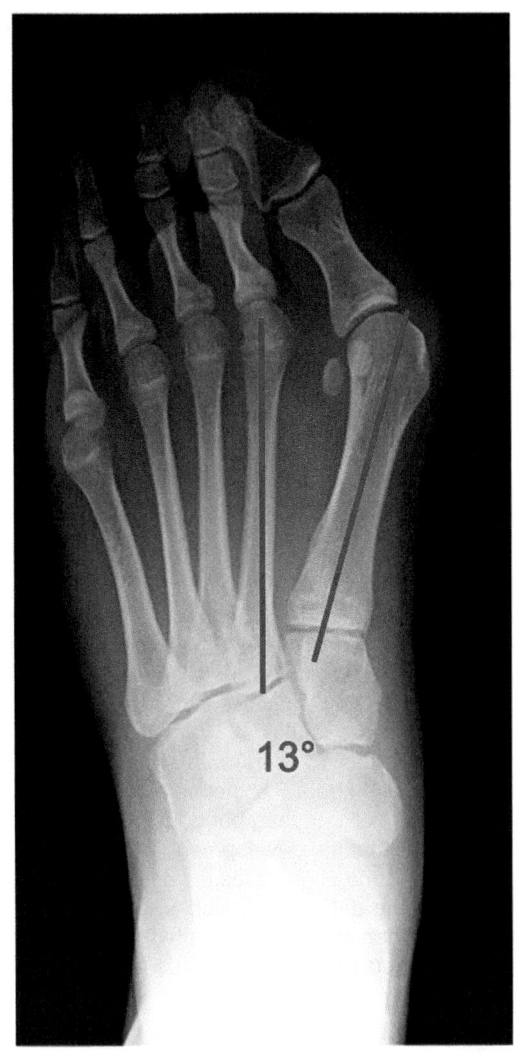

Fig. 4. IMA. The angle between a line drawn down the axis of the first metatarsal compared to a line drawn down the axis of the second metatarsal. Typically, in normal feet, this is less than 10°.

procedures.[4] Conversely, if the MTPJ is incongruent, then the joint needs to be aligned, and soft tissue realignment needs to be part of the surgical plan; in JHV, this is typically done in addition to bony procedures.

Surgical Options

A recent systemic review of treatment for JHV revealed that most of the literature is retrospective case reviews, in which the treatments are heterogeneous but generally effective.[33] Short-term complication rates are low but with only medium-term follow-up at best[33] making it difficult to predict long-term the likelihood of recurrence. More than 150 different procedures have been described for treating hallux valgus[34] although these have largely been pioneered in the adult population. The recurrence

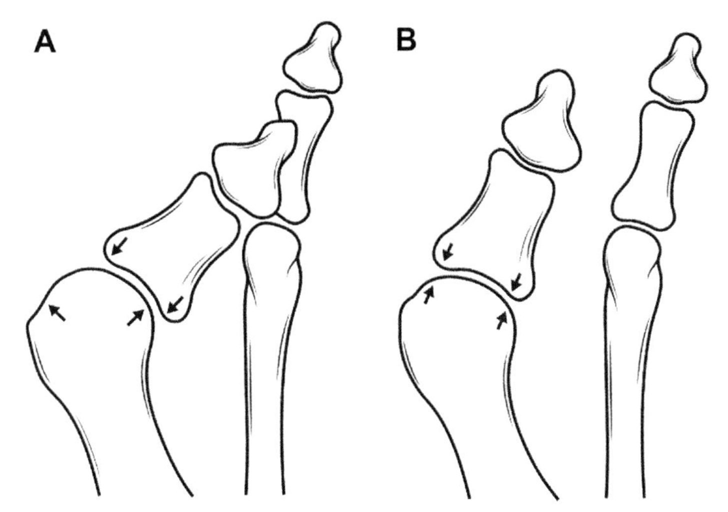

Fig. 5. Metatarsophalangeal joint congruency. Edges of the joint are noted by the arrows. In (*A*), the arrows and the joint do not align and are incongruent; in (*B*), the arrows and the joint are in alignment and this is congruent.

rate remains around 20% in most recent studies[35] with true long-term recurrence difficult to predict. With such a multitude of options, there is no clear best procedure, and this has added to the confusion and difficulty of treating this condition.

When considering treatment for JHV, there are 6 basic categories, which are described elaborately in the following subsections: (1) proximal metatarsal osteotomy (can also include medial cuneiform osteotomy); (2) distal metatarsal osteotomy; (3) soft tissue procedures; (4) combined procedures[5]; (5) arthrodesis, either metatarsal cuneiform joint (also known as a "Lapidus") or MTPJ; and (6) guided growth. Minimally invasive options are contained in these categories but will also be discussed separately.

Proximal metatarsal osteotomies, including medial cuneiform osteotomy

Several types of proximal metatarsal or cuneiform osteotomies have been used to treat JHV. A proximal metatarsal osteotomy can involve a Scarf type, a crescentic, closing or opening wedge osteotomy, a Ludloff or a chevron osteotomy.

- The Scarf osteotomy is a longitudinal coronal cut in the first metatarsal and a translation of the distal portion of the metatarsal more laterally; this has been shown to also improve the DMAA in patients.[36,37] Scarf osteotomy has had some success for treatment of JHV[36,37]; however, others have found a high recurrence rate in the pediatric population with this operation.[35,38]
- Opening wedge osteotomies are technically easier to perform but have the disadvantage of lengthening the metatarsal.[39]
- Closing wedge osteotomies are more difficult to perform in the small space of the proximal metatarsal and are not commonly performed.
- Crescentic osteotomies are length stable (they do not shorten or lengthen the metatarsal) and can be performed with either a special curved saw blade, or with multiple drill hole techniques; it can be difficult to obtain satisfactory fixation using this technique.[40]
- A Ludloff osteotomy is an oblique osteotomy with lateral rotation of the distal fragment and has the advantage of ease of fixation while still length neutral.[41]
- Proximal chevron osteotomies can also be used in a similar manner.

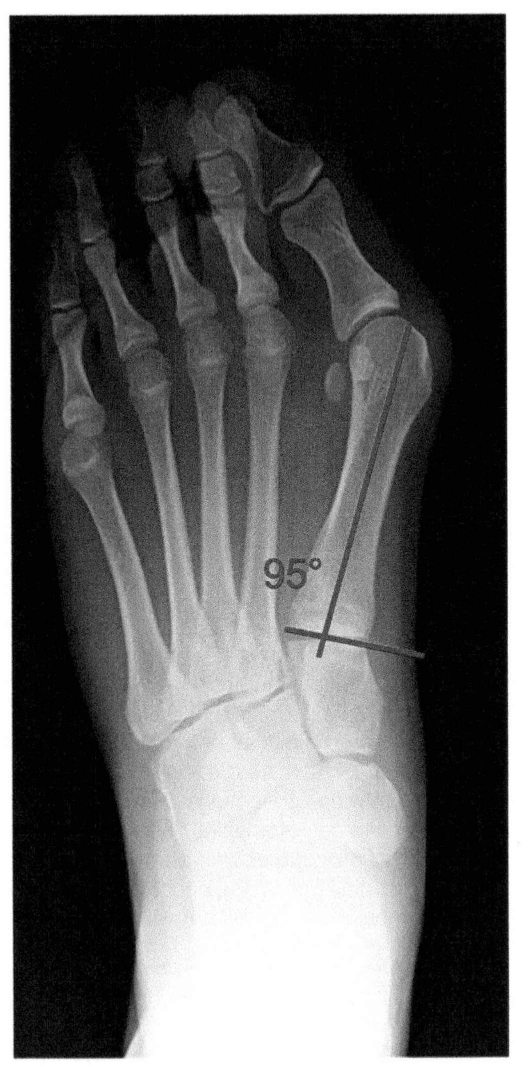

Fig. 6. MCA. This is the angle formed between the long axis of the first metatarsal and the articular surface of the medial cuneiform.

- Medial cuneiform osteotomies can also be performed for the treatment of JHV.[42] This is particularly appealing in patients with significant cuneiform obliquity[10,12] and could be used in the presence of open physes as the first metatarsal physis would not be at risk with a cuneiform osteotomy. Although there have been occasional notes in the literature of cuneiform medial-based opening wedge osteotomy for the treatment of JHV,[42] there does not appear to be uniform acceptance of this procedure. There may also be unintentional multiplanar effects from this osteotomy because of ligamentous and capsular tethering.[43] This suggests that consistent satisfaction with this procedure has not been achieved.

Distal metatarsal osteotomies

Various distal metatarsal osteotomies have been described, classically the chevron and Mitchell osteotomies. This group also includes a more recent minimally invasive option, coined "Simple Effective, Rapid and Inexpensive" (SERI). Modulation of the DMAA can typically be achieved in well-executed distal metatarsal osteotomies.

- The Chevron osteotomy is a V-shaped distal metatarsal osteotomy initially described for adults[44] but has been also used successfully in the treatment of JHV.[45] There have been concerns for avascular necrosis to the metatarsal head[46] with this procedure, particularly when it is accompanied with a lateral release; however, with more recent techniques, it is felt that this can be safely avoided.[47–49] This also has minimally invasive options that have had some cautionary initial success.[50] The chevron osteotomy can also be combined with proximal metatarsal osteotomies for correction of moderate to severe deformities but with a high complication rate.[51]
- The Mitchell osteotomy is a combination of biplanar distal metaphyseal osteotomies, which achieves shortening of the first metatarsal and lateral and plantar displacement of the distal fragment.[52] A notch is created in the distal fragment, which is then reduced and fixed on the more proximal fragment. The original Mitchell has been modified for improved results. Results in treatment of JHV have been generally mixed[52–54] and are in the older literature; this procedure does not appear to be used in more recent reports.
- SERI—This procedure was coined "Simple, Effective, Rapid and Inexpensive" (SERI) by the surgeon who developed it. It involves a minimally invasive osteotomy of the distal metatarsal with medial translation and a percutaneous pin to hold the reduction during healing.[28,55,56] Initial series by the author were very encouraging but other surgeons have had difficulty reproducing the excellent results as consistently. More recently, this is being used in the treatment of JHV without a consistent published series but encouraging anecdotal results so far. See additional discussion below.

Soft tissue procedures

Soft tissue procedures typically include medial capsulorrhaphy with possible exostectomy (when present, rare in JHV). This can also include a lateral release. Generally, soft tissue procedures should be performed only when the MTPJ is incongruent or it may destabilize a congruent joint.[57]

- Medial soft tissue capsulorrhaphy is typically less critical in JHV than in AHV. Certainly, the correction of the JHV should not depend on the medial soft tissue repair or the correction will surely fail. Overtightening the medial capsule could also lead to incongruency of the joint, which can cause further stiffness and ongoing pain.[4,5,32]
- Lateral soft tissue release has been a part of surgical treatment in AHV[41,47] but because of the predominance of bony deformity in JHV, this is typically less of a component of treatment.[47] The DMAA in JHV is typically elevated and the joint is congruent, so soft tissue release is not indicated and would potentially destabilize the joint. However, in some severe JHV, there is both elevated DMAA and an incongruent joint. These can be particularly difficult because operating on both sides of the joint has some concerns, particularly historically, for causing avascular necrosis of the head of the metatarsal head.[49,58] In the situation of both elevated DMAA that needs to be addressed with bony correction and incongruence of the MTPJ, a lateral soft tissue release should be considered in addition to the bony correction. A lateral soft tissue release can restore the balance of the soft tissues, including the capsular, muscular, and ligamentous components, to provide longstanding correction of the bunion.[47] Anatomic studies[46] and

clinical studies[44,48,59,60] have shown that this can be performed along with a bony procedure provided proper care is taken during both the osteotomy and release. Before performing a lateral release, an important understanding of the anatomy of the lateral side of the MTPJ as well as the deforming structures is critical. It is important to release the (1) deep metatarsal ligament, (2) the attachment of the adductor hallucis muscle, (3) the lateral collateral ligament, and the (4) lateral metatarsosesamoid suspensory ligament, with the latter structure considering the key to a successful lateral release.[47] (**Fig. 7**).

Common combinations (including phalangeal osteotomies)

In treating JHV, typically combination surgery is necessary. In the setting of a congruent joint, a double metatarsal osteotomy can address both the 1 to 2 metatarsal angle and the elevated DMAA. In the setting of an incongruent joint, a proximal metatarsal osteotomy with a lateral release may be necessary.

- Double osteotomy (or triple when phalangeal osteotomy is included) of the first metatarsal is tempting in JHV to correct both the IMA and the DMAA while improving the HVA.[61,62] Although this can provide powerful results often with generally good outcomes,[63,64] there can be a high rate of complications including over and under correction,[51] as well as phalangeal stiffness and recurrence.[65]
- Proximal metatarsal osteotomy with a lateral soft tissue release is a satisfying solution in the setting of an elevated IMA and an incongruent joint.[41]
- Proximal phalangeal osteotomies, often called the "Akin" osteotomy, can be necessary to achieve the final satisfactory appearance of the hallux. This procedure alone is typically not sufficient for the treatment of JHV although is used often in combination of soft tissue procedures for the treatment of AHV or with other bony procedures in JHV.[35] This is also the treatment of choice for hallux interphalangeus.[66] In long-standing JHV, the proximal phalanx is often not square and a proximal phalangeal can address this often-subtle deformity (**Fig. 8**).

Arthrodesis either of the MTPJ or metatarsocuneiform joint

Arthrodesis can be considered in rare situations of JHV.

- Arthrodesis of the MTPJ can be performed in select low-demand patients. It is often recommended in the setting of JHV associated with Down's syndrome, other hyperflexible states, and cerebral palsy[20,21,67] and other neuromuscular

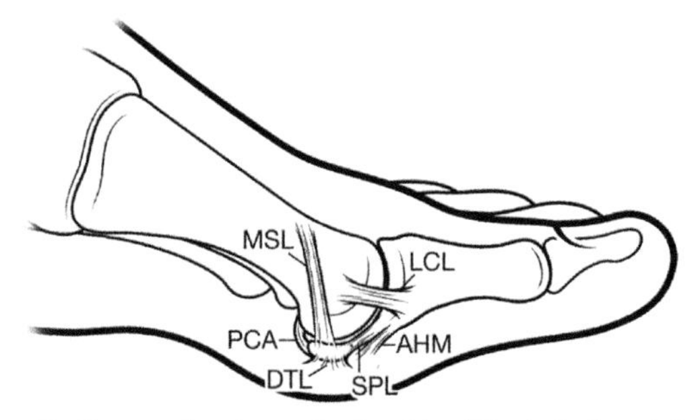

Fig. 7. The lateral soft tissues structures to be identified during lateral release. AHM, adductor hallucis muscle; DTL, deep transverse metatarsal ligament; LCL, lateral collateral ligament; MSL, lateral metatarsosesamoid suspensory ligament; PCA, plantar capsular attachment; SPL, lateral short sesamophalangeal ligament. (Adapted with permission from Schneider 2013.)

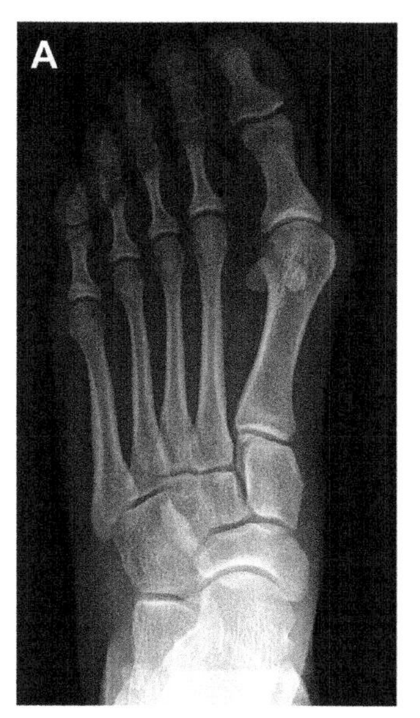

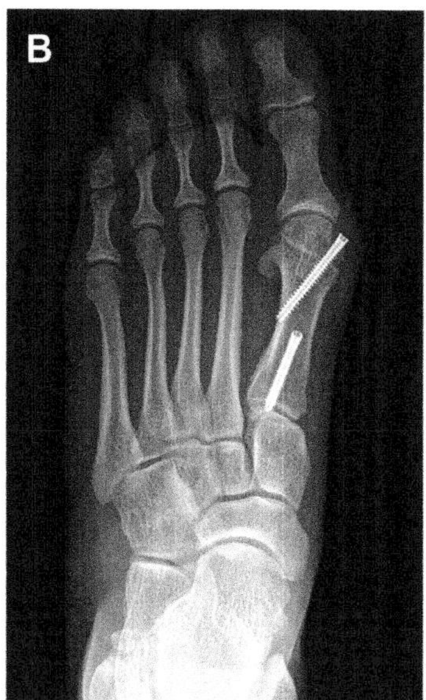

Fig. 8. (*A*) Moderate hallux valgus with elevated distal metatarsal articular angle and congruent joint. (*B*) This was treated with proximal metatarsal osteotomy ("Ludloff") and distal osteotomy. Some residual valgus of the proximal phalanx was noted.

conditions.[22] Interestingly, when MTPJ fusion is performed in this setting, the 1 to 2 IMA is typically improved despite not addressing that aspect of the deformity specifically[22,68] (**Fig. 9**).

- Arthrodesis of the first metatarsal-cuneiform joint (often called a "Lapidus" procedure) can be used in severe cases of JHV, when hyperlaxity is noted, or for salvage operations.[69] The Lapidus procedure also includes an acute correction of the 1 to 2 IMA. This does not address the elevated DMAA often seen in JHV, which would need to be addressed separately.

Guided growth using lateral hemiepiphysiodesis

- Guided growth is very useful in the treatment of limb deformity in the pediatric population. Lateral first metatarsal hemipiphysiodesis[70,71] can be used in the still growing child to address the increased IMA by stopping the growth on the lateral side of the first metatarsal physis and allowed the medial side to continue growing.[72] The intervention needs to occur while the foot is still skeletally immature (age 9–11 years optimally). Unfortunately, children are often not symptomatic from their hallux valgus at the optimal age for treatment so often the window of opportunity to benefit from this is lost. Furthermore, while hemiepiphysiodesis of the lateral first metatarsal can be effective to decrease the clinical symptoms (at least temporarily) and decrease the IMA,[70] it does not address the elevated DMAA often seen in JHV. The hemiepiphysiodesis can either be done through the drill and curettage technique, as initially described by Davids and colleagues,[72] but has also been described more recently using a screw hemiepiphysiodesis[71] which has the advantage of being reversible. Typically, further procedures are needed after skeletal maturity to address the residual deformity including elevated DMAA.

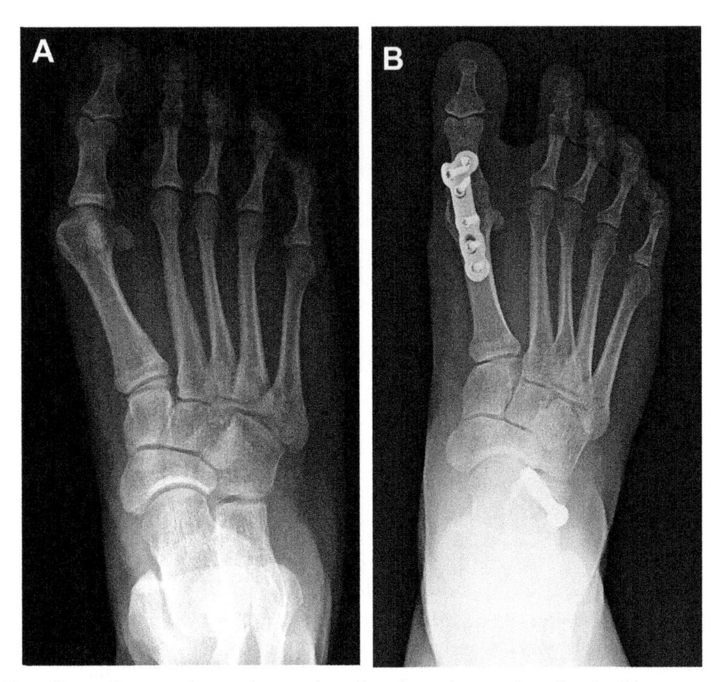

Fig. 9. (*A*) Hallux valgus and pes planovalgus in a low-demand patient with severe developmental disabilities. (*B*) She did well with a metatarsophalangeal joint fusion and subtalar extra-articular screw arthroereisis for treatment of her symptomatic pes planovalgus.

MINIMALLY INVASIVE CONSIDERATIONS

Recent attention to minimally invasive techniques for the treatment of hallux valgus has been considered.[34] The advantages of these techniques potentially include reduced surgical time, decreased cost, easier recovery, and less stress to the patient, in addition to less scarring to both skin and deeper structures.[34] Initially, minimally invasive procedures involved the same operations and equipment but with smaller skin incisions, and these were not uniformly successful.[73] More recent modern techniques for minimally invasive surgery use special operative equipment that needs further training and have some significant learning curve associated with it.[73]

Although most of the studies were originally described for AHV, some treatments have been used in JHV with encouraging success. Several systemic reviews of percutaneous and minimally invasive osteotomies in hallux valgus found a large variety of surgical techniques, which qualified, but with generally low evidence of efficacy as most were retrospective reviews or case series.[34,73,74] Generally, the HVA and clinical outcomes improved, but with variable complications and studies with generally poor levels of evidence. Some studies have shown minimally invasive techniques to be an improvement over open techniques,[50] whereas others have not[75]; so, some skepticism about these minimally invasive options needs to remain.

The SERI technique was described by Giannini and colleagues[55] and involves preoperative stretching of the toe and lateral capsule, a 1-cm incision at the level of the first metatarsal neck, an oblique osteotomy at the level of the metatarsal neck, and a long k-wire that stabilizes the osteotomy and comes out the tip of the toe.[55] Their initial series of over 600 patients had a decrease in mean HVA from 32° to 13°, mean IMA from 14° to 7°, and mean DMAA from 13° to 6°. AOFAS scores improved from mean 47 preoperatively to 89 points at follow-up (scale with a maximum of 100). They also compared the SERI procedure to the scarf technique, and it came out favorably.[56] Although the SERI results from the original author are quite encouraging, not all surgeons have had similar results and there have been problems with lack of fixation and infection after this procedure.[73] However, the SERI may have more usefulness in JHV with the improved bone healing potential seen in the pediatric population, but the original studies were of adults (youngest was age 20 years). The SERI procedure was described in children with hallux valgus and PPV as combined with subtalar arthroereisis implantation.[28] Although we have not used this type of arthroereisis implant in children, the SERI can be combined with the subtalar extra-articular screw arthroereisis (SESA).[76]

Screw for minimally invasive treatment of JHV and PPV in children with encouraging initial results; however, this has yet to be published (**Fig. 10**).

COMPLICATIONS

Unfortunately, any invasive procedure has complications, and the treatment of JHV is not different. Recurrence of the deformity is the most common complication, particularly with inadequate bony correction and in the setting of skeletal immaturity.[5] Hallux varus is an iatrogenic complication from overcorrection or overbalancing of the deformity, and particularly in the setting of removal of the lateral sesamoid, which is contraindicated for this reason.[77] Avascular necrosis of the metatarsal head is a devastating complication, particularly in a younger population.[59] It usually occurs as the result of a combined distal metatarsal osteotomy and distal soft tissue procedure which threatens the intraosseous blood supply to the metatarsal head, although this can be avoided with more modern techniques.[47] Closing wedge osteotomies have also been associated with shortening and transfer metatarsalgia.[78]

TREATMENT ALGORITHM FOR JHV

Each individual foot needs careful assessment of the deformity and only then can a complete surgical plan be created to address that particular combination of deformities.

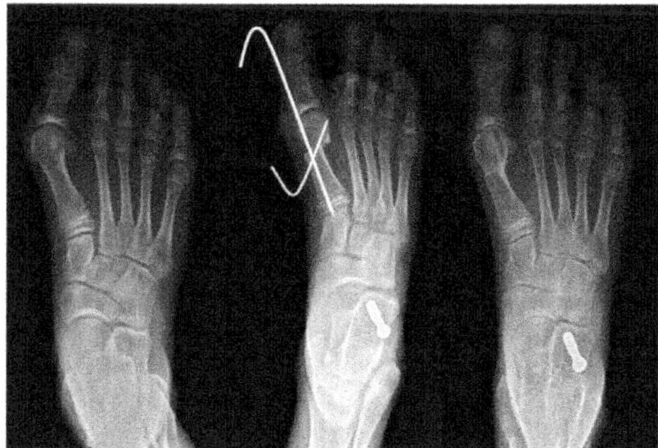
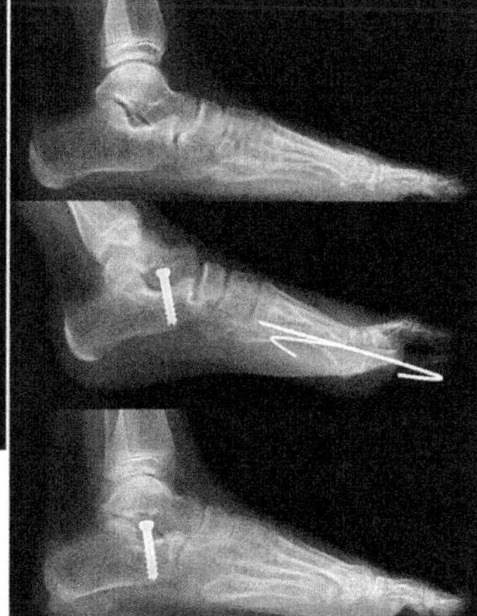

Fig. 10. Combined SESA and SERI technique. Including preoperative, 2 weeks postoperative, and 9 months postoperative.

General principles:

- Operate only on painful feet when conservative measures have been exhausted.
- Delay surgery until skeletally mature if possible. If corrective surgery is performed before skeletal maturity, be sure to select the procedure that does not put the first metatarsal physis at risk of unintentional growth arrest.
- Assess carefully the congruency of the MTPJ. If the MTPJ is congruent, then do not perform soft tissue procedures which may make the joint incongruent; do not rely on soft tissue procedures to correct a bony deformity[3]
- Know your patient—systemic factors can affect your treatment outcomes and should influence your treatment choices.

We have proposed a treatment algorithm for surgical treatment of JHV (**Fig. 11**). When assessing a patient for consideration of surgical treatment of their JHV, it is imperative to have good quality standing AP and standing lateral radiographs of the involved foot. Skeletal maturity is the first consideration, and this is based on the patency of the proximal first metatarsal physis. If this physis is still open, then the patient is considered "skeletally immature" and if this physis is closed, then they are "skeletally mature."

For the skeletally immature patient, there is extra emphasis on consideration of nonoperative treatment until maturity is met as there is a higher recurrence rate in the skeletally immature population.[4,5] If surgery is nonetheless to be pursued, then avoiding osteotomies of the proximal first metatarsal physis is necessary to avoid unintended growth arrest. Lateral first metatarsal hemiepiphysiodesis can be considered if there is satisfactory growth remaining (typically at least 2 years more of growth). A medial cuneiform osteotomy with possible distal metatarsal osteotomy (if MTPJ is congruent and the DMAA is elevated) or soft tissue realignment (if MTPJ is incongruent and DMAA is normal). Finally, a SERI is a reasonable choice in the immature foot and creates minimal scarring in case further procedures are needed in the future.

For the skeletally mature patient, the next key consideration is the status of the patient. For adolescents who have hyperlaxity states (eg, Down's Syndrome or Ehlers-Danlos) or neuromuscular considerations (eg, cerebral palsy) and are low demand, then an MTPJ arthrodesis provides satisfactory and reliable correction. However, if patients are more normal in their soft tissue balance and are high demand, then the next key consideration is the congruency of the MTPJ. If the joint is congruent (almost assuredly with an elevated DMAA), then only bony procedures should be considered, or there is potential for making the joint incongruent. Then, if the IMA is elevated (which is typical), either multiple osteotomies, a Scarf osteotomy, or the SERI can be considered. If the IMA is low, then a distal only metatarsal osteotomy or the SERI could be considered. For very severe hallux valgus with a congruent joint, multiple osteotomies or a metatarsocuneiform arthrodesis (also known as a "Ludloff") are the available options. If the MTPJ is incongruent, the DMAA is low, and the deformity is relatively mild, then a proximal metatarsal osteotomy with a soft tissue lateral release is sufficient. However, in more severe cases of hallux valgus and incongruency, multiple osteotomies combined with distal soft tissue lateral release are recommended with the possibility of considering an arthrodesis in some cases.

AUTHOR'S PREFERRED METHODS

When conservative measures for the treatment of hallux valgus fail and surgical treatment is recommended, we generally follow the treatment algorithm proposed earlier. If the patient is skeletally immature, we have used the SERI with very satisfactory results although our long-term series is still in process. In patients with symptomatic PPV, this can also be combined with the SESA for a minimally invasive approach to the whole foot (see **Fig. 10**). The most common JHV patient with skeletal maturity has a congruent MTPJ, elevated DMAA, and elevated IMA. If they have only moderate deformity, then this can be addressed with either multiple or distal only osteotomies (eg,

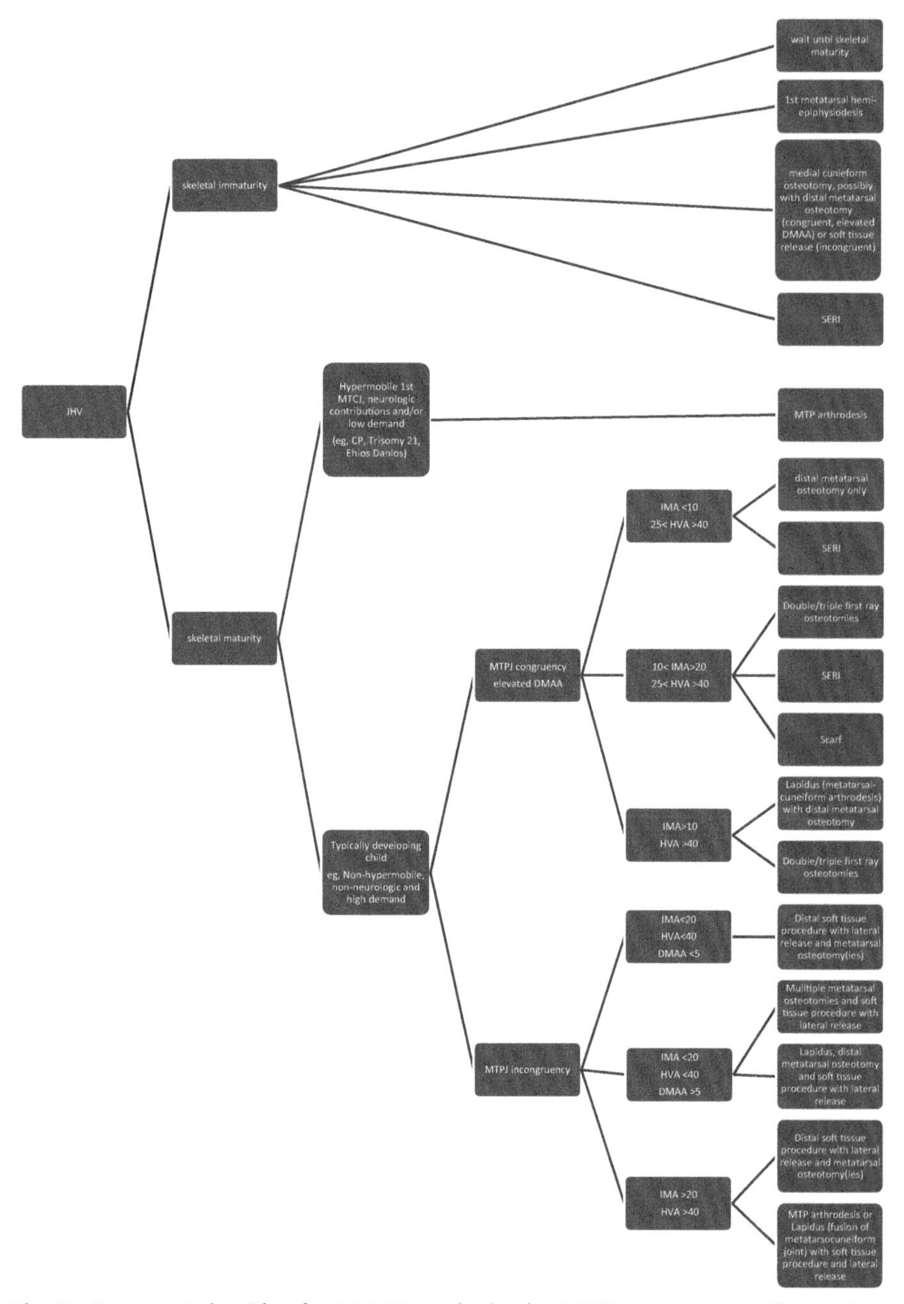

Fig. 11. Treatment algorithm for JHV. CP, cerebral palsy; MTCJ, metatarsocuneiform joint.

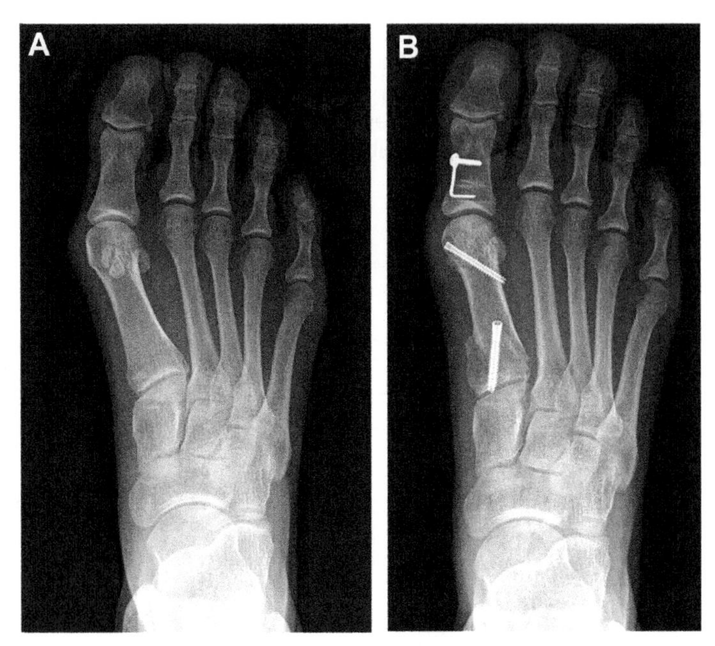

Fig. 12. (*A*) Treatment of moderate JHV with proximal metatarsal osteotomy, distal metatarsal osteotomy, and proximal phalanx osteotomy. (*B*) Satisfactory alignment was achieved.

SERI). More severe JHV typically needs either multiple osteotomies, and, if the MTPJ is incongruent, then a lateral release is necessary.[47] In this more severe JHV, one must measure the parallelism of the proximal phalanx because residual valgus of that bone left unaddressed can leave persistent, usually asymptomatic, deformity after correction is completed (**Fig. 12**).

CLINICS CARE POINTS

- Nonoperative care should be exhausted before procedural care. Delay surgical care until after skeletal maturity when possible. If surgical care is needed before skeletal maturity, be sure to use techniques that avoid unintended physeal injury.
- A thorough examination and understanding of the whole patient is necessary to appreciate systemic factors that may influence the outcome.
- When procedural care is determined necessary, proper imaging should be obtained and carefully measured. Careful assessment of the congruency of the metatarsophalangeal joint before surgical correction is imperative. Do not perform soft tissue procedures on bony-only deformity!
- Many surgical options are available and not all are appropriate in all situations. Understand the uniqueness of each foot and treat appropriately.
- More recent minimally invasive techniques show promise for improving outcomes and decreasing complications.

DISCLOSURE

The authors have nothing to disclose.

REFERENCES

1. Durlacher L. Art. XXVI.—A treatise on corns, bunions, and the diseases of nails, and the general management of the feet. Am J Med Sci 1846;7(21):183.
2. Stephens MM. Pathogenesis of hallux valgus. Foot Ankle Surg 1994;1(1):7–10.
3. Coughlin MJ. Hallux valgus. J Bone Joint Surg Am 1996;78(6):932–66.
4. Coughlin MJ. Roger A. Mann Award. Juvenile hallux valgus: etiology and treatment. Foot Ankle Int 1995;16(11):682–97.
5. Chell J, Dhar S. Pediatric hallux valgus. Foot Ankle Clin 2014;19(2):235–43.
6. Nix S, Smith M, Vicenzino B. Prevalence of hallux valgus in the general population: a systematic review and meta-analysis. J Foot Ankle Res 2010;3:21.
7. Coughlin MJ, Jones CP. Hallux valgus: demographics, etiology, and radiographic assessment. Foot Ankle Int 2007;28(7):759–77.
8. Piqué-Vidal C, Solé MT, Antich J. Hallux valgus inheritance: pedigree research in 350 patients with bunion deformity. J Foot Ankle Surg 2007;46(3):149–54.
9. Perera AM, Mason L, Stephens MM. The pathogenesis of hallux valgus. J Bone Joint Surg Am 2011;93(17):1650–61.
10. Kaiser P, Livingston K, Miller PE, et al. Radiographic evaluation of first metatarsal and medial cuneiform morphology in juvenile hallux valgus. Foot Ankle Int 2018; 46(3). 1071100718789696.
11. Banks A, Hsu Y, Mariash S, et al. Juvenile hallux abducto valgus association with metatarsus adductus. J Am Podiatr Med Assoc 1994;84(5):219–24.
12. Vyas S, Conduah A, Vyas N, et al. The role of the first metarsocuneiform joint in juvenile hallux valgus. J Pediatr Orthop B 2010;19(5):399–402.
13. Haines RW, McDougall A. The anatomy of hallux valgus. J Bone Joint Surg Br 1954;36-B(2):272–93.
14. Wilson DW. Treatment of hallux valgus and bunions. Br J Hosp Med 1980;24(6): 548–9.
15. Mortier J-P, Bernard J-L, Maestro M. Axial rotation of the first metatarsal head in a normal population and hallux valgus patients. Orthop Traumatol Surg Res 2012; 98(6):677–83.
16. Carl A, Ross S, Evanski P, et al. Hypermobility in hallux valgus. Foot Ankle Int 1988;8(5):264–70.
17. McNerney J, Johnston W. Generalized ligamentous laxity, hallux abducto valgus and the first metatarsocuneiform joint. J Am Podiatr Med Assoc 1979;69(1): 69–82.
18. Clark H, Veith R, Hansen S. Adolescent bunions treated by the modified Lapidus procedure. Bull Hosp Jt Dis Orthop Inst 1987;47(2):109–22. Available at: http://europepmc.org/abstract/MED/2825872.
19. Coughlin MJ. Hallux valgus in men: effect of the distal metatarsal articular angle on hallux valgus correction. Foot Ankle Int 1997;18(8):463–70.
20. Davids JR, Mason TA, Danko A, et al. Surgical management of hallux valgus deformity in children with cerebral palsy. J Pediatr Orthop 2001;21(1):89–94.
21. Sung W, Kluesner AJ, Irrgang J, et al. Radiographic outcomes following primary arthrodesis of the first metatarsophalangeal joint in hallux abductovalgus deformity. J Foot Ankle Surg 2010;49(5):446–51.
22. Wood EV, Walker CR, Hennessy MS. First metatarsophalangeal arthrodesis for hallux valgus. Foot Ankle Clin 2014;19(2):245–58.
23. Dietze A, Bahlke U, Martin H, et al. First ray instability in hallux valgus deformity: a radiokinematic and pedobarographic analysis. Foot Ankle Int 2013;34(1):124–30.

24. Barouk LS. The effect of gastrocnemius tightness on the pathogenesis of juvenile hallux valgus: a preliminary study. Foot Ankle Clin 2014;19(4):807–22.
25. Sung KH, Kwon S-S, Park MS, et al. Natural progression of radiographic indices in juvenile hallux valgus deformity. Foot Ankle Surg 2018;25(3):378–82.
26. Kim HW, Park KB, Kwak YH, et al. Radiographic assessment of foot alignment in juvenile hallux valgus and its relationship to flatfoot. Foot Ankle Int 2019;40(9):1079–86.
27. Kilmartin TE, Wallace WA. The significance of pes planus in juvenile hallux valgus. Foot Ankle 1992;13(2):53–6.
28. Faldini C, Nanni M, Traina F, et al. Surgical treatment of hallux valgus associated with flexible flatfoot during growing age. Int Orthop 2016;40(4):737–43.
29. Kilmartin TE, Barrington RL, Wallace WA. A controlled prospective trial of a foot orthosis for juvenile hallux valgus. J Bone Joint Surg Br 1994;76(2):210–4.
30. Groiso JA. Juvenile hallux valgus. A conservative approach to treatment. J Bone Joint Surg Am 1992;74(9):1367–74.
31. Coughlin MJ, Freund E. Roger A. Mann award. The reliability of angular measurements in hallux valgus deformities. Foot Ankle Int 2001;22(5):369–79.
32. Coughlin MJ, Mann RA. The pathophysiology of the juvenile bunion. Instr Course Lect 1987;36:123–36.
33. Harb Z, Kokkinakis M, Ismail H, et al. Adolescent hallux valgus: a systematic review of outcomes following surgery. J Child Orthop 2015;9(2):105–12.
34. Bia A, Guerra-Pinto F, Pereira BS, et al. Percutaneous osteotomies in hallux valgus: a systematic review. J Foot Ankle Surg 2018;57(1):123–30.
35. Agrawal Y, Bajaj SK, Flowers MJ. Scarf-Akin osteotomy for hallux valgus in juvenile and adolescent patients. J Pediatr Orthop B 2015;24(6):535–40.
36. John S, Weil L, Weil LS, et al. Scarf osteotomy for the correction of adolescent hallux valgus. Foot Ankle Spec 2010;3(1):10–4.
37. Farrar NG, Duncan N, Ahmed N, et al. Scarf osteotomy in the management of symptomatic adolescent hallux valgus. J Child Orthop 2012;6(2):153–7.
38. George HL, Casaletto J, Unnikrishnan PN, et al. Outcome of the scarf osteotomy in adolescent hallux valgus. J Child Orthop 2009;3(3):185–90.
39. Glazebrook M, Copithorne P, Boyd G, et al. Proximal opening wedge osteotomy with wedge-plate fixation compared with proximal chevron osteotomy for the treatment of hallux valgus: a prospective, randomized study. J Bone Joint Surg Am 2014;96(19):1585–92.
40. Petratos DV, Anastasopoulos JN, Plakogiannis CV, et al. Correction of adolescent hallux valgus by proximal crescentic osteotomy of the first metatarsal. Acta Orthop Belg 2008;74(4):496–502.
41. Chiodo CP, Schon LC, Myerson MS. Clinical results with the Ludloff osteotomy for correction of adult hallux valgus. Foot Ankle Int 2004;25(8):532–6.
42. Lynch FR. Applications of the opening wedge cuneiform osteotomy in the surgical repair of juvenile hallux abducto valgus. J Foot Ankle Surg 1995;34(2):103–23.
43. Mortimer JA, Bouchard M, Acosta A, et al. The biplanar effect of the medial cuneiform osteotomy. Foot Ankle Spec 2020;13(3):250–7.
44. Pochatko DJ, Schlehr FJ, Murphey MD, et al. Distal chevron osteotomy with lateral release for treatment of hallux valgus deformity. Foot Ankle Int 1994;15(9):457–61.
45. Grill F, Hetherington V, Steinböck G, et al. Experiences with the chevron (V) osteotomy on adolescent hallux valgus. Arch Orthop Trauma Surg 1986;106(1):47–51.

46. Jones KJ, Feiwell LA, Freedman EL, et al. The effect of chevron osteotomy with lateral capsular release on the blood supply to the first metatarsal head. J Bone Joint Surg Am 1995;77(2):197–204.
47. Schneider W. Distal soft tissue procedure in hallux valgus surgery: biomechanical background and technique. Int Orthop 2013;37(9):1669–75.
48. Shariff R, Attar F, Osarumwene D, et al. The risk of avascular necrosis following chevron osteotomy: a prospective study using bone scintigraphy. Acta Orthop Belg 2009;75(2):234–8.
49. Resch S, Stenström A, Gustafson T. Circulatory disturbance of the first metatarsal head after chevron osteotomy as shown by bone scintigraphy. Foot Ankle Int 1992;13(3):137–42.
50. Kaufmann G, Dammerer D, Heyenbrock F, et al. Minimally invasive versus open chevron osteotomy for hallux valgus correction: a randomized controlled trial. Int Orthop 2019;43(2):343–50.
51. Braito M, Dammerer D, Hofer-Picout P, et al. Proximal opening wedge osteotomy with distal chevron osteotomy of the first metatarsal for the treatment of moderate to severe hallux valgus. Foot Ankle Int 2019;40(1):89–97.
52. McDonald MG, Stevens DB. Modified mitchell bunionectomy for management of adolescent hallux valgus. Clin Orthop Relat Res 1996;332:163–9.
53. Canale PB, Aronsson DD, Lamont RL, et al. The Mitchell procedure for the treatment of adolescent hallux valgus. A long-term study. J Bone Joint Surg Am 1993;75(11):1610–8.
54. Weiner BK, Weiner DS, Mirkopulos N. Mitchell osteotomy for adolescent hallux valgus. J Pediatr Orthop 1997;17(6):781–4.
55. Giannini S, Faldini C, Nanni M, et al. A minimally invasive technique for surgical treatment of hallux valgus: simple, effective, rapid, inexpensive (SERI). Int Orthop 2013;37(9):1805–13.
56. Giannini S, Cavallo M, Faldini C, et al. The SERI distal metatarsal osteotomy and scarf osteotomy provide similar correction of hallux valgus. Clin Orthop Relat Res 2013;471(7):2305–11.
57. Coughlin MJ. Hallux valgus. Instr Course Lect 1997;46:357–91.
58. Meier PJ, Kenzora JE. The risks and benefits of distal first metatarsal osteotomies. Foot Ankle Int 1985;6(1):7–17.
59. Easley ME, Kelly IP. Avascular necrosis of the hallux metatarsal head. Foot Ankle Clin 2000;5(3):591–608.
60. Bai LB, Lee KB, Seo CY, et al. Distal chevron osteotomy with distal soft tissue procedure for moderate to severe hallux valgus deformity. Foot Ankle Int 2010;31(8):683–8.
61. Coughlin MJ, Carlson RE. Treatment of hallux valgus with an increased distal metatarsal articular angle: evaluation of double and triple first ray osteotomies. Foot Ankle Int 1999;20(12):762–70.
62. Smith BW, Coughlin MJ. Treatment of hallux valgus with increased distal metatarsal articular angle: use of double and triple osteotomies. Foot Ankle Clin 2009;14(3):369–82.
63. Jochymek J, Peterková T. Double osteotomy of the first metatarsal for treatment of juvenile hallux valgus deformity - our experience. Acta Chir Orthop Traumatol Cech 2016;83(1):32–7 [in Czech].
64. Johnson AE, Georgopoulos G, Erickson MA, et al. Treatment of adolescent hallux valgus with the first metatarsal double osteotomy: the denver experience. J Pediatr Orthop 2004;24(4):358–62.

65. Marshall TJ, Shung JR, Khoury JG. Adolescent hallux valgus revisited. Orthopedics 2014;37(8):531–5.
66. Shannak O, Sehat K, Dhar S. Analysis of the proximal phalanx size as a guide for an Akin closing wedge osteotomy. Foot Ankle Int 2011;32(4):419–21.
67. Herring JA. Disorders of the foot. In: Herring JA, Tachdjian MO, editors. Tachdjian's pediatric orthopaedics, vol. 2, 4th edition. Philadelphia: Saunders/Elsevier; 2007. p. 1166–72.
68. Mann RA, Katcherian DA. Relationship of metatarsophalangeal joint fusion on the intermetatarsal angle. Foot Ankle Int 1989;10(1):8–11.
69. Grace D, Delmonte R, Catanzariti AR, et al. Modified lapidus arthrodesis for adolescent hallux abducto valgus. J Foot Ankle Surg 1999;38(1):8–13.
70. Sabah Y, Rosello O, Clement JL, et al. Lateral hemiepiphysiodesis of the first metatarsal for juvenile hallux valgus. J Orthop Surg (Hong Kong) 2018;26(3). 2309499018801135.
71. Schlickewei C, Ridderbusch K, Breyer S, et al. Temporary screw epiphyseodesis of the first metatarsal for correction of juvenile hallux valgus. J Child Orthop 2018; 12(4):375–82.
72. Davids JR, McBrayer D, Blackhurst DW. Juvenile hallux valgus deformity: surgical management by lateral hemiepiphyseodesis of the great toe metatarsal. J Pediatr Orthop 2007;27(7):826–30.
73. Jeyaseelan L, Malagelada F. Minimally invasive hallux valgus surgery—A systematic review and assessment of state of the art. Foot Ankle Clin 2020;25(3):345–59.
74. Malagelada F, Sahirad C, Dalmau-Pastor M, et al. Minimally invasive surgery for hallux valgus: a systematic review of current surgical techniques. Int Orthop 2019;43(3):625–37.
75. Frigg A, Pellegrino A, Maquieira G. Minimally invasive versus open hallux valgus surgery. Foot Ankle Orthop 2018;3(3). 2473011418S00053.
76. De Pellegrin M, Moharamzadeh D, Strobl WM, et al. Subtalar extra-articular screw arthroereisis (SESA) for the treatment of flexible flatfoot in children. J Child Orthop 2014;8:479–87.
77. Schwitalle M, Karbowski A, Eckardt A. Hallux valgus in young patients: long-term results after McBride operation. Arch Orthop Trauma Surg 1997;116(6):412–4.
78. Resch S, Stenström A, Egund N. Proximal closing wedge osteotomy and adductor tenotomy for treatment of hallux valgus. Foot Ankle Int 1989;9(6): 272–80.

Ilizarov Technique in Severe Pediatric Foot Disorders

Alexander Kirienko, MD, Emiliano Malagoli, MD*

KEYWORDS

- Ilizarov • External fixator • Deformity correction • Foot disorders • Clubfoot
- Charcot-Marie-Tooth • Arthrogryposis

KEY POINTS

- The correct application of the Ilizarov technique starts from understanding and identifying the disorders.
- Ilizarov technique is usually used in relapsing deformities, in which there is poor soft-tissue quality or shortening of bone tissue.
- Ilizarov technique involves two strategies of treatment: closed or open progressive correction.
- Complications during treatment with Ilizarov method are frequent; however, in most cases, they do not compromise the result of the treatment.

INTRODUCTION

Typically, treatment with the Ilizarov method in pediatric foot disorders is reserved for those more complex, relapsing deformities or if there is a need for lengthening.[1–6]

The origin of the deformity can be different. They can be epiphenomena of syndromic diseases, isolated, congenital, or acquired, in the context of musculoskeletal, neuromuscular, and connective tissue disease or in posttraumatic pathologies.[7,8]

A complex deformity is typically multiplanar involving coronal, sagittal, and transverse planes. Foot disorders can be associated with deformities and shortening of the entire lower limb, which represent a simultaneous involvement followed by a treatment at different levels of deformity[9] (**Fig. 1**).

Surgical toolbox permits several approaches. The approaches can be roughly divided into two groups: soft tissue or bony surgery procedures.[2,10]

In cases of congenital clubfoot (CF), soft-tissue procedures using a circular external fixator can be applied in combination with the Ponseti method in relapsed CF in older children.[1] Thanks to spreading of the Ponseti method, the cases which need more aggressive surgery are considerably decreased in the last 20 years, but there are still

External Fixation Unit, Humanitas Clinical and Research Center IRCCS, Via Manzoni 56, Rozzano, Milan 20089, Italy
* Corresponding author.
E-mail address: emiliano.malagoli@gmail.com

Foot Ankle Clin N Am 26 (2021) 829–849
https://doi.org/10.1016/j.fcl.2021.07.009
1083-7515/21/

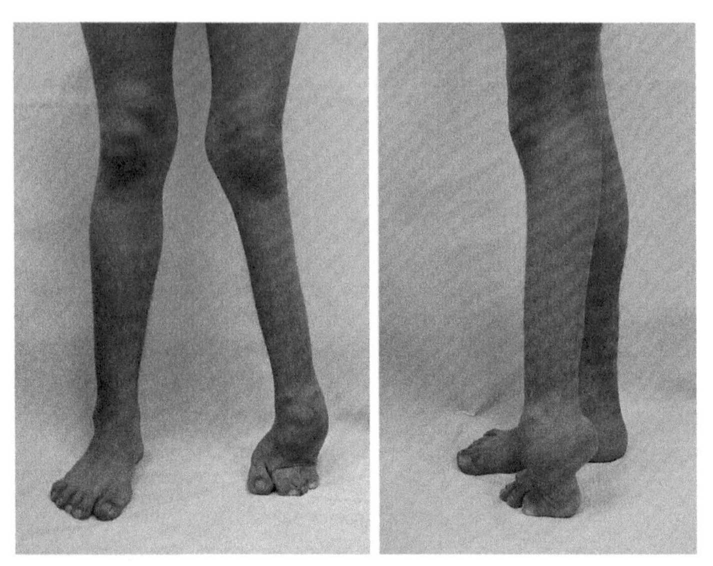

Fig. 1. Multiplanar foot deformity with more than one foot deformity and deformities and shortening of the entire associated lower limb.

patients who unfortunately show up for recurrence, residual deformities, or neglected CF which all have poor soft-tissue quality because of scarring of previous surgery.[1]

Conventional bone surgical corrections (eg, talectomy) often lead to foot shortening and joint stiffness.[11]

In this delicate background, the use of Ilizarov's method finds its space as the best treatment.[1,12]

The advantages of ring external fixation for correction of complex deformities of the foot and ankle include the possibility to correct severe deformities, perform gradual correction, modify treatment during correction, and minimize neurovascular damage. External fixation can provide opportunities to operate on scarred and contracted tissues, preserve joints and joint function, maintain or gain foot length, and allow weight-bearing during treatment.[13–15]

We are aware that a best treatment derives first from an accurate study and evaluation of pathology including clinical history.

We agree with Mosca reporting that the decision to operate is more important than the incision (ie, the surgical technique) and that a "well-executed" operation for the right indication is far better for the patient than the "most skillfully executed operation in the history of surgery" for the wrong indication.[16]

CLINICAL EVALUATION AND IMAGING

Clinical Evaluation

Although the foot and ankle examination of pediatric population is essentially similar to that of the adult patient, there are subtle differences that are unique of a child's examination.[17]

Clinical evaluation of the musculoskeletal system should include 2 steps in both adults and children: the first on weight-bearing and analyzing gait, and the second without weight-bearing.

The examination should begin with gait assessment with a patient walking with and without shoes, followed by visual observation of the gait pattern which results in normal, antalgic, or indicative of neuromuscular disease.[18]

During knee examination, the patella should be evaluated resulting in straight position during midstance. An in-toe type of gait shows a negative angle of gait or adduction of the foot in the transverse plane relative to the line of progression.[19]

During gait analysis, we should evaluate if toe walking is present. Toe walking is commonly seen in early walkers because of the ankle allowing 20° to 30° of dorsiflexion. This dorsiflexion decreases to approximately 10° in adults. Abnormalities in this progression are most seen as gastrocnemius, soleus, or gastrosoleus equinus; bony/cartilaginous ankle block; pseudoequinus; or cavus deformity.[20]

In the presence of a decreased dorsiflexion, an assessment is important to differentiate true ankle equinus from a forefoot plantar flexion position (plantarflexion of first and fifth rays across the midfoot).

Deformities in one or more districts of the lower limb can develop, and a compensatory adjustment in adjacent joints is a common phenomenon.[21,22] During the non-weight-bearing examination, it is important to evaluate patients' joint position and range of motion. Muscle strength should be assessed to all muscle groups: plantarflexors, dorsiflexors, inverters, and everters of the foot.

The inspection could reveal the presence of important signs such as coffee and milk spots expression of neurofibromatosis type 1 or retracting scars deriving from burns or previous surgery. A thorough neurologic examination should be performed on every pediatric patient (**Fig. 2**).

Patients should be evaluated for any signs of or lower motor neuron lesion.[19]

Imaging

Imaging is a key component of diagnosis and follow-up.[23]

Five views are performed to allow appropriate preoperative planning and postoperative evaluation. These are standard anteroposterior (AP) and lateral projection of foot and ankle plus one special projection (Saltzman or Cobey).

In Saltzman projection of the foot, the calcaneus appears foreshortened compared with the long axial view of the same foot. This view allows an evaluation of the ankle joint as well as the calcaneus and tibia.[24,25]

Recent studies for radiographic assessment of hindfoot alignment recommended the long axial hindfoot view (Cobey's view) in bilateral stance.[25,26]

In each patient, the key angles have to be evaluated on radiographic images and compared with normal range values (N.V.): talocalcaneal, Kite angle, (N.V. 25°–45° on AP and 30°–50° on lateral view), calcaneal inclination angle, (N.V. 20°–30° on lateral view), Meary angle (N.V. 0°–4° on lateral view), and tibiocalcaneal angle (N.V. <90°).[23,25,27] In AP projection, the bisection of the calcaneus should be parallel to the middiaphyseal line and lateral to it by 5 to 10 mm[6,27] (**Fig. 3**).

After an accurate clinical physical examination and evaluation of X-ray imaging, the patient could undergo a computerized tomography (CT) to assess bone structures or MRI to better assess soft tissues.

Images in CT studies can be manipulated on computer to enhance tissue separations. CT allows a combined reconstruction of frontal, sagittal, and transverse planes to get a 3D model of the foot and ankle. Complex deformities can be evaluated through plastic models based on CT studies to fully understand preoperative situation[28] (**Fig. 4**).

MRI is very useful to identify the cartilage, blood vessels, and soft tissues, thanks to its superior contrast and spatial resolution. The disadvantages of MRI are the long-term acquisition of the sequences, the necessity of patients to collaborate, and the high costs of the examination. Anyway MRI is perfect to assess soft-tissue structures and joints and has become for some authors the examination of choice to further

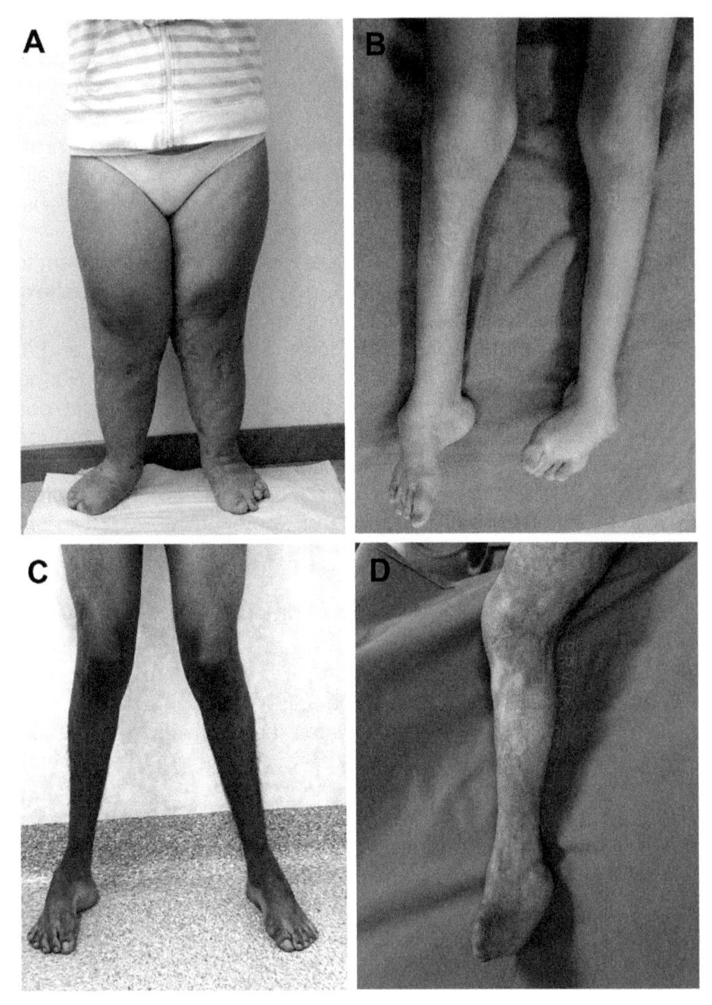

Fig. 2. Different foot pathologies and deformities in four patients. Typical flat foot deformity after leg lengthening in Ellis Van Creveld Syndrome. (*A*) Equinus-cavus-varus deformity in Arthrogryposis. (*B*) Equinus-cavus-varus deformity in Charcot-Marie-Tooth disease. (*C*). Foot deformity in burn contractures and scars (*D*).

evaluate patients with foot and ankle complaints and fully understand three-dimensionally the deformity.[29,30] One of the most popular abnormalities is tarsal-coalition in which the cartilaginous components are not always easy to detect.[31]

CLASSIFICATION OF FOOT DEFORMITY

Medical history and clinical and radiological evaluation allow the surgeon to choose the strategy of treatment as well as type of osteotomy.

Catagni and colleagues identified 5 treatment groups, and each corresponds to a particular construct with respect to the type of osteotomy. An advantage of this classification is undoubtedly the practical aspect; however, it lacks a specific reference to the type of deformity.[9]

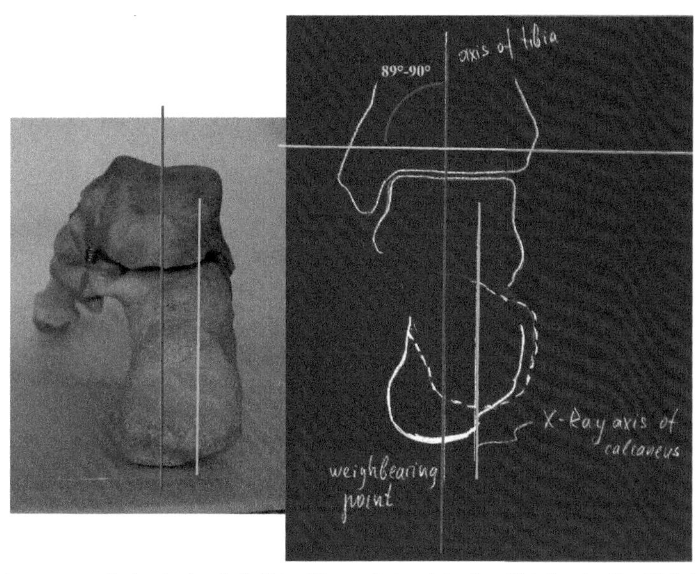

Fig. 3. Calcaneus radiological axis is 5 to 10 mm lateral to the tibial axis, the tibial anatomic axis instead corresponding to the weight-bearing point of the calcaneus.

Shalaby and Hefny developed their algorithm treatment.[21] Although the origin of the deformity may derive from different pathologies, they show convergence on the same patterns in which the treatment strategy is the same. Most of the severe long-standing deformities will fit the criteria for a V-osteotomy.[21]

Once again, it is imperative to perform an accurate assessment of each segmental deformities of the foot and ankle before planning the treatment steps. Anatomy of the deformities of foot segment and relative joints is analyzed as follows[16]:

1. Forefoot: pronated or supinated; plantar flexed (equinus) or dorsiflexed
2. Midfoot: abducted or adducted

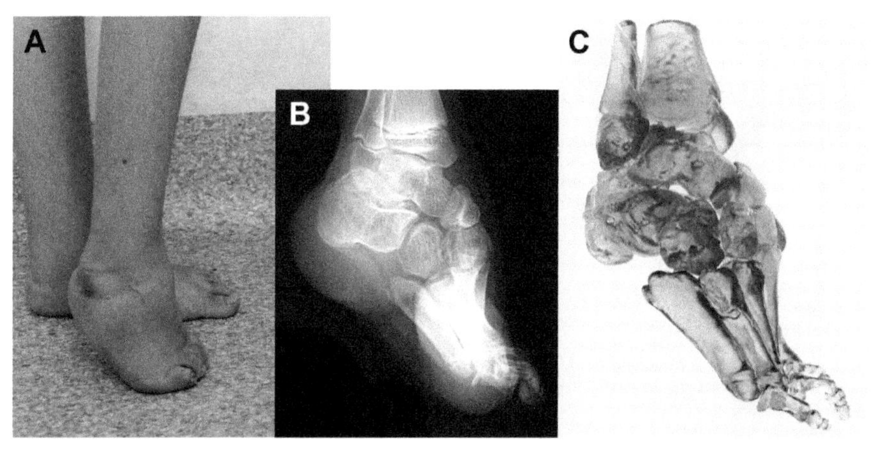

Fig. 4. Equinus-cavus-varus deformity, clinical view (*A*), X-ray (*B*), 3D printed model based on the CT study (*C*).

3. Hindfoot: varus/inverted or valgus/everted
4. Ankle: varus or valgus, plantar flexed (equinus) or dorsiflexed (calcaneus)

An ankle joint deformity may coexist with a foot deformity, or it may be an isolated deformity.

The deformity may involve bones or joints.[14]

THE ILIZAROV METHOD

Since the spread of the Ilizarov method in the world, the concepts of deformity correction and lengthening have been profoundly changed.

The advantages of ring external fixation include the possibility to correct severe deformities of foot and ankle, performing gradual correction, modifying treatment during correction, and minimizing neurovascular damage. External fixation technique allows foot correction on scarred and contracted tissues, preserving joints' structure and function, maintaining or gaining foot length, and allowing weight-bearing during treatment[13] (**Fig. 5**).

Principles and Treatment Strategies

The basic difference between the method of Ilizarov and others relates to the recognition that growth of a bone, previously cut in a minimally invasive manner, can be influenced by frequency and rate of distraction. This rate and frequency (1 mm/d divided in four times, 0.25 mm) did not exceed the physiologic limits for normal bone growth simulation.[13,32–35] The application of Ilizarov method to bones induces a rearrangement of soft tissues too; in fact, due to the distraction applied on bones, skin, vessels, nerves, connective tissue, and ligaments also reorganize their structure. This process is called distraction histogenesis and permits longitudinal elongation of these structures by cell proliferation.[32–36]

The aim of each treatment is to achieve a plantigrade, stable, and painless foot with a good function. Treatment strategies essentially depend on four factors: the age of

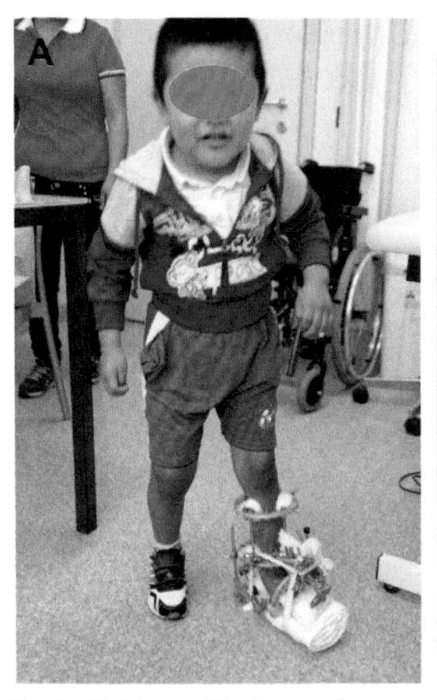

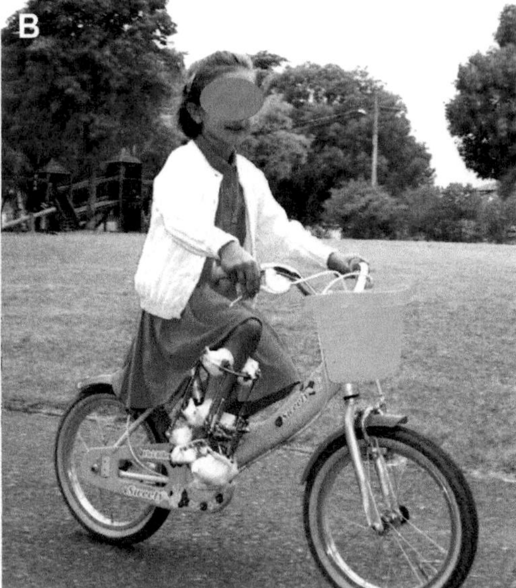

Fig. 5. Children with Ilizarov frame walking without crutches (*A*) and riding bicycle (*B*).

the child, the severity of the deformity, the stiffness of foot and ankle joints, and the etiology of the condition. There are three approaches to correct foot deformities in children with the Ilizarov frame: closed correction (based purely on distraction histogenesis), closed correction with soft-tissue release. and correction with osteotomy.[36]

Closed Correction and Closed Correction with Soft-Tissue Release

In the close correction method, the deformity is corrected by distracting the foot joints and their soft tissues, thus avoiding compressive forces across the joints. Differential distraction of soft tissues is a powerful technique to achieve correction. It can be used in younger patients (younger than 10 years) with mainly soft-tissue and joint contractures, rather than major bone deformities (**Fig. 6**). In these patients, the remaining potential of bone deformities remodeling achieving joints congruity is thought to occur by activation of the circumferential physis of these bones.[6,36]

In some patients, it could be necessary to associate distraction to the release of involved tendons.

For the correction of an equinus deformity, for example, Achilles tendon lengthening could be necessary.

Correction With Osteotomy

With this technique, the deformity is corrected directly through the osteotomy. Osteotomy distraction is preferred in children usually older than 10 years, in patients with neuromuscular imbalance in whom tendon transfers alone would not maintain correction, in severe stiff feet, and in case of previous fusions or nonunions.

Four basic distraction foot osteotomy levels have been described for correction of foot deformity: (1) supramalleolar (**Fig. 7**), (2) hindfoot, (3) midfoot, and (4) forefoot and combined hind and midfoot.[6,9,16,22] Supramalleolar osteotomies are indicated when there is a supramalleolar deformity; it can also be used for derotation and limb lengthening[6,9,22](**Fig. 8**).

Hindfoot osteotomies include osteotomies that involve the posterior region of calcaneus alone or below the subtalar joint, osteotomies between talus and calcaneus such as scythe-shaped talocalcaneal osteotomies (U osteotomies), Y osteotomies, the V-shaped osteotomy, and anterior talocalcaneal osteotomies (**Fig. 9**). Midfoot osteotomies are navicular-cuboid and cuboid-cuneiform osteotomies (**Fig. 10**). Forefoot osteotomies involve metatarsal bones and phalanges (**Table 1**).

Scythe-shaped talocalcaneal osteotomies, described by Ilizarov[32] and afterward by Paley,[36,37] passed under the subtalar joint through the superior part of the calcaneus and across the sinus tarsi through the neck of the talus. The osteotomy is performed using a 5–6-cm curved chisel. The indication for this type of osteotomy is the correction of equinus deformity with a rigid tibiotalar joint. Correction of supination or pronation of the foot associated with equinus deformity can also be achieved by medial or lateral lengthening osteotomy.

The scythe-shaped osteotomy is theoretically promising but is a difficult procedure to perform and can have significant complications.[3] The large size of the osteotomy may cause rapid consolidation due to the high friction during gliding of the bone fragments, which makes gradual correction difficult, and it does not lengthen the foot as the V osteotomy does.

The *V-shaped osteotomy* is a double osteotomy, proximally across the body of the calcaneus and distally across the neck of the talus or the midfoot. The two osteotomy cuts intersect at an acute angle of 60° to 70° at the plantar tip on the lower surface of the calcaneus. V osteotomy is indicated when there are deformities between the

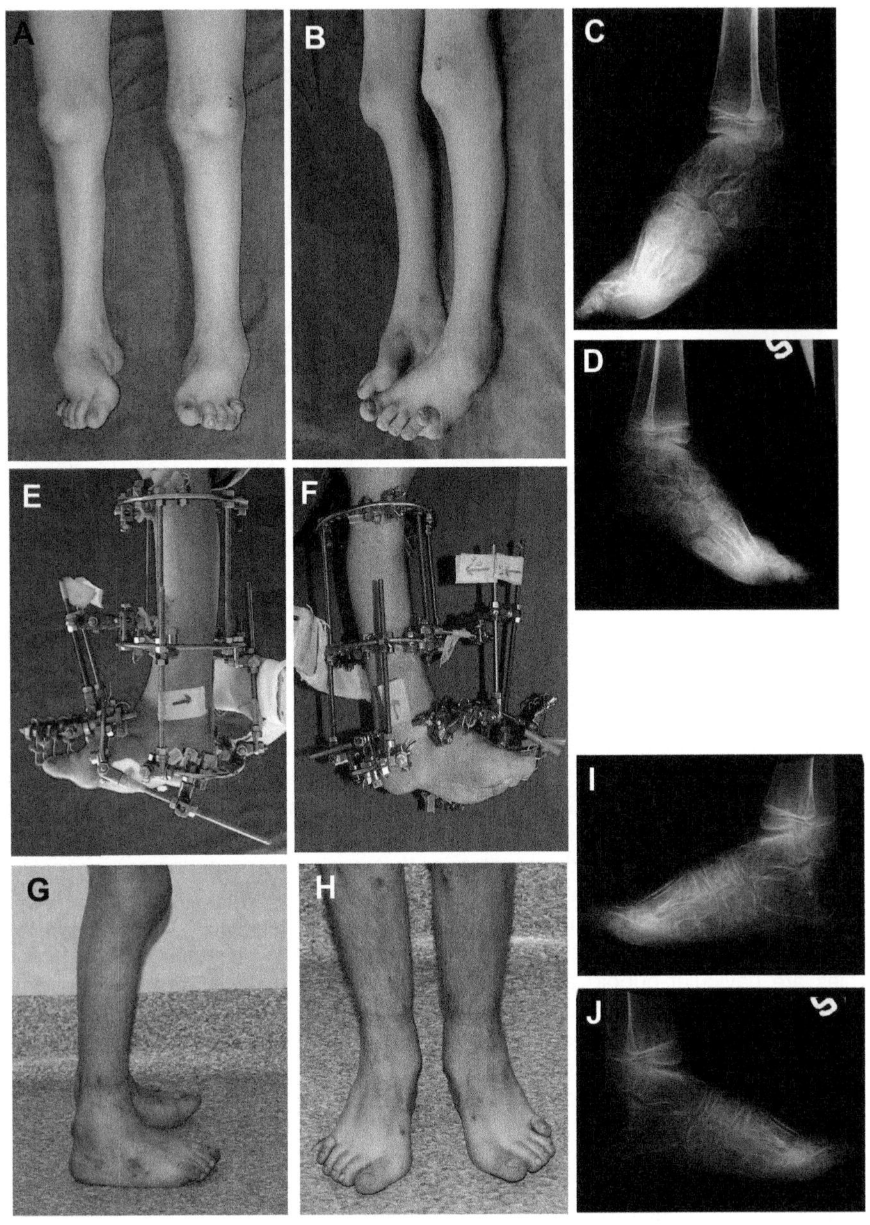

Fig. 6. Seven-year-old child with arthrogryposis. Severe, complex deformity of the right and left foot. Clinical view of right and the left foot before treatment (*A*, *B*). X-ray of the right (*C*) and left foot (*D*) before surgery. Progressive closed correction of both feet deformities (*E*, *F*). Clinical view of the feet after treatment (*G*, *H*). X-ray of right (*I*) and left foot (*J*) after treatment.

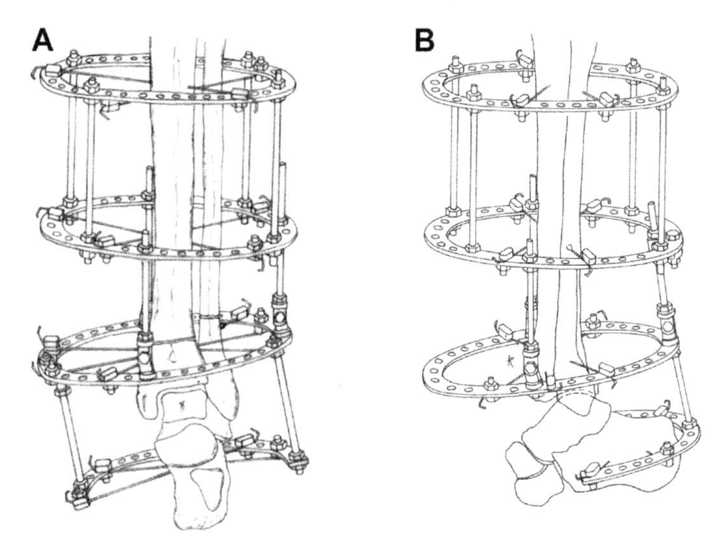

Fig. 7. Supramalleolar osteotomy. Frame construction for correction of valgus deformity of the ankle (*A*) and of procurvatum deformity (*B*). (With Permission of Taylor & Francis Group LLC – Books.)

hindfoot and forefoot. Essentially, all foot deformities can be corrected through this osteotomy[21] (**Fig. 11**).

The Y osteotomy is similar to V osteotomy but differs from it because the osteotomies of the calcaneus and the talar neck meet at an angle in the anterior calcaneus, forming a Y. This osteotomy is appropriate for the same clinical indications of the V osteotomy, but it avoids excessive lengthening of the foot.[6] Moreover, healing time is shorter because less bony regeneration is required.

The last two osteotomies both cross the subtalar joint and, hence, potentially stiffen it and should, therefore, only be performed if the subtalar joint is already stiff or fused. However, most subtalar joints in severe deformities are stiff or ankylosed anyway.

In performing an osteotomy, it is important to minimize thermal necrosis and periosteal damage by avoiding the use of motorized saws. The multiple drill hole and osteotome technique is commonly used in the calcaneus and neck of the talus.

An alternative way, particularly in midfoot, to avoid complications of neurovascular damage in open wedge osteotomy is to use the Gigli saw.[38]

The success of correction does not depend only on the final shape of the osteotomy but also on the realignment of the normal biomechanical angles of the foot and ankle. The osteotomy is a means of restoring these biomechanical angles. The relationship of these angles to one another must be considered when determining the success of correction.[6,39,40]

Operative Technique

Without doubt, the success of the Ilizarov method of treatment derives from the possibility of three-dimensional correction.[41] If the elongation capacity is added to the correction defined by the 3 anatomic planes, the use of the circular fixator as a joystick potentially allows to correct any deformity. Ilizarov developed components, which together act as a fulcrum. The positioning, orientation, and number of hinges are critical factors for deformity correction. The hinges, used in combination with distraction-

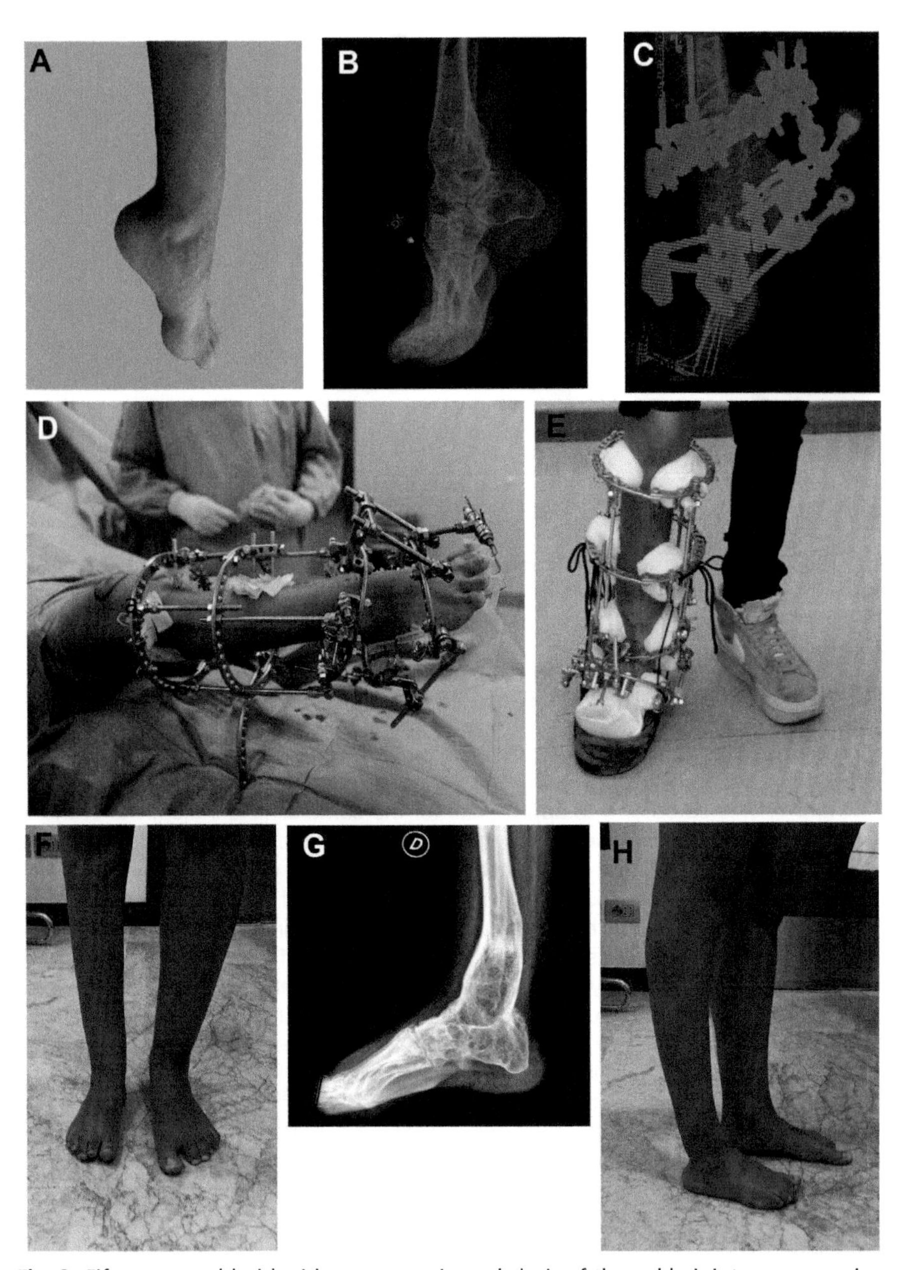

Fig. 8. Fifteen-year-old girl with postoperative ankylosis of the ankle joint, severe equinus and cavus deformity of the foot. Lateral view of the foot before surgery (*A*). X-rays showing tibiotalar arthrodesis (*B*). X-rays with Ilizarov frame after surgery (*C*). Ilizarov external fixator during correction of foot deformity and simultaneous leg lengthening (*D*). Walking patient with frame and sole at the end of correction (*E*). Frontal clinical view after correction (*F*). Radiological evaluation after 6 months at follow-up (*G*). Lateral clinical view showing plantigrade foot (*H*).

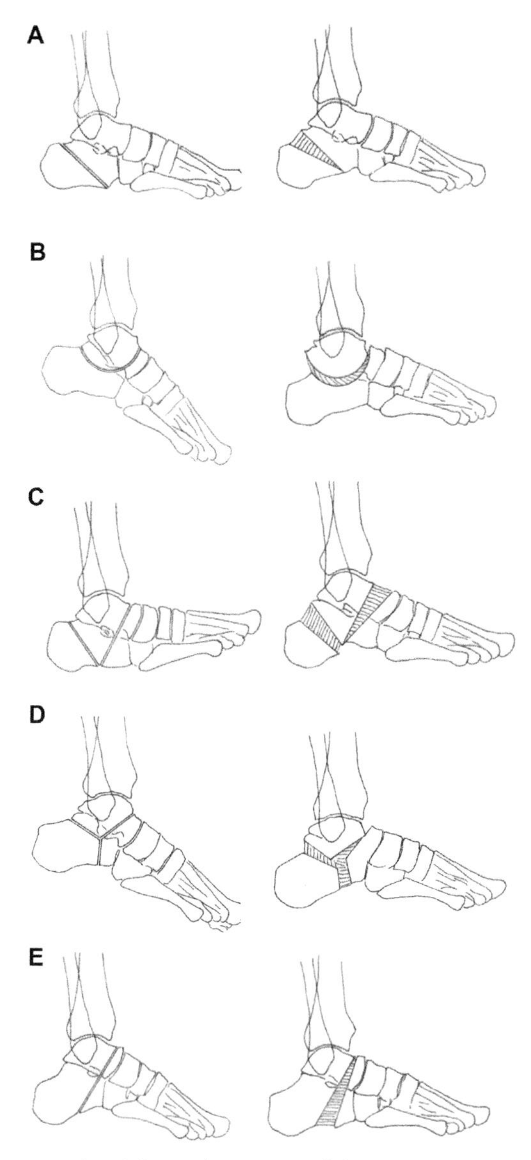

Fig. 9. Hindfoot osteotomies. Calcaneal osteotomy (*A*). Scythe-shaped talocalcaneal osteotomy (*B*). V osteotomy (*C*). Y osteotomy (*D*). Anterior talocalcaneal osteotomy (*E*). (With Permission of Taylor & Francis Group LLC – Books.)

compression devices (graduated telescopic rods), lead to gradual correction of deformities, with simultaneous transformation of the bones and soft tissues. The position of the hinges typically correspond to what was subsequently called Paley CORA (center of rotation of angulation)[22]

To follow, we described two techniques to correct similar deformities.

The first is a closed treatment of a combination of two deformities: cavus and equinus foot. Closed treatment is more suitable for complex cases in younger patients and for recurrence after previous surgical treatment.

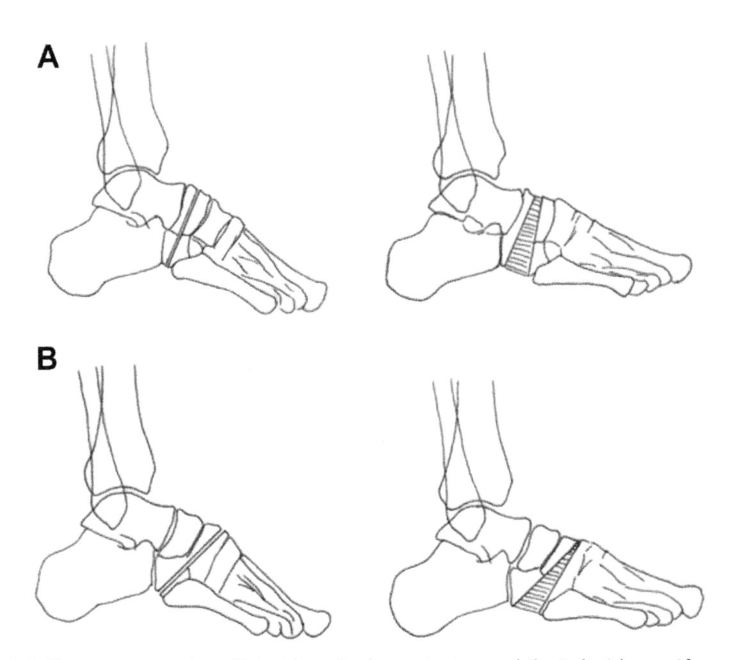

Fig. 10. Midfoot osteotomies. Cuboid-navicular osteotomy (*A*). Cuboid-cuneiform osteotomy (*B*). (With Permission of Taylor & Francis Group LLC – Books.)

The medial and lateral plantar rods are lengthened 1 mm per day. The cavus deformity is corrected by distraction of the foot bones between the two-half rings. The posterior rod is lengthened 1 mm per day while the two middle rods are kept static so that the equinus hindfoot is corrected. The anterior rods can be compressed up to 3 mm per day. The effect of the tractional forces causes the rotation of the talus into a dorsiflexed position. The difference between the calcaneal distraction and the anterior compression corrects the cavus deformity. Once the calcaneal half ring is at a right angle to the tibia, the posterior lengthening is stopped. The correction of anterior cavus deformity goes on by lengthening of the medial and lateral plantar rods by 1 mm and continuing the anterior compression of 2 mm per day. The forces in the metatarsals are transmitted to the talus through the midfoot with only the extremities fixed (calcaneus and metatarsals); the intermediate elements are mobile (talus and midfoot). Once correction has been achieved, the usual treatment protocol is resumed. Clinical example is described in **Fig. 12**.

The second approach is an open treatment for severe combined cavus and equinus deformity.

Open treatment is needed for rigid deformities in adolescents and adults. Correction is necessary using osteotomies that have been described before. An oblique calcaneus osteotomy is used to lengthen and correct a vertical talus deformity while a cuneiform-cuboid osteotomy is used to correct cavus and equinus deformity of the forefoot (**Fig. 13**). The osteotomy should be performed by percutaneous technique with a straight osteotome from two small lateral incisions. Cut olive K-wire (Rein wires) are inserted inside osteotomy for multiple reasons. Rein wires are useful to fix bone fragments of the cuboid and cuneiform, to guarantee the distraction of osteotomy site, and to prevent both premature consolidation and diastasis of Chopart and Lisfranc joints. There are no differences in the frame assembly between open and closed treatment. Two opposing olive wires or one wire and one half-pin are placed into the

Table 1
Classification of foot osteotomies

Calcaneal osteotomies	• Osteotomies of the posterior calcaneus • Osteotomy below the subtalar joint
Talocalcaneal osteotomies	• Anterior talocalcaneal osteotomies • Scythe-shaped talocalcaneal osteotomies • V osteotomies • Y osteotomies
Midfoot osteotomies	• Navicular-cuboid osteotomies • Cuneiform-cuboid osteotomies
Forefoot osteotomies	• Metatarsal osteotomies • Phalanges osteotomies

talus body and attached to the leg support. Pinning of the toes with K-wires should be performed to prevent claw-toe deformity.

Correction is initiated on the third or fourth day after surgery. The appropriate rods between the leg support and the half rings should be lengthened 1 to 1.5 mm per day; the rods between the leg support and the metatarsal half ring should be compressed 1 to 1.5 mm per day. The goal is to distract the osteotomies to create the space necessary for corrective movement of the bony segments and to prevent premature consolidation. After 1 week, radiographs are taken to evaluate how the distraction is progressing and the tibiotalar joint for possibly occurring subluxations. The period of fixation lasts approximately 45 days. The frame is removed as soon as consolidation occurs, then progressive weight-bearing with crutches is initiated.

NEW MODIFICATIONS OF ILIZAROV TECHNIQUE

The development of the Taylor spatial frame (TSF) in 1994 (Smith and Nephew, Memphis, TN) used the principles of the Stewart Gough platform incorporating six struts of adjustable length that could allow simultaneous six-axis deformity correction.[42] There are now several hexapod systems on the market. The concept of placement of a virtual hinge and the ability to rerun correction programs have resulted in an extremely versatile weapon in the limb reconstruction surgeon's armory. The spatial frame was stated to be more stable than a "4-threaded rod" Ilizarov frame during axial, bending, and torsional force testing. There are some limitations in the system, including fixed position of the fast-fix struts and reduced stability associated with lower strut angles.[43–45] There are other hexapod fixators that enable the struts to have a greater variation in position on the rings, such as the TL-Hex system (Orthofix, Verona, Italy).[4] Since the turn of the century, the literature has confirmed the worldwide appeal of the TSF.[43–47] There is a universal agreement that the hexapod offers versatility and is tolerated by the patient with accurate deformity correction. Based on the mechanical advantages, most authors demonstrated excellent results using only two-ring construct and a combination of wires and half-pins. Sluga and colleagues specifically commented that no instability was noted in their patient constructs.[46] One limitation highlighted by Eidelman and colleagues is the inability to dynamize the frame.[47] Removal of one of the struts results in loss of frame stability. They suggested replacing the struts with Ilizarov threaded rods which would enable dynamization and gradual reduction of frame stability, if required, during the bone consolidation period.[15]

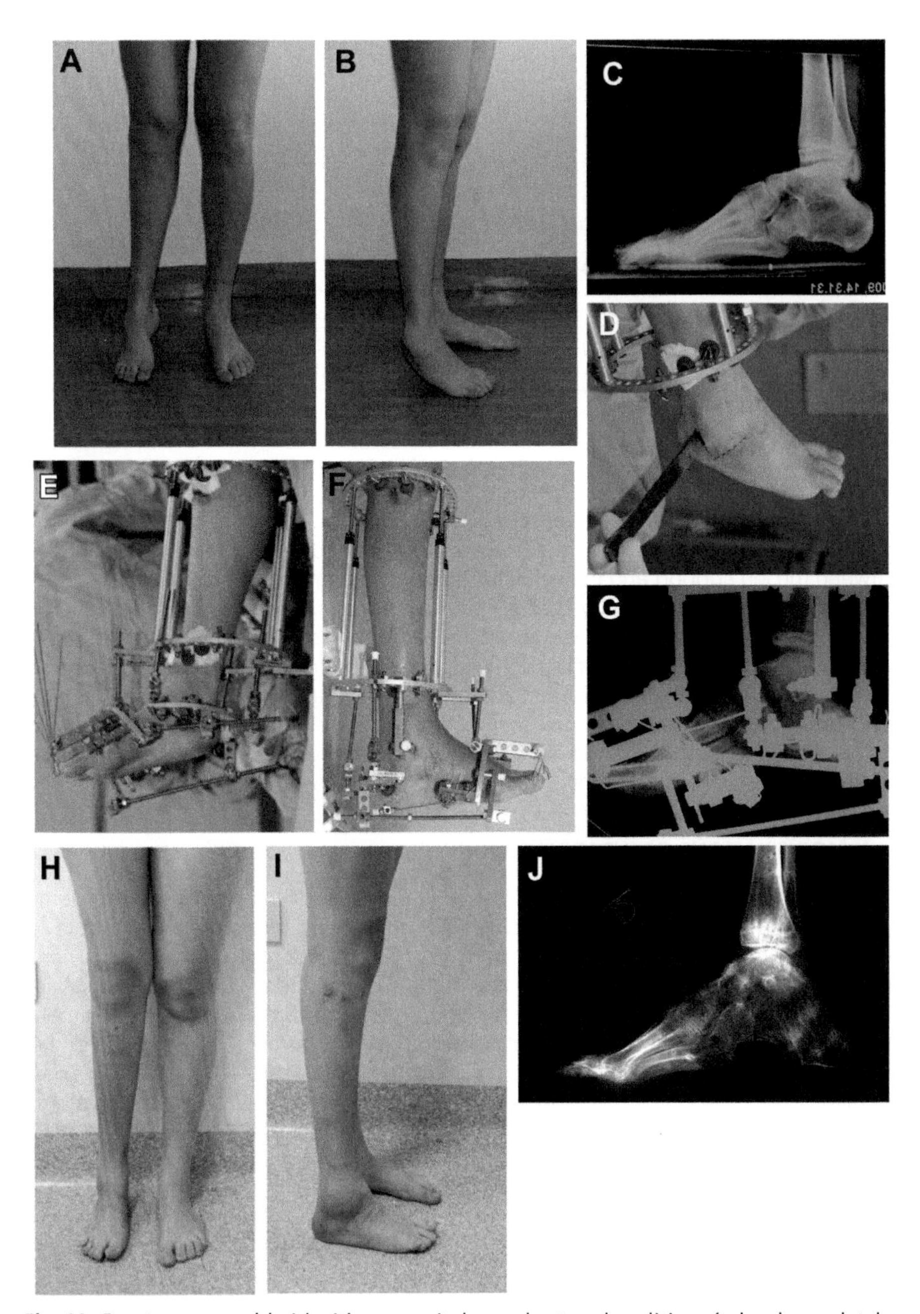

Fig. 11. Fourteen-year-old girl with congenital complex tarsal coalitions (talocalcaneal, talonavicular, and calcaneal-cuboid). Clinical view before treatment (*A*, *B*). X-ray (*C*). Intraoperative approach with osteotome and external fixator (*D*). Clinical view at the end of surgical procedure (*E*) and at follow-up (*F*). Radiological evaluation during distraction phase achieving deformity correction and foot lengthening (*G*). Clinical (*H*, *I*) and radiological (*J*) outcome.

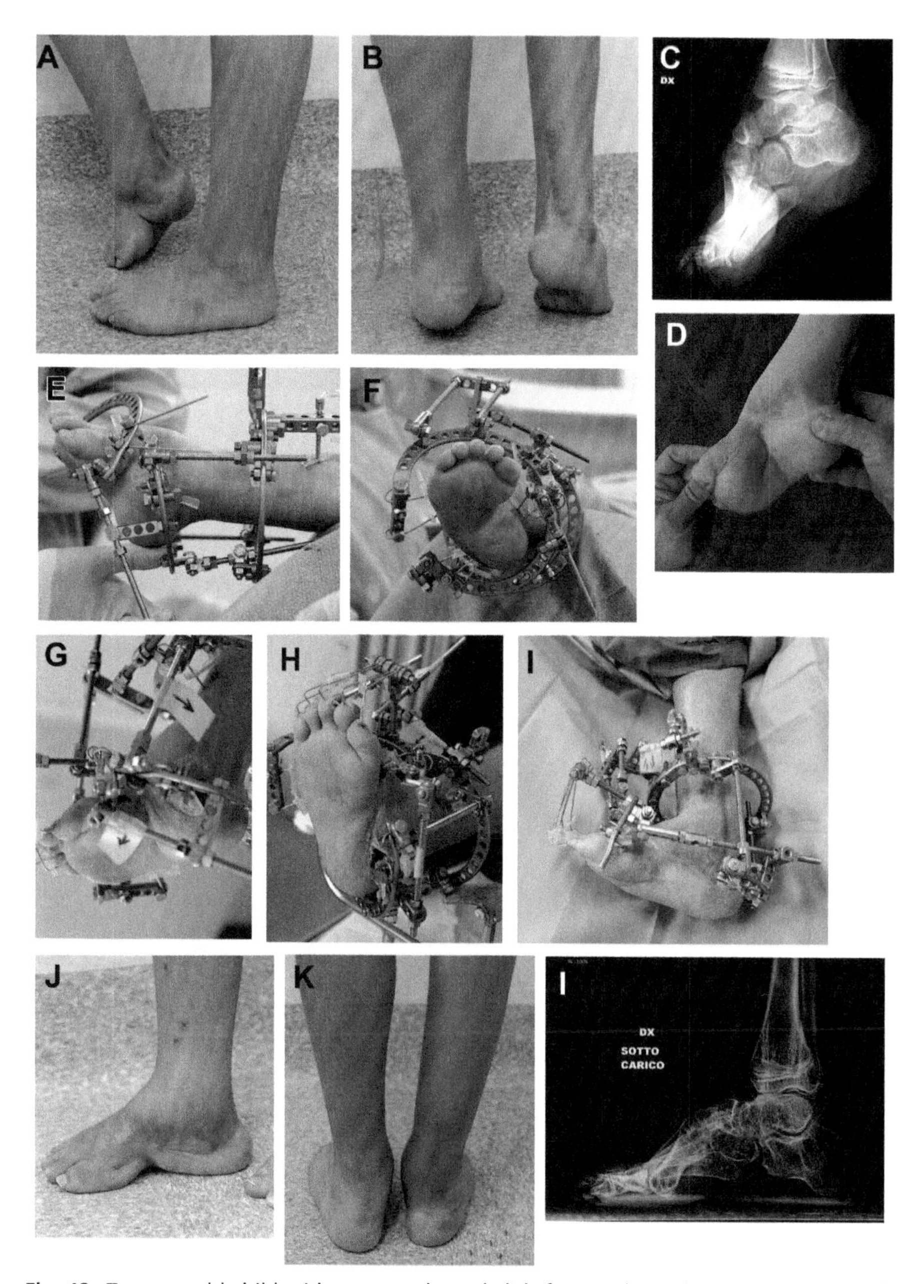

Fig. 12. Ten-year-old child with severe relapsed club foot and massive postoperative soft-tissue scars. Closed correction. Clinical (*A*, *B*) and radiological (*C*) view of the right foot before treatment. Maximum passive correction of adduction before surgery (*D*). Closed gradual correction of the foot deformities with hinged constrain frame (*E*, *F*). Planned over-correction of all components of the deformity (*G*, *H*). Note the distracted and lengthened scars medially (*I*). Clinical view (*J*, *K*) and weight-bearing X-ray (*L*) after treatment.

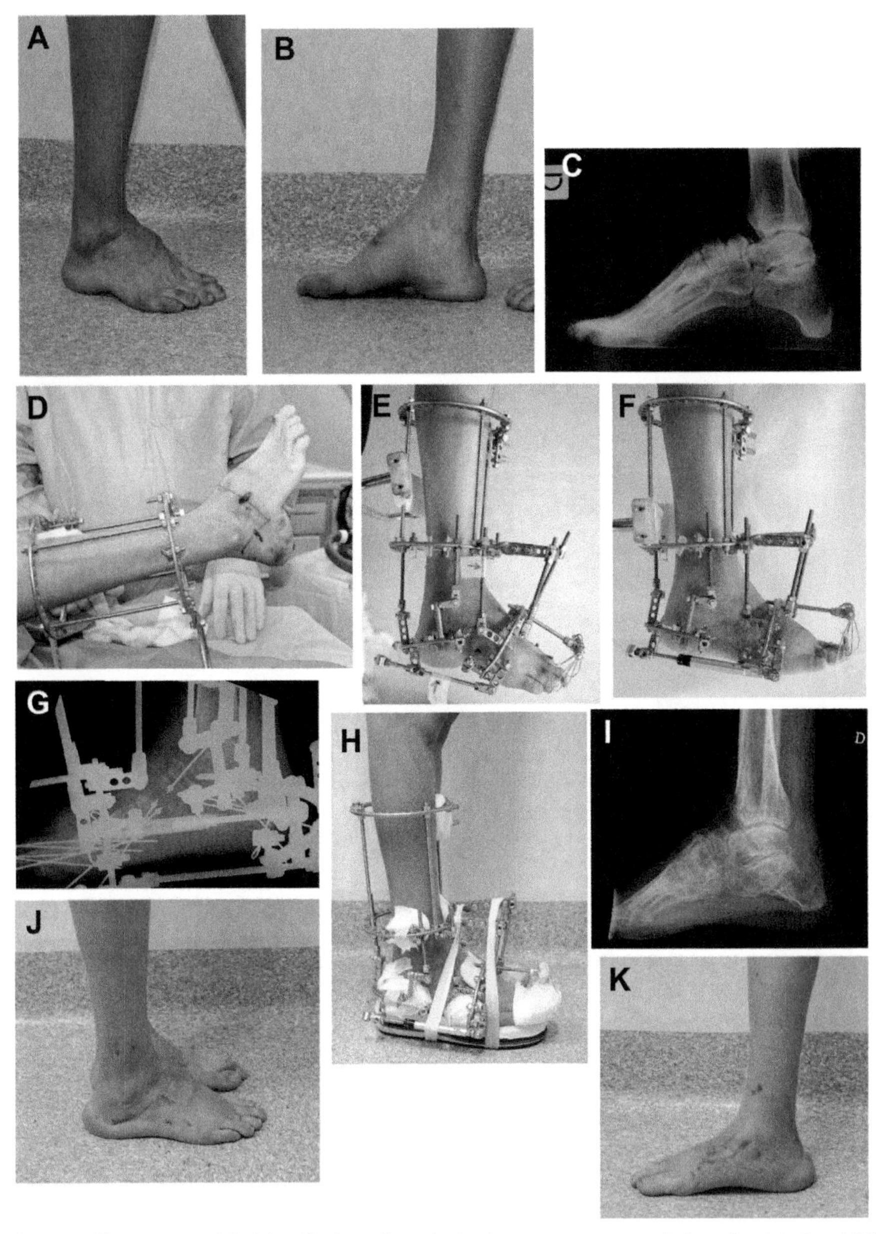

Fig. 13. Fifteen-year-old girl suffering of vertical calcaneus, cavus, and short foot. Lateral (*A*) and medial (*B*) view of the foot before surgery. Lateral X-ray showing vertical calcaneus and cavus deformity at the level of midfoot (*C*). Small skin incisions for calcaneus and cuboid-cuneiform osteotomy (*D*). Ilizarov frame after 10 days of distraction (*E*) and at the end of foot deformity correction and lengthening (*F*). Lateral X-ray during correction; note the cut rein olive wires inside of cuboid-cuneiform osteotomy (*G*). Patient during treatment with sole for walking at the end of correction (*H*). Radiological lateral view of the foot at 4-month follow-up (*I*). Lateral and medial clinical view at follow-up showing plantigrade foot (*J*, *K*).

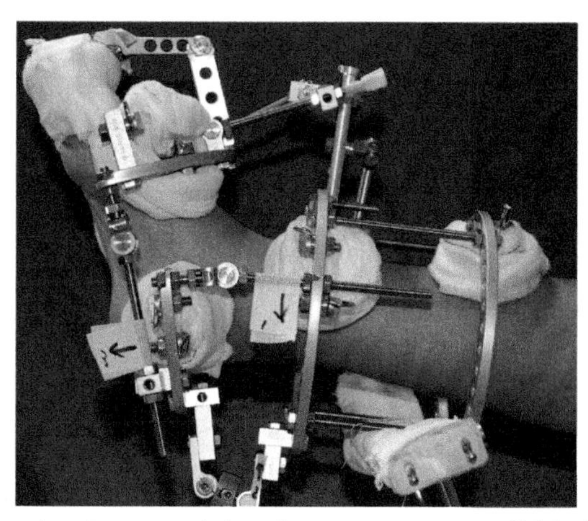

Fig. 14. Compressive dressing around the wires to prevent superficial wires infection.

The hexapod system of external fixation seeks to simplify the principles underlying the Ilizarov method. However, in dealing with a complex deformity, it is essential to master the basic principles of deformity correction beyond the hardware that you prefer to use to obtain the result.

In the specific case, the treatment of complex deformities in pediatric age, besides the circular external fixation with hexapod, requires very often bulky constructs.[4]

COMPLICATIONS

Many complications may arise during the long course of treatment with the Ilizarov technique.

Most complications, however, are preventable or correctable and will not interfere with successful results of treatment.[36,48] Complications of the Ilizarov technique can be classified as (1) general, due to the method; (2) specific, related to technique; and (3) inflammatory.[41]

According to Paley, complications can be divided into 2 groups, problems and obstacles.[48] The first arises during distraction or fixation period which is fully resolved by the end of treatment by nonoperative means. The second is fully resolved by operative treatment at the end of distraction or fixation period by operative means[48]

By timing criteria, the complications can be immediate or delayed. The immediate ones are generally related to a surgical act (eg, vascular-nerve injuries due to the penetration of a wire). Intraoperative neurovascular injury can be avoided by following safe anatomic windows while inserting wires.[49] Complications that occur late usually after the patient is discharged may be due to surgery (eg, incomplete osteotomy with premature healing) or correction (nerve injury due to excessive stretching). Some authors suggest preventive execution of tarsal canal release during equine and varus deformity correction.[50] For these reasons, it is mandatory to check the patient periodically every 2 weeks at least until the correction phase is over.

One of the most frequent complications is certainly the superficial infection of wires. This may be due to both an incorrect skin tension during the surgery and, more frequently, the tension generated by the correction.

Paley in his case series on treatment of foot deformity with external fixator reported that one pin-track infection of superficial nature occurred in every patient during their

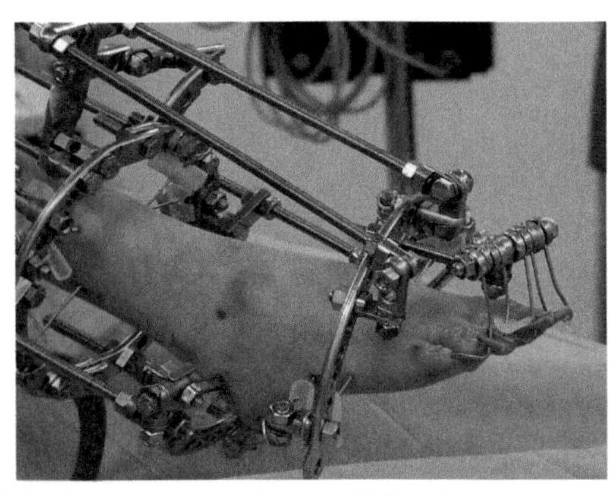

Fig. 15. Pinning of the toes to prevent claw toe deformity.

treatment. Pin-tract problems are related to major areas of tension at the interface with skin, often observed in the metatarsal wires. Superficial pin-tract infections are managed with regular pin-site care (**Fig. 14**) and oral antibiotics.[36]

Muscle contracture due to imbalance of agonist-antagonist muscle strength could generate new deformities (eg, the development of claw fingers due to the correction of a deformity in cavus). For this reason, the advice is to perform prophylactic K-wiring of the toes which helps to reduce this complication (**Fig. 15**). Epiphysiolysis is rare and often noted in rigid deformities. Choi and colleagues advocated a transepiphyseal wire to prevent it, but there is a risk of septic arthritis caused by pin-tract infection.[51]

Particular attention during assembling of apparatus should be given to speed of correction in equinus deformity to avoid subluxation of ankle.[6]

The possibility of complications must be explained fully to the patient before treatment is begun. This is especially important because the patients (or their parents) actively participate in the process of treatment.

DISCLOSURE

The authors have nothing to disclose.

REFERENCES

1. Eidelman M, Kotlarsky P, Herzenberg JE. Treatment of relapsed, residual and neglected clubfoot: adjunctive surgery. J Child Orthop 2019;13(3):293–303.
2. Uglow MG, Kurup HV. Residual clubfoot in children. Foot Ankle Clin 2010;15(2):245–64.
3. Dhar S. Ilizarov external fixation in the correction of severe pediatric foot and ankle deformities. Foot Ankle Clin 2010;15(2):265–85.
4. Riganti S, Coppa V, Nasto LA, et al. Treatment of complex foot deformities with hexapod external fixator in growing children and young adult patients. Foot Ankle Surg 2019;25(5):623–9.
5. Matar HE, Beirne P, Bruce CE, et al. Treatment of complex idiopathic clubfoot using the modified Ponseti method: up to 11 years follow-up. J Pediatr Orthop B 2017;26(2):137–42.
6. Kirienko A, Villa A, Calhoun JH. Ilizarov technique for complex foot and ankle deformities. New York: Marcel Dekker; 2004. p. 461.

7. Seaman TJ, Ball TA. Pes Cavus. In: StatPearls [Internet]. Treasure Island (FL: StatPearls Publishing; 2020.
8. Dobbe AM, Gibbons PJ. Common paediatric conditions of the lower limb. J Paediatr Child Health 2017;53(11):1077–85.
9. Catagni MA, Guerreschi F, Manzotti A, et al. Treatment of foot deformities using the Ilizarov method. Foot Ankle Surg 2000;6(4):207–37.
10. Chen ZY, Wu ZY, An YH, et al. Soft tissue release combined with joint-sparing osteotomy for treatment of cavovarus foot deformity in older children: analysis of 21 cases. World J Clin Cases 2019;7(20):3208–16.
11. Langan T, Lalli TAJ, Smith CN, et al. Talectomy as part of chronic foot and ankle deformity correction procedure: a retrospective study. J Foot Ankle Surg 2020; 59(1):16–20.
12. Tecimel O, Öçgüder A, Doğan M, et al. Ilizarov external fixator for correction of complex foot deformities. Eklem Hastalik Cerrahisi 2013;24(2):72–6.
13. Grant AD, Atar D, Lehman WB. The Ilizarov technique in correction of complex foot deformities. Clin Orthop Relat Res 1992;280:94–103.
14. Beaman DN, Gellman R. The basics of ring external fixator application and care. Foot Ankle Clin 2008;13(1):15–27, v.
15. Calder PR, Faimali M, Goodier WD. The role of external fixation in paediatric limb lengthening and deformity correction. Injury 2019;50(Suppl 1):S18–23.
16. Mosca VS. Principles and management of pediatric foot and ankle deformities and malformations. Philadelphia: Lippincott Williams & Wilkins; 2014.
17. Uden H, Scharfbillig R, Causby R. The typically developing paediatric foot: how flat should it be? A systematic review. J Foot Ankle Res 2017;10:37.
18. Warnock AM, Raducanu R, DeHeer PA. Lower extremity pediatric history and physical examination. Clin Podiatr Med Surg 2013;30(4):461–78.
19. Valmassy RL. Clinical biomechanics of the lower extremities. St Louis (MO): Mosby; 1996. p. 149. Chapter 7, Gait evaluation in clinical biomechanics, by C.C. Southerland Jr.
20. Whitney AK, Green DR. Pseudoequinus. J Am Podiatry Assoc 1982;72(7): 365–71.
21. Shalaby H, Hefny H. Correction of complex foot deformities using the V-osteotomy and the Ilizarov technique. Strateg Trauma Limb Reconstr 2007;2(1):21–30.
22. Paley D. Principles of deformity correction. New York: Springer-Verlag Berlin Heidelberg; 2002.
23. Winfeld MJ, Winfeld BE. Management of pediatric foot deformities: an imaging review. Pediatr Radiol 2019;49(12):1678–90.
24. Saltzman CL, el-Khoury GY. The hindfoot alignment view. Foot Ankle Int 1995; 16(9):572–6.
25. Reilingh ML, Beimers L, Tuijthof GJ, et al. Measuring hindfoot alignment radiographically: the long axial view is more reliable than the hindfoot alignment view. Skeletal Radiol 2010;39(11):1103–8.
26. Cobey JC. Posterior roentgenogram of the foot. Clin Orthop Relat Res 1976;118: 202–7.
27. Mendicino RW, Catanzariti AR, Reeves CL, et al. A systematic approach to evaluation of the rearfoot, ankle, and leg in reconstructive surgery. J Am Podiatr Med Assoc 2005;95(1):2–12.
28. Staheli LT. Fundamentals of pediatric orthopedics. Philadelphia: Lippincott Williams & Wilkins; 2008.
29. Harty MP, Hubbard AM. MR imaging of pediatric abnormalities in the ankle and foot. Magn Reson Imaging Clin N Am 2001;9(3):579–602, xi.

30. Hintermann B. What the orthopaedic foot and ankle surgeon wants to know from MR Imaging. Semin Musculoskelet Radiol 2005;9(3):260–71.
31. Lucas P, Kaplan P, Dussault R, et al. MRI of the foot and ankle. Curr Probl Diagn Radiol 1997;26(5):209–66.
32. Ilizarov GA. The principles of the Ilizarov method. Bull Hosp Jt Dis Orthop Inst 1988;48(1):1–11.
33. Ilizarov GA. The tension-stress effect on the genesis and growth of tissues. Part I. The influence of stability of fixation and soft-tissue preservation. Clin Orthop Relat Res 1989;(238):249–81.
34. Ilizarov GA. The tension-stress effect on the genesis and growth of tissues: Part II. The influence of the rate and frequency of distraction. Clin Orthop Relat Res 1989;(239):263–85.
35. Paley D. Current techniques of limb lengthening. J Pediatr Orthop 1988;8(1): 73–92.
36. Paley D. The correction of complex foot deformities using Ilizarov's distraction osteotomies. Clin Orthop Relat Res 1993;(293):97–111.
37. Gourdine-Shaw MC, Lamm BM, Paley D, et al. Distraction osteogenesis for complex foot deformities: U-osteotomy with external fixation. J Bone Joint Surg Am 2012;94(15):1420–7.
38. Lamm BM, Gourdine-Shaw MC, Thabet AM, et al. Distraction osteogenesis for complex foot deformities: gigli saw midfoot osteotomy with external fixation. J Foot Ankle Surg 2014;53(5):567–76.
39. Solomin LN, Ukhanov KA, Kirienko AP, et al. Foot deformity correction planning in the sagittal plane based on the vitruvian foot first metatarsal anatomic axis. J Foot Ankle Surg 2020;59(4):774–80.
40. Solomin LN, Ukhanov KA, Kirienko AP, et al. New sagittal plane reference parameters for foot deformity correction planning: the vitruvian foot. J Foot Ankle Surg 2019;58(5):865–9.
41. Golyakhovsky V, Frankel VH. Textbook of Ilizarov surgical techniques: bone correction and lengthening. India: Jaypee Brothers Publishers; 2010.
42. Taylor JC, Paley D. Six axis deformity analysis and correction. New York: Springer-Verlag; 2002.
43. Hawkins R, Calder P, Goodier D. Anatomical considerations and limitations of wire placement using the taylor spatial frame. In Orthopaedic Proceedings 2006;88(SUPP_I):170-1.
44. Henderson ER, Feldman DS, Lusk C, et al. Conformational instability of the taylor spatial frame: a case report and biomechanical study. J Pediatr Orthop 2008; 28(4):471–7.
45. Barker A, Smitham PJ, Scarsbrook C, et al. What Is A Safe Angle For Struts On A Hexapod Frame? Defining The Limitations Of Different Hexapod Frames And A Potential Novel Solution To Frame Instability. In Orthopaedic Proceedings 2013;95(SUPP_23):13-13.
46. Sluga M, Pfeiffer M, Kotz R, et al. Lower limb deformities in children: two-stage correction using the Taylor spatial frame. J Pediatr Orthop B 2003;12(2):123–8.
47. Eidelman M, Bialik V, Katzman A. Correction of deformities in children using the Taylor spatial frame. J Pediatr Orthop B 2006;15(6):387–95.
48. Paley D. Problems, obstacles, and complications of limb lengthening by the Ilizarov technique. Clin Orthop Relat Res 1990;(250):81–104.
49. Nayagam S. Safe corridors in external fixation: the lower leg (tibia, fibula, hindfoot and forefoot). Strateg Trauma Limb Reconstr 2007;2(2–3):105–10.

50. Lamm BM, Paley D, Testani M, et al. Tarsal tunnel decompression in leg lengthening and deformity correction of the foot and ankle. J Foot Ankle Surg 2007; 46(3):201–6.
51. Choi IH, Yang MS, Chung CY, et al. The treatment of recurrent arthrogrypotic club foot in children by the Ilizarov method: a preliminary report. J Bone Joint Surg Br 2001;83(5):731–7.

Benign and Malignant Tumors in Child Foot

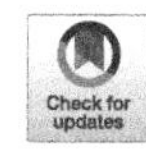

Domenico Andrea Campanacci, MD*, Guido Scoccianti, MD

KEYWORDS

- Bone tumors • Musculoskeletal oncology • Foot diseases • Pediatric foot

KEY POINTS

- Bone tumors affecting the child foot are rare, and most lesions are benign, but a thorough diagnostic evaluation is crucial to rule out a malignant lesion.
- Tumors affecting the foot clinically behave analogous to tumors in other skeletal sites and must be treated according to the same protocols.
- In benign lesions, a conservative treatment is the treatment of choice with curettage or mininvasive techniques.
- In malignant lesions, a wide resection must be performed, and reconstructive procedures should aim to mechanical stability and long-lasting results.
- In foot malignant tumors, amputation is a viable choice because it offers a quick functional recovery and often a better result than complex reconstructive attempts with a high risk of complications.

INTRODUCTION AND GENERAL EPIDEMIOLOGY

Foot and ankle tumors represent about 3% of all bone tumors in general population.[1] In the last few decades, several articles addressed the characteristics of bone tumors at the foot, confirming the peculiarities in this anatomic region both for epidemiology and treatment options.[2–7] While these pathologies in children are rarely reported, most of the lesions are benign, with malignant tumors accounting for approximately one-fifth of the whole number. In a series of 981 cases, 20.59% of the lesions were malignant.[6] Similar findings were reported by other authors, with a percentage of malignant tumors ranging from 13% to 25%.[2,5,7]

In comparison with the general prognosis of malignant bone and soft-tissue tumors, a less aggressive behavior of tumors distally occurring at the ankle and foot, with an inferior rate of distant metastases, was speculated by some authors.[3,8,9] Proposed possible explanations of apparent better prognosis include an

Department of Orthopaedic Oncology and Reconstructive Surgery, Careggi University Hospital, Largo Brambilla 3, Firenze 50134, Italy
* Corresponding author:
E-mail address: domenicoandrea.campanacci@unifi.it

Foot Ankle Clin N Am 26 (2021) 851–871
https://doi.org/10.1016/j.fcl.2021.07.010

earlier diagnosis, due to subcutaneous or quite superficial location of the bone segments, a usually smaller tumor volume, a more limited blood supply, and maybe also a lower temperature due to the distal anatomic location.[8] In contrast with the hypothesis of an earlier diagnosis in the foot, Brotzmann and colleagues[9] found a significant delay in diagnosis of foot malignant bone tumors in comparison to other anatomic sites. The authors attributed this finding to a possible specific biological behavior of the tumors, which at this location would present a lower growing rate and aggressiveness; this lower progression rate would be demonstrated by the fact that survival of the patients did not seem to be affected by the long delay in diagnosis.[9] Data from other authors do not confirm this hypothesis. In a review of 23 cases of high-grade osteosarcoma of the foot by the Cooperative Osteosarcoma Study Group, outcome and prognostic factors were similar as osteosarcoma of other sites.[10] Similar findings had previously been reported by Anninga and colleagues,[11] who examined 19 osteosarcomas of the foot; these authors found a higher rate of low-grade osteosarcoma at the foot (29%) than usually expected from general data at all sites, but, when the analysis was limited to high-grade tumors, a similar outcome as osteosarcomas at other skeletal locations was detected. Similarly, in a large series of 975 Ewing sarcomas, a prognostic advantage for location at the foot in comparison with other non-axial locations was not evident.[12]

From these findings, malignant bone tumors cannot be considered less harmful when occurring at the foot than in other anatomic sites and must be treated with the same protocols and therapeutic aggressiveness.

CLINICAL PRESENTATION

Presentation of foot bone tumors can be quite variable. While soft-tissue tumors usually present with a lump, this does not always happen in bone tumors. Even if a clinically evident lump can occur in any bone tumor, it is particularly frequent in osteochondromas, aggressive giant cell tumors, aneurysmal bone cysts (ABCs), and Ewing sarcomas with extraosseous extension.

Pain is often a presenting symptom in foot osseous tumors, frequently occurring in many histotypes, including osteoid osteoma (OO), ABC, giant cell tumor, chondroblastoma (CBL), and chondromyxoid fibroma among benign lesions and osteosarcoma and Ewing sarcoma among malignant lesions.

Limp can be part of an already overt clinical presentation but can be also the first sign, particularly in very young children.

Some tumors, usually in the benign group, can be completely silent and are incidentally detected in imaging diagnostics performed for other causes, most often trauma.

DIAGNOSTIC WORKUP

First-line approach examinations are standard x-ray and ultrasound, which are usually already performed when the patient presents at a specialized bone and soft-tissue tumor center.

While these procedures can be sufficient for a limited number of benign lesions (similar to some osteochondromas or bone cysts without radiological patterns of aggressiveness and without symptoms, often detected as incidental findings in examinations performed for trauma or other reasons), second-line diagnostics is mandatory in all other situations of a suspected bone tumor.

MRI is usually the first choice, and on the basis of its findings, the following diagnostic procedures are determined. A gadolinium-enhanced MRI is indicated in most cases, except for lesions with benign characteristics such as bone cysts and osteochondromas without x-ray signs of suspicion for malignant degeneration. A CT scan can be useful in better defining osseous contours of the lesion and confirming the presence of calcifications or an ossifying pattern of the tumor. A CT scan can also be the first examination to perform if an OO is suspected because of the better CT definition of the "nidus" in comparison with MRI.

Nuclear medicine examinations, including both Tc99 bone scan or fluorodeoxyglucose (^{18}FDG) positron emission tomography, can complete the diagnostic procedure in selected cases, to better define lesions' location, grade of activity, and systemic staging. Particularly, in pediatric patients, nuclear medicine examinations must be reserved to specific and limited situations, such as staging in osteosarcoma or Ewing sarcoma.

After all the diagnostic paths have been completed, biopsy remains the fundamental step for diagnosis, unless a benign lesion is univocally indicated at imaging, suggesting clinical observation ("leave me alone" lesions) or direct excision with postoperative histologic examination.

In most lesions, a tru-cut biopsy can be performed under CT guidance. As in all anatomic sites, in foot pathology, a fine needle biopsy should be avoided in bone lesions because of the difficulty in histologic examination in most histotypes and the consequent need for the pathologist to have an adequate amount of tissue to analyze.

The biopsy is the first step of our treatment and can importantly affect subsequent treatment options because of the need of excising also the biopsy tract in case of malignant lesions. Therefore, biopsy must be performed along the surgical incision which will be used in definitive surgery, and consequently it must be carried out in specialized sarcoma centers.

If a malignant tumor is detected, diagnostic workup is thereafter completed with systemic evaluation by chest and abdomen contrast-enhanced CT scan. FDG PET or TC99 bone scan is included for patients with osteosarcoma and Ewing sarcoma. FDG PET is the examination of choice in patients with lymphoma.

MOST RELEVANT HISTOTYPES

Simple Bone Cyst

Simple bone cysts, also called unicameral bone cysts, are benign lesions filled with serous fluid. They rarely affect the bones of the foot unless for the calcaneus, which is the affected site in 2% to 3% of all simple bone cysts.[13] Different pathogenetic mechanisms were proposed, and the debate is still ongoing, as well summarized by Noordin and colleagues,[14] with blockage in the venous drainage and increased internal bone pressure as the most favored mechanism.[15] A combination of x-ray and MRI imaging is usually diagnostic, with the finding of a nonaggressive radiolucent central lesion on radiographs and homogeneous fluid signal on MRI (low intensity on T1-weighted images and high intensity on T2-weighted images). At the calcaneus, the cyst is usually located just inferior to the angle of Gissane,[16] where it must be differentiated from intraosseous lipomas, frequently occurring at the same site, and also from physiologic rarefaction of cancellous bone trabeculae which often is present in this area.

Most simple bone cysts are asymptomatic and do not need any treatment. Surgical treatment must be reserved to symptomatic patients or when the bone is at fracture risk, especially in young and active patients (**Fig. 1**). Many different treatments were advocated by different authors, from percutaneous techniques, including both injection (steroids, demineralized bone matrix, concentrated autologous bone marrow)

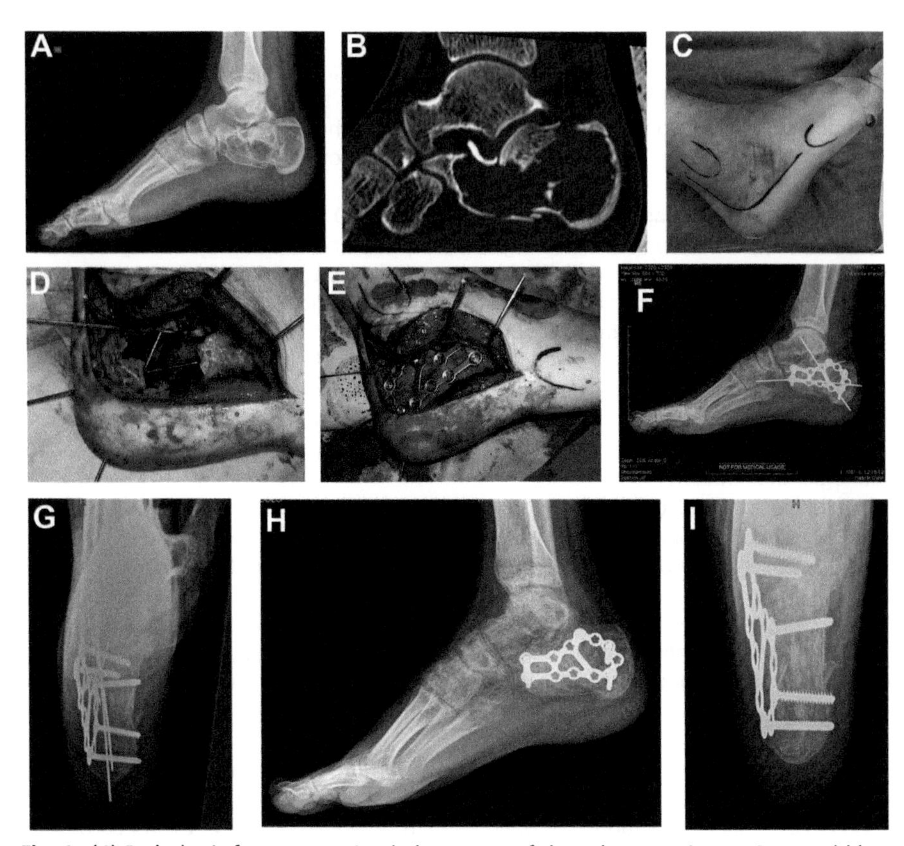

Fig. 1. (*A*) Pathologic fracture on simple bone cyst of the calcaneum in an 18-year-old boy. The patient was asymptomatic before fracture, occurred during sport activity. (*B*) Sagittal reconstruction of CT scan shows fracture's comminution and thin residual cortical bone. A lateral extended approach was performed (*C*). And after fragment reduction and temporary fixation with Kirshner wires (*D*), the defect was filled with autologous bone grafts from iliac crest, and reconstruction plate was used for definitive fixation (*E*). Wires fixation of subtalar and calcaneocuboid joint and subtalar fragments was maintained for 4 weeks (*F, G*). Fracture healing and remodeling of bone grafts were evident after 6 months (*H, I*).

and decompression procedures, to open surgery. Owing to the little volume of simple bone cysts of the foot and the minor procedure requested for curettage and bone grafting in this anatomic region, our preference is open surgery as the first choice, to avoid multiple procedures often necessary in percutaneous treatments.

Aneurysmal Bone Cyst

ABCs are hemorrhagic and often expansive bone lesions, occurring as primary lesions or associated to other oncological diseases such as giant cell tumor, CBL, fibrous dysplasia, or even osteosarcoma. Secondary ABC account for about 30% of all ABCs.[17] After being considered for a long time as derived from intraosseous arteriovenous abnormalities, at present, an oncological nature of the disease is mainly claimed for primary lesions, after the discovery of rearrangement of USP6 oncogene on chromosome 17.[18] Actually, etiology of ABC is likely to be multivariate, as suggested by the variability of their clinical behavior and the occurrence of secondary ABC associated to other diseases.

In a multicentric review of 408 primary ABCs in pediatric patients (aged<17 years), 13 lesions affected the hindfoot or midfoot, accounting for 3% of the total, with the calcaneus as the bone most often involved.[19]

In contrast to simple bone cysts, ABC usually presents with pain and sometimes a bump because of expansion of involved bone. MRI is usually diagnostic, showing the characteristic multiloculated fluid-fluid levels (**Fig. 2**), but a high index of suspicion for different diagnosis must always be applied because of the possibility of a secondary ABC associated to other tumoral lesions, including malignant ones.

Even in ABC, several different treatment regimens have been proposed, and treatment of this entity is still under debate, ranging from arterial selective embolization, percutaneous or minimally invasive treatments, aggressive curettage with or without grafting, and even wide resection in selected cases.[20]

In our experience, in the foot, curettage is the treatment of choice, in accordance with reports from other authors.[21] Bone grafting is used in larger lesions, while it can be avoided in minor lesions. In very aggressive and repeatedly recurrent lesions, a wide resection and consequent reconstruction can be needed, but this is a very rare occurrence.

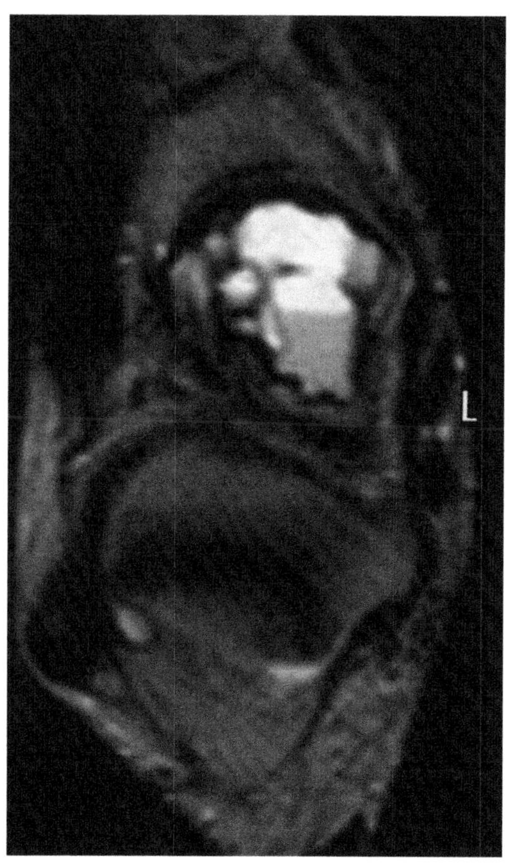

Fig. 2. Aneurysmal bone cyst of the talus showing the characteristic fluid-fluid levels in T2-weighted MRI view.

Chondroblastoma

CBL is a locally aggressive cartilaginous bone tumor; although generally benign, it is included in the category of intermediate, rarely metastasizing tumors in the 2013 World Health Organization classification of bone tumors[22] because of the reported rare occurrence of lung metastases. In a recent review of 130 CBLs in pediatric age, focused on the metastatic potential of the tumor, no distant metastases were observed at an average follow-up of 50 months; authors, therefore, speculated that metastasizing potential could be very low in pediatric age in comparison to all age series, reporting 2% - 3% of metastatic rate.

It most often affects the epiphysis or the apophysis of the long bones but can occur in any bone segment. The second decade is the most affected age, but CBL can occur also in the first decade or in adulthood. In a large series of 332 cases, 42 (13%) occurred in the foot, with calcaneus and talus accounting together for 88% of the lesions.[23] In this series, patients affected by lesions in the foot presented an older mean age than the whole series, with no case occurring in patients younger than 14 years and only 6 (14%) presenting in skeletally immature individuals. A similar finding was reported also by other authors.[24] In a series of 87 CBLs, all in pediatric age, only 5% occurred in the foot, affecting tarsal bones.[25] CBL, which is mainly a tumor of the young age, in the foot seems, therefore, to occur more rarely in pediatric age than expected for localizations in long bones.

Pain is the most common complaint at presentation, sometimes combined with local swelling.

Similar to giant cell tumor of bone (GCTB), on the basis of imaging diagnostics, CBL can be staged as latent, active, or aggressive, following Musculoskeletal Tumor Society benign bone tumor staging system.

Both radiographically and histologically, a secondary ABC component is a frequent finding in CBLs, with a rate of about 25%.[24–26]

Treatment of CBL is surgical excision, which can be usually performed with curettage and bone grafting. In particularly aggressive lesions, a wide excision and consequent reconstruction can be required (**Fig. 3**); even complex reconstructions with vascularized bone transfer were reported for aggressive CBLs in pediatric feet.[27,28] Local adjuvant treatment, such as cryosurgery, can be applied during curettage procedures, to decrease the risk of local recurrence.[29] In recent literature, successful minimally invasive treatment of CBL with percutaneous radiofrequency ablation or cryoablation has been reported.[30]

Local recurrence after surgical treatment is not infrequent, but data are quite inhomogeneous in literature with a reported rate ranging from 2% to 32%.[24–26,31,32]

Giant Cell Tumor of Bone

Commonly considered a tumor affecting the mature skeleton, GCTB can occur also in skeletally immature individuals. In a series of 326 GCTBs, 1.8% affected patients had open growth plates.[33] Despite its rarity during childhood, GCTBs must be considered in differential diagnosis when approaching a lytic aggressive bone lesion even in pediatric age, including the first decade of life. GCTBs affecting the foot in patients younger than 10 years were reported by different authors, mostly involving the metatarsals[34–37] and occurring in patients as young as 3 years old.[34]

Symptoms at presentation usually include pain and swelling. Radiological evaluation shows a lytic bone lesion, frequently expanding the cortical bone and presenting ill defined borders; the same pattern is confirmed at MRI, where the lesion usually presents a low signal in T1 sequences, a high signal in T2, and a strong gadolinium

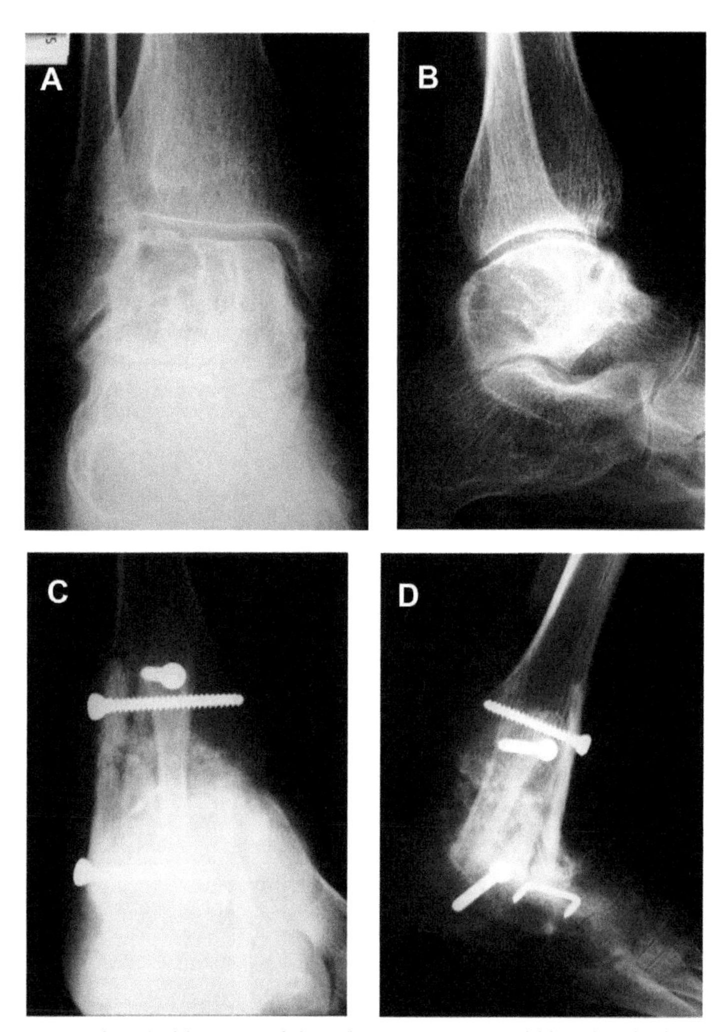

Fig. 3. Recurrent chondroblastoma of the talus in an 18-year-old boy (*A, B*). The patient underwent talectomy and ankle arthrodesis with autologous and allogenic bone grafts (*C, D*).

enhancement. Sometimes a secondary ABC component is present. The lesion is staged as latent, active, or aggressive according to its radiological features and aggressiveness.[38]

GCTBs can be rarely multicentric, with multiple lesions occurring either synchronous or metachronous. The mean age of this particular subset of patients appears to be lower than that of the general population of GCTB patients with more than one-half diagnosed before 20 years of age.[39] Foot bones involvement in multicentric giant cell tumors in pediatric age was reported by different authors.[39,40]

Even if benign, GCTB has a low metastasizing potential to the lung. A chest radiological investigation must therefore be performed at presentation and once a year during follow-up.

As in CBL, surgical treatment is mostly performed with curettage and bone grafting (**Fig. 4**), but particularly aggressive lesions may need wide resection and complex reconstructions. The use of local adjuvants after curettage (phenol, hydrogen-peroxide, cryosurgery) is recommended, although their efficacy is still under debate.[41]

Local recurrence is a frequent finding with a recurrence rate of 15% to 20% after curettage and bone grafting using local adjuvants.

Chondromyxoid Fibroma

Chondromyxoid fibroma is a very rare tumor (<1% of all bone tumors), which can occur at any age, most frequently in the first three decades. Usually located eccentrically in the metaphysis or metaepiphysis when affecting a long bone, it can be centrally located, occupying also the entire width when in small bones like in the foot.[42] The lesion is radiolucent with usually a peripheral thin sclerotic rim and sometimes a trabecular pattern inside. Enlarging of the involved bone with inflating, thinning, and interruption of the cortex can be seen. Most cases present with pain and local swelling.

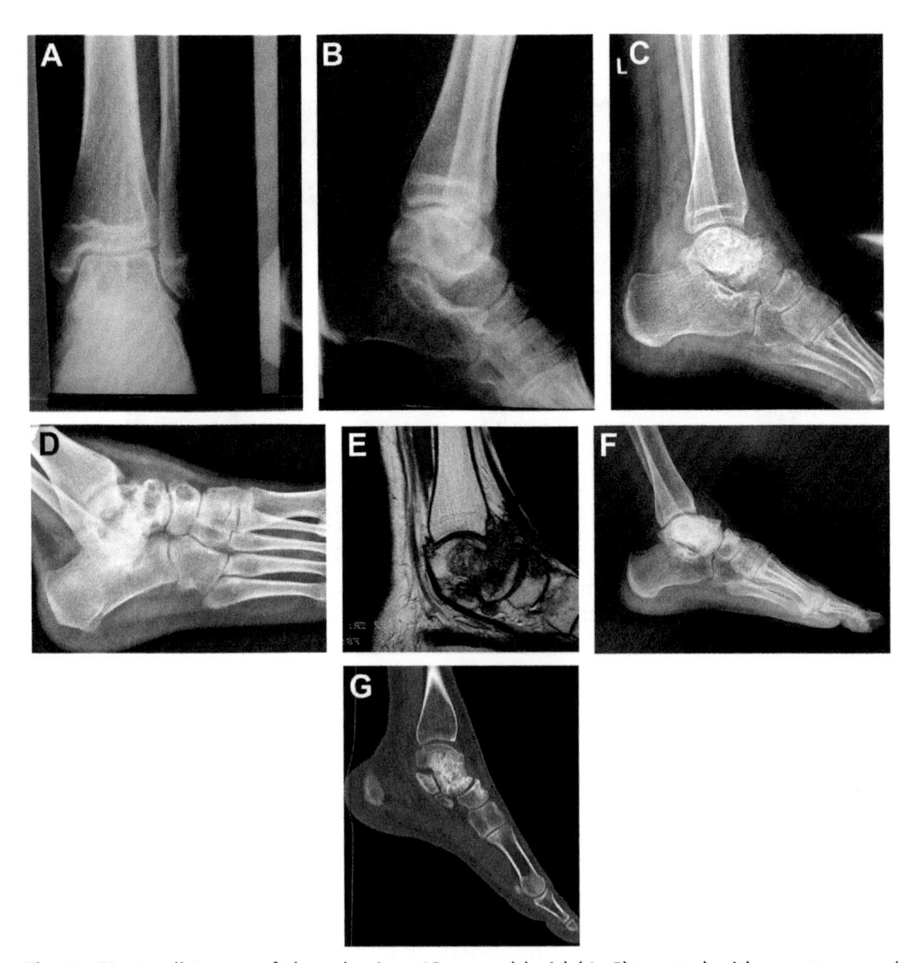

Fig. 4. Giant cell tumor of the talus in a 13-year-old girl (*A, B*) treated with curettage and bone grafting in another center (*C*). Local recurrence 6 months later with a satellite lesion in the scaphoid (*D, E*). Radiograph and CT scan after 2 years from curettage and allogenic bone grafting with bisphosphonate augmentation (*F, G*).

Owing to its rarity, only small series were reported in literature except for a large series (278 cases) from Mayo Clinic.[43] In this series, 14% of the lesions occurred in the foot with the metatarsals and phalanxes as the most often involved segments (only one-quarter of the cases affected the hindfoot).

Surgical excision is the treatment of choice, usually performed with aggressive curettage and bone grafting. In some cases, a wide excision and reconstruction can be necessary.

About one-quarter of the patients will experience a local recurrence.[43,44]

Osteoid Osteoma

OO is a benign bone-forming skeletal neoplasm, accounting for about 12% of primary benign bone tumors.[45] According to a large review of 94 published studies, which included data about 223 OOs in the foot, the talus is the most frequently affected bone, followed by the calcaneus and the phalanges; the occurrence in the metatarsals, scaphoid, cuboid, and cuneiforms is more rare.[46] OOs can occur at any age, but most patients are aged between 15 and 30 years, with a lower incidence below 14 and above 30 years and exceptional under 5 and over 40 years. Classic presentation is a long-standing pain with nocturnal worsening, relieved by nonsteroidal anti-inflammatory drugs (NSAIDs). Pain is caused by synthesis and release of prostaglandins in the nidus[47] and concomitant presence of nerve endings and abundant vascularity. Another typical clinical sign of OO arising in the foot toes is evident macrodactyly, capable to return to a normal aspect after excision in the growing child (**Fig. 5**). Not infrequently, patients undergo a long series of physical and medical treatments before the correct diagnosis is made.

The tumor can be cortical, cancellous, or periosteal according to its location. Cancellous and periosteal cases are often more challenging to ascertain because of less evident alterations in imaging diagnostics. MRI, usually performed as second-line imaging in pediatric patients, can be misleading in OO, showing diffuse alterated signal due to edema and inflammatory reaction, often failing to identify the nidus. In cancellous and periosteal tumors, often a gadolinium-enhanced MRI is useful to confirm the diagnostic hypothesis. The most efficient, and usually sufficient, diagnostic examination is a direct CT, which shows the characteristic radiolucent nidus surrounded by bone sclerosis. Bone scan can be used to confirm diagnosis of OO, showing the typical hot spot, even though nuclear medicine should be used with caution in pediatric patients.

CT-guided percutaneous treatment (radiofrequency thermoablation or cryosurgery) has become the treatment of choice in most OOs, including pediatric patients[48–51] and specifically also cases affecting the foot.[49,51] When the tumor affects the little bones of the midfoot and forefoot, an open excision can be recommended because of possible complications of ablation procedures in a similar setting. In particular locations, such as the neck of the talus, an arthroscopic excision was proposed first by Resnick[52] and reported thereafter also by other authors.

Osteoblastoma

Histologically quite similar to OO, osteoblastoma presents a different radiological and clinical behavior, characterized by a larger and slowly growing lesion surrounded by a thin sclerotic shell with less reactive bone sclerosis than in OO. Pain is usually present but lacking the characteristic nocturnal pattern and response to NSAIDs, which is in accordance with the absence of demonstrable increased production of prostaglandins found in OO.

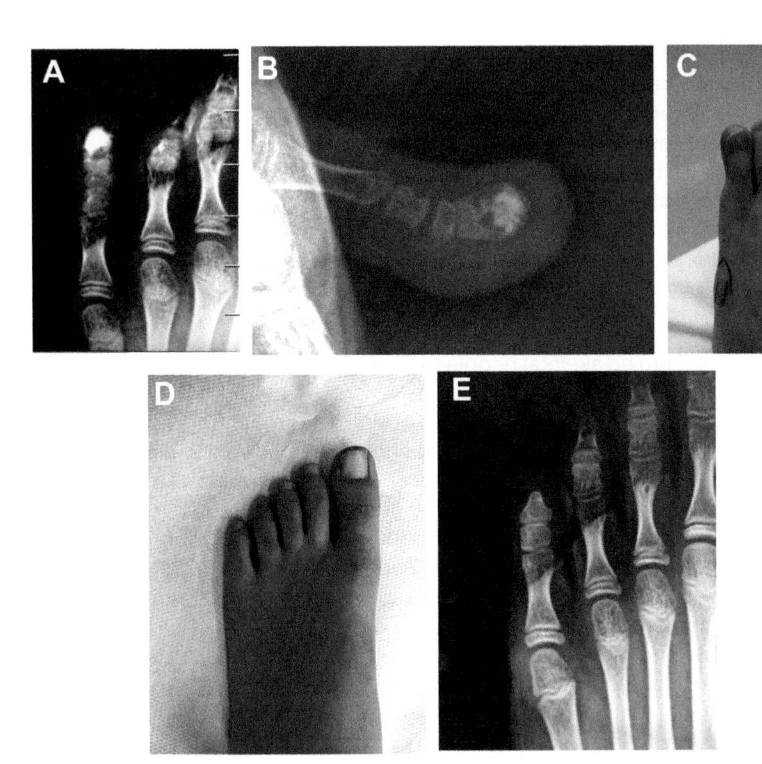

Fig. 5. Osteoid osteoma of fifth toe distal phalanx in a 9-year-old girl (*A, B*) causing the typical macrodactyly, evident at clinical examination (*C*). Two years after curettage, both radiographic (*D*) and clinical control (*E*) show complete remodeling and normal aspect of the toe.

Foot and ankle region is the first site of occurrence for osteoblastoma after the spine and the femur; the second and third decades of life are the most affected period, followed by the first one, with cases reported also in the first years of life; the talus is most frequently affected, but osteoblastoma can be found in any bone of the foot.[53]

Surgical excision with bone grafting is usually the treatment of choice, but also other minimally invasive procedures were proposed for osteoblastoma including hindfoot locations, such as percutaneous cryoablation[54] (**Fig. 6**). In more aggressive cases, wider excision and consequent reconstructions can be necessary.

A preliminary histologic examination from a biopsy is mandatory to confirm the diagnosis and to exclude an osteoblastoma-like osteosarcoma, a rare type of osteosarcoma first described by Bertoni and colleagues[55] with a series of cases over 17 years not affecting the foot, but reported thereafter by other authors also with occurrence in the foot[56] and specifically in the pediatric foot.[57]

Eosinophilic Granuloma and Langerhans Cell Histiocytosis

Langerhans cell histiocytosis and its localized single-bone condition, eosinophilic granuloma, are a still not well-understood proliferative disorder of the reticuloendothelial system containing cells with the characteristics of Langerhans cell. Typical of childhood and young adults (<20 years), it frequently occurs in very young children. The most frequent site of bone involvement is the skull, followed by femur, pelvis, vertebrae, and ribs.[58] Foot bones involvement is quite rare, but it can occur (**Fig. 7**). The

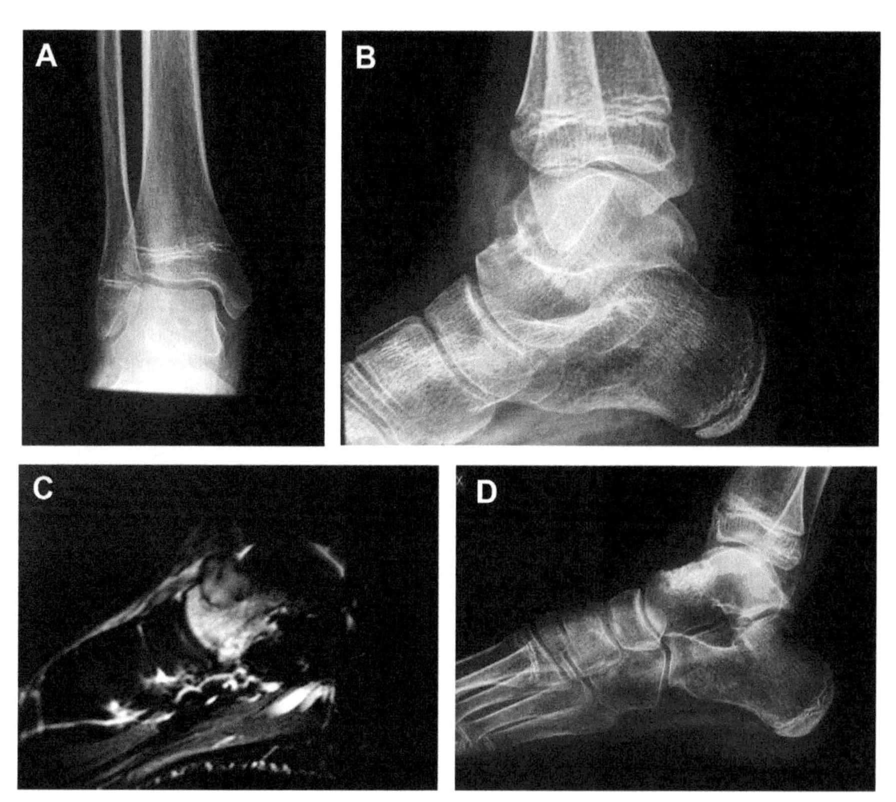

Fig. 6. Osteoblastoma of the talus in an 11-year-old boy (*A, B*). Sagittal MRI view showing the round lesion on the neck of the talus and perilesional edema extending to the talar head and neck (*C*). Radiographic control after 1 year from curettage and allogenic bone grafting (*D*).

lesion can be unifocal or multifocal, involving more than one bone segment. The disease can be single-system (affecting only the skeleton) or multisystem (involving both skeleton and other organs). Radiological presentation is usually characterized by an aggressive radiolucent lesion with not well-demarcated margins and surrounding edema, resembling Ewing sarcoma or also osteomyelitis, which must be considered

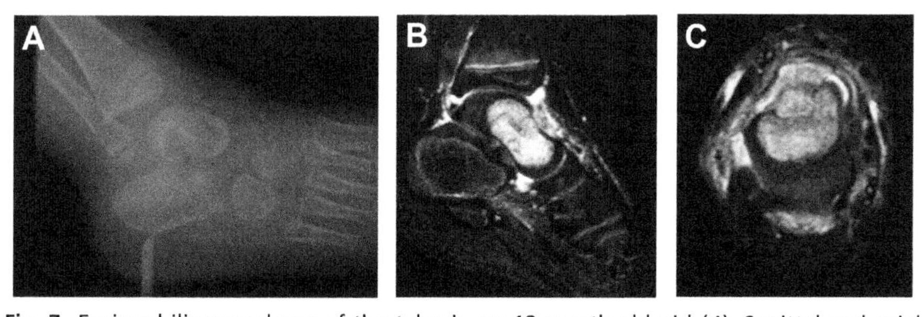

Fig. 7. Eosinophilic granuloma of the talus in an 18-month-old girl (*A*). Sagittal and axial MRI view showing subtotal involvement of the talus (*B, C*). Complete healing was observed after simple curettage.

in differential diagnosis. In unifocal lesions, a conservative approach is advised, from simple observation[59] to percutaneous injection of steroids.[60] In multifocal and multisystem diseases, a systemic medical therapy (chemotherapy + cortisone) is necessary.

Osteosarcoma

Osteosarcoma is the most frequent primary malignant bone tumor in childhood, accounting for 3% to 6% of all pediatric malignancies.[11]

Anninga and colleagues[11] found only 27 cases of osteosarcoma of the foot out of a series of 4221 osteosarcomas (0.64%). If osteosarcoma of the foot bones is generally rare, it seems to be even rarer in pediatric patients because age of presentation in osteosarcoma of the foot is generally older than that in osteosarcoma of other sites.[10,11,61] No patients younger than 17 years were present in the series of Anninga and colleagues[11]; even if patients in the first or initial second decade of life were reported by Choong and colleagues[61] and Schuster and colleagues,[10] these authors reported the mean age of osteosarcoma of the foot as older than expected from general osteosarcoma epidemiology. Osteosarcoma can affect any bone of the foot, from the hindfoot to the phalanges. Tarsal bones are more often affected with calcaneus as the most frequent tumor location in the foot.[10,11,61] Main presenting symptom is pain[10,11] with swelling reported in about two-third of the cases.[10]

Most radiological characteristic features are a mixed lytic-sclerotic lesion with signs of abnormal ossifying areas, often invading the extraosseous space. Periosteal reaction is usually seen, even if the classical features of sunburst appearance or Codman's triangle are often difficult to observe in the small bones of the foot.

Most osteosarcomas are high-grade tumors, but in a minority of cases, the lesion can present with a low-grade pattern. A possible higher incidence of low-grade tumors in the foot in comparison to other sites was reported.[11,62] In low-grade tumors, surgical wide resection without adjuvant systemic therapies is the treatment of choice. In high-grade osteosarcomas, in the foot as in any other location, treatment must include surgery with wide margins and preoperative and postoperative multiagent chemotherapy. Reconstruction can be achieved with a wide range of different techniques, according to location and extension of the tumor and consequent resection (**Fig. 8**).

Owing to the high aggressiveness of the disease, achievement of wide surgical margins is of paramount importance. In a complex location such as the foot, wide margins are not always easy to obtain, and reconstruction is often very challenging. In this setting, in selected cases, amputation (partial or of the entire foot) must be considered, in view of the excellent recovery of function provided by an external prosthesis after a below-knee amputation, sometimes better than what can be achieved after a very complex reconstruction.

Ewing Sarcoma

Ewing sarcoma is the second bone malignancy affecting childhood in order of frequency, but it is more frequently observed than osteosarcoma in the pediatric foot, especially in the first decade of life, as older age of presentation is not reported for the foot as in osteosarcoma.

In a large series of 975 Ewing sarcomas of bone, location at the foot accounted for 2% to 4% of cases.[12] Calcaneus and metatarsals are the bones most frequently affected in the foot, while other bones seem to be quite more rarely affected.[63,64] Multifocal Ewing sarcomas of the foot have been exceptionally reported.[63,65]

Clinical presenting symptoms are pain, usually combined with swelling, which is very frequent because of extraosseous expansion of the tumor. A limp can also be

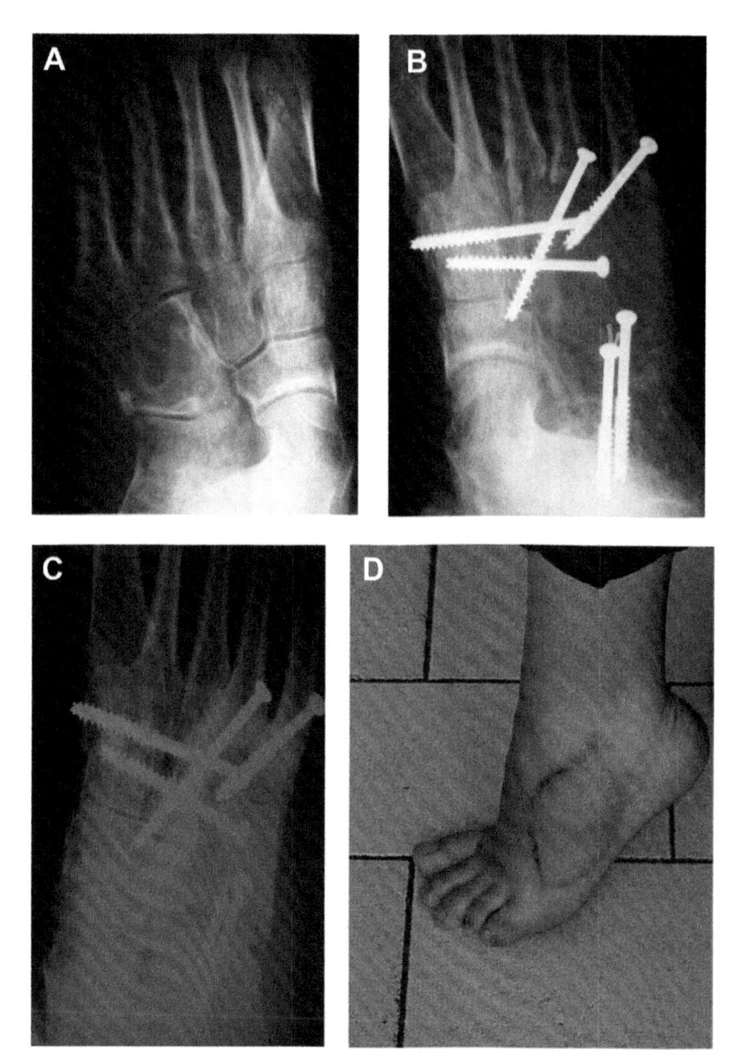

Fig. 8. Osteosarcoma of the cuboid in a 16-year-old girl (*A*). After preoperative chemotherapy, a wide resection including a skin island was performed, and the reconstruction was performed using an autologous structural iliac crest and a latissimus dorsi free flap (*B*). Radiographic control after 4 years shows complete fusion and remodeling of the graft (*C*). Clinical image showing excellent function and esthetical result of the flap (*D*).

present. In a few cases, systemic symptoms, such as fever, can be found. Also, some laboratory parameters can be altered, such as lactate dehydrogenase and erythrocyte sedimentation rate.

Imaging diagnostics usually show an aggressive osteolytic lesion with expansive pattern and periosteal onion peel appearance. A soft-tissue mass surrounding the bone is often present, which usually greatly decreases or even disappears after preoperative multiagent chemotherapy. If resection must consider prechemotherapy or postchemoterapy extension of the tumor is still a subject of debate.[66–68]

Similar to osteosarcoma, a surgery with wide margins must be achieved, and surgical considerations are similar as for osteosarcoma (see the previous paragraph)

(**Fig. 9**). Preoperative and postoperative multiagent chemotherapy are mandatory as Ewing sarcoma must be considered as a systemic oncological disease, even in the absence of evident further lesions besides the primary tumor.

Differently from osteosarcoma, Ewing sarcoma is sensitive to radiotherapy, and this gives one more therapeutic option to the clinician either as a unique local treatment, in nonoperable tumors, or after surgery in case of inadequate margins.[69,70] Nonetheless, in the growing foot of a child, radiotherapy can have severe long-term negative effects, and the use of radiotherapy in this setting must be reserved to highly selected cases.

Cartilaginous Tumors

Cartilaginous tumors include central (enchondroma, central chondrosarcoma, clear cell chondrosarcoma) and peripheral (osteochondroma, periosteal chondroma,

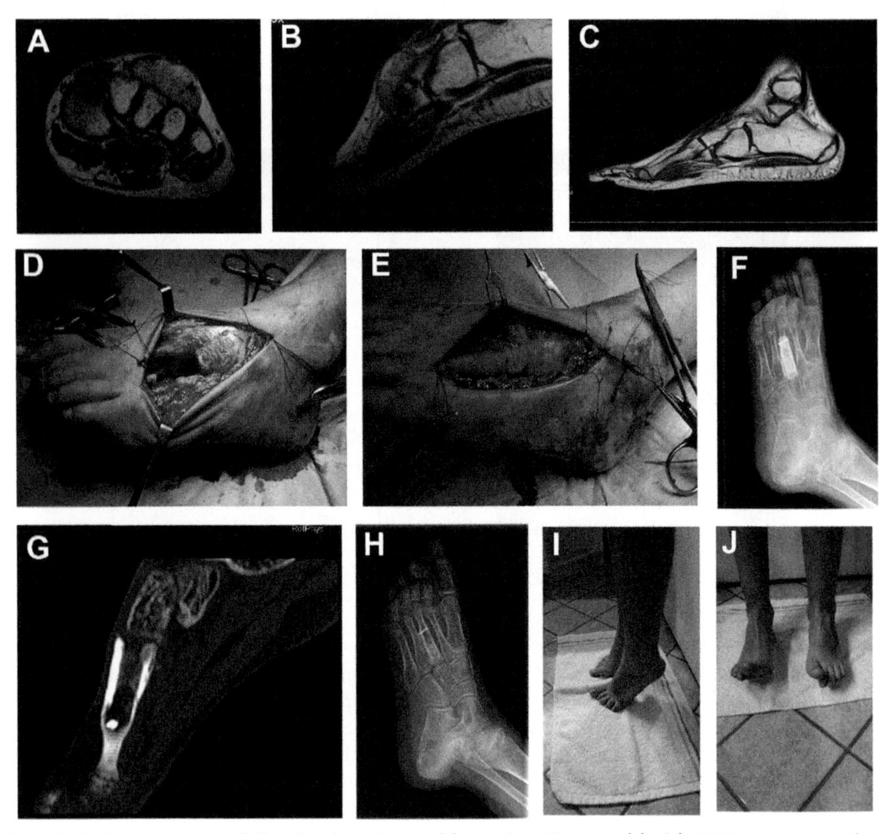

Fig. 9. Ewing sarcoma of the third metatarsal bone in a 7-year-old girl; MRI at presentation (*A, B*). The tumor was excised without previous biopsy in a nonspecialized center. After diagnosis, chemotherapy was started in a neoadjuvant setting before a re-excision surgical procedure; MRI after preoperative chemotherapy (*C*). Resection of the proximal portion of the third metatarsal together with extensor tendons of the second, third, and fourth ray and previous incision scar was performed (*D*). Reconstruction was accomplished with an allograft fixed with one screw to the residual metatarsal; cuneometatarsal joint was reconstructed with an interpositional arthroplasty (autologous fascia lata) (*E, F*). Extensor tendons were reconstructed with tendon allografts. CT scan at 20 months shows good osteointegration of the graft (*G*). X-ray (*H*) and functional result (*I, J*) at 3 years. The patient is now continuously disease free at 5 years.

peripheral chondrosarcoma, periosteal chondrosarcoma) entities. A description of these entities is not possible in this review. Chondral malignancies are usually a disease of adulthood, but they can very seldom occur in pediatric age. A particular expertise is necessary in histologic evaluation of samples from chondromas in pediatric age, particularly if affecting the hand and foot, because the activity of the lesion and histologic characteristics can mimic a low-grade chondrosarcoma also in absolutely benign lesions.[71] In a national series of 311 chondrosarcomas in Norway, no tumors before the age of 10 years were found, and only 0.8% of the series occurred in the second decade of life.[72] Chondrosarcomas can nonetheless occur also in the first decade as reported by large population studies[73] or case reports. Favoring factors are genetic diseases such as Ollier's disease, Maffucci syndrome, and Hereditary Multiple Exostoses disease. Particular attention must be applied in monitoring of these patients, particularly when pain presents at a particular anatomic site.

CLINICS CARE POINTS

Approach to Oncological Diseases in the Pediatric Foot

Dealing with tumors of the pediatric foot require not only a solid oncological experience but also a thorough understanding of complex foot biomechanics, the awareness to work on a structure in evolution, a complete knowledge of reconstructive options, and often a fair amount of creativity. Orthopedic oncologist can benefit from consulting an experienced foot and ankle surgeon, at least in the planning phase, to define the best excisional and reconstructive procedures. Highly successful procedures can be performed only if an adequately wide tumoral excision will be followed by a biomechanically valid reconstruction.

Furthermore, a keystone of the treatment of any oncological patient is the multidisciplinary approach involving, in any decision, the complete team: the surgeon, medical oncologist, pathologist, radiologist, and radiotherapist. All these figures must be experienced in musculoskeletal oncology because of the specific complexity and rarity of bone tumors.

Is It a Tumor or Osteomyelitis?

Clinical and imaging presentation of osteomyelitis can mimic a tumor and vice versa. Osteolysis, surrounding edema, periosteal reaction can be present also in infection of bone, resembling a tumor, and sometimes tumors with permeative patterns, especially Ewing sarcoma, lymphoma, and eosinophilic granuloma, can resemble an osteomyelitis.[74] A high index of suspicion must always be kept, and a histologic examination must always be performed also when an osteomyelitis is supposed from imaging diagnostics and clinical presentation. To underline the importance of avoiding a misdiagnosis between infection and tumor, due to the sometimes-overlapping presentation features, an old aphorism in orthopedic oncology suggests to "biopsy the infection and culture the tumor," as the only way not to miss the correct diagnosis on the sampling setting during a biopsy procedure.

Preoperative Evaluation

A complete diagnostic workup must be accomplished before choosing and performing any surgical treatment in an oncological patient. The diagnostic path must be defined by an oncological orthopedic surgeon together with a radiologist with experience in musculoskeletal oncology to avoid useless examinations (reducing the diagnostic burden for the patient) and, at the same time, to guarantee that all the necessary examinations are performed (giving the best chances to get to the right diagnosis and to the right treatment selection). In particular, in malignant tumors, imaging workup should aim to detect tumoral bone and soft-tissue extension and to precisely assess which structures need to be removed and what can be preserved. Ascertaining if a tumor has an intracompartmental or extracompartmental extension is of utmost importance. A bone tumor can remain confined to bone (intracompartmental) or involve surrounding soft tissues, becoming extracompartmental. In this case, a precise definition of which of the four compartments of the foot (three plantar and one dorsal) is affected is necessary to plan the excision. Unfortunately, the complex anatomy of the foot, the thin fascial layers and septae which divide the compartments, and the presence of several fascial defects where tendons pass through[75] make a multicompartmental tumor spread quite easy and frequent. On the basis of this evaluation, an accurate resection planning is carried out, aiming to obtain negative margins and to preserve as much as possible the healthy tissues. In primary malignant bone tumors undergoing neoadjuvant chemotherapy, local and systemic imaging studies are repeated before surgical treatment.

Minimally Invasive Versus Wide

In the last few decades, mini-invasive surgery has gained more and more popularity among both surgeons and patients. Mini-invasive procedures can be successfully performed also in foot oncological surgery when dealing with benign tumors. Cryosurgery, radiofrequency thermal ablation, high-intensity focused ultrasound, and radiowave ablation, together with percutaneous infiltration procedures, are important and efficient techniques to be used for the right targets. In malignant bone tumors, wide resection is mandatory, with or without subsequent reconstruction.

Also in the era of limb-salvage surgery, amputation must remain an option to be always considered in locally advanced aggressive malignant tumors, both to allow tumor-free surgical margins and to avoid multiple subsequent revision procedures, as it can happen when reconstruction is too complex. This is particularly true at the foot, where an amputation, either at the foot or at the leg, allows a very good functional recovery with an external prosthesis, sometimes better than what can be obtained with a too daring conservative reconstruction. In the forefoot, malignant tumors of middle metatarsal bone or toes can be successfully managed with ray or multiple ray amputations, preserving an adequate functional and esthetic result.

More than in other anatomic locations and similar as the hand, in the foot (and in the pediatric foot even more), percutaneous procedures are not always feasible because of the small available space to operate and the proximity of structures (nerves, vessels, articular cartilage) which could be damaged by the ablation procedure. In this setting, in many cases, an open excision can be less invasive than a mini-invasive technique.

Stability, Motion, Growth: Which Characteristics of the Pediatric Foot Can Be Restored in Reconstruction after Resection and Which Should Be Addressed First?

Stability and motion are both fundamental functional properties of the foot provided by its complex anatomy. Furthermore, the foot in pediatric age is also a growing structure, increasing challenges for the surgeon facing a reconstruction after oncological resection. All these issues should be theoretically addressed in planning the reconstruction, but there is a priority order which must guide surgeons's choices. Stability is the first issue to address, and its restoration cannot be missed. Differently from the hip and the knee, motion loss in the foot and ankle is well tolerated and compatible with a good functional result. Arthrodesis is, therefore, the best choice in many cases, either in the hindfoot or the midfoot and forefoot. Arthrodesis after bone loss due to resection of the tumor can be accomplished with massive bone grafts either autologous (usually from the fibula or the iliac crest of the patient) or homologous (fresh frozen grafts from the bone bank)[76]; recently also heterologous custom-made bone substitutes with bioactive polymers were introduced. Usually, the iliac crest is the most-fitting donor site for reconstructions of the hindfoot, while fibula is better suited for reconstructions of the midfoot and forefoot. Alternatively, a joint-restoring reconstruction can be performed with the implant of an osteoarticular graft or composite arthroplasty in the small joints of the forefoot and midfoot, but a balance between the advantage of restoring motion and the risk of instability must always be considered. Growth is another complex issue in the child foot. After the first report in the late 1970s,[77] a growing number of reports and series has shown that, after resection of the epiphysis of a growing bone, transfer of an autologous vascularized epiphysis is a viable procedure, which can restore joint function and, at the same time, the growth capacity of the affected bone segment. The most consolidated and used option as a donor site is the proximal fibula, even if other sites, such as the iliac crest and the distal scapula, were proposed; in case of reconstruction of small segments, as for the rays of the hand, vascularized epiphyseal transfer can be accomplished with the metatarsal as the donor site.[78] In the last decades, the technique of vascularized epiphyseal transfer, mainly using the proximal fibula, was applied mostly to pediatric reconstructions in the upper limb (proximal humerus, distal radius) but also in the lower limb (proximal femur, distal fibula). Shenaq and Dinh in 1989[79] reported a vascularized growing iliac bone transfer to reconstruct the heel, but vascularized epiphyseal transfer to the foot seems to have been quite rarely performed according to the lack of reports in literature. Till now, the foot has been usually used as a donor and not as the recipient for such a procedure because always a balance has to be made between advantages and disadvantages of similar procedures, particularly for donor site morbidity, and this evidently questions any possible indication in reconstruction of foot bone segments. Nevertheless, we cannot exclude that in very rare and highly selected complex reconstructions of large defects of the hindfoot in a pediatric patient, a vascularized epiphyseal transfer could be evaluated as a possible option.

Postoperative Follow-up

Postoperative follow-up must include not only oncological and functional evaluation but also biomechanical evaluation (with the frequent need of the use of custom foot orthoses after major reconstructions) and psychological evaluation. Minor growth disturbances after treatment are usually well tolerated in the foot, but more substantial alterations can require further treatments.

DISCLOSURE

The authors have nothing to disclosure.

REFERENCES

1. Unni KK, Dahlin DC. Dahlin's bone tumors: general aspects and data on 11,087 cases. 5th edition. Philadelphia: Lippincott-Raven; 1996.
2. Murari TM, Callaghan JJ, Berrey BH Jr, et al. Primary benign and malignant osseous neo- plasms of the foot. Foot Ankle 1989;10:68–80.
3. Özdemir HM, Yildiz Y, Yilmaz C, et al. Tumors of the foot and ankle: analysis of 196 cases. J Foot Ankle Surg 1997;36(6):403–8.
4. Bakotic B, Huvos AG. Tumors of the bones of the feet: the clinicopathologic features of 150 cases. J Foot Ankle Surg 2001;40(5):277–86.

5. Chou LB, Ho YY, Malawer MM. Tumors of the foot and ankle: experience with 153 cases. Foot Ankle Int 2009;30(9):836–41.
6. Ruggieri P, Angelini A, Jorge FD, et al. Review of foot tumors seen in a university tumor institute. J Foot Ankle Surg 2014;53(3):282–5.
7. Toepfer A, Harrasser N, Recker M, et al. Distribution patterns of foot and ankle tumors: a university tumor institute experience. BMC Cancer 2018;18:735–44.
8. Zeytoonjian T, Mankin HJ, Gebhardt MC, et al. Distal lower extremity sarcomas: frequency of occurrence and patient survival rate. Foot Ankle Int 2004;25(5): 325–30.
9. Brotzmann M, Hefti F, Baumhoer D, et al. Do malignant bone tumors of the foot have a different biological behavior than sarcomas at other skeletal sites? Sarcoma 2013.
10. Schuster AJ, Kager L, Reichardt P, et al. High-Grade Osteosarcoma of the Foot: Presentation, Treatment, Prognostic Factors, and Outcome of 23 Cooperative Osteosarcoma Study Group COSS Patients. Sarcoma 2018.
11. Anninga JK, Picci P, Fiocco M, et al. Osteosarcoma of the hands and feet: a distinct clinico-pathological subgroup. Virchows Arch 2013;462(1):109–20.
12. Cotterill SJ, Ahrens S, Paulussen M, et al. Prognostic factors in Ewing's tumor of bone: Analysis of 975 patients from the European Intergroup Cooperative Ewing's Sarcoma Study Group. J Clin Oncol 2000;18:3108–14.
13. Carbonara PN, Neer CS 2nd, Francis KC, et al. Treatment of unicameral bone cyst. J Bone Joint Surg Am 1966;48:731–45.
14. Noordin S, Allana S, Umer M, et al. Unicameral bone cysts: Current concepts. Ann Med Surg 2018;34:43–9.
15. Komiya S, Inoue A. Development of a solitary bone cyst–a report of a case suggesting its pathogenesis. Arch Orthop Trauma Surg 2000;120(7):455–7.
16. Moreau G, Letts M. Unicameral bone cyst of the calcaneus in children. J Pediatr Orthop 1994;14:101–4.
17. Martinez V, Sissons HA. Aneurysmal bone cyst. A review of 123 cases including primary lesions and those secondary to other bone pathology. Cancer 1988;61: 2291–304.
18. Nielsen GP, Fletcher JA, Oliveira AM. Aneurysmal bone cyst. In: Fletcher BJA, Hogendoorn PCW, Mertens F, editors. WHO classification of tumours of soft tissue and bone. Lyon: IARC; 2013. p. 348–9.
19. Cottalorda J, Kohler R, Sales de Gauzy J, et al. Epidemiology of aneurysmal bone cyst in children: A multicenter study and literature review. J Pediatr Orthop B 2004;13(6):389–94.
20. Rapp TB, Ward JP, Alaia MJ. Aneurysmal bone cyst. J Am Acad Orthop Surg 2012;20:233–41.
21. Chowdhry M, Chandrasekaar CR, Mohammed R, et al. Curettage of aneurysmal bone cysts of the feet. Foot Ankle Int 2010;31(2):131–5.
22. WHO classification of tumours of soft tissue and bone. In: Fletcher CDM, Bridge JA, Hogendoorn PCW, et al, editors. World health organization classification of tumours, vol. 5, 4th edition. Lyon (France): IARC Press; 2013. p. 240.
23. Fink BR, Temple HT, Chiricosta FM, et al. Chondroblastoma of the foot. Foot Ankle Int 1997;18:236–42.
24. Angelini A, Arguedas F, Varela A, et al. Chondroblastoma of the foot: 40 cases from a single institution. J Foot Ankle Surg 2018;57(2):1105–9.
25. Sailhan F, Chotel F, Parot R. Chondroblastoma of bone in a pediatric population. J Bone Joint Surg Am 2009;91:2159–68.

26. Laitinen MK, Stevenson JD, Evans S, et al. Chondroblastoma in pelvis and extremities—a signle centre study of 177 cases. J Bone Oncol 2019;17:100248.
27. Hassenpflug J, Ulrich HW, Liebs T, et al. Vascularized iliac crest bone graft for talar defects: case reports. Foot Ankle Int 2007;28(5):633–7.
28. Wagener J, Schweizer C, Horn Lang T, et al. Vascularized bone autograft for the treatment of chondroblastoma of the talus at imminent risk of joint breakdown: three case reports. J Foot Ankle Surg 2019;58(2):363–7.
29. Van der Geest ICM, Van Noort MP, Schreuder HWB, et al. The cryosurgical treatment of chondroblastoma of bone: long-term oncologic and functional result. J Surg Oncol 2007;96(3):230–4.
30. Xie C, Jeys L, James SLJ. Radiofrequency ablation of chondroblastoma: long-term clinical and imaging outcomes. Eur Radiol 2014;25(4):1127–34.
31. Ebeid WA, Hasan BZ, BAdr IT, et al. Functional and oncological outcome after treatment of chondroblastoma with intralesional curettage. J Pediatr Orthop 2019;39(4):e312–7.
32. Arkader A, Williams A, Binitie O, et al. Pediatric chondroblastoma and the need for lung staging at presentation. J Pediatr Orthop 2020;40(9):e894–7.
33. Picci P, Manfrini M, Zucchi V, et al. Giant-cell tumor of bone in skeletally immature patients. J Bone Joint Surg Am 1983;65(4):486–90.
34. Aaron AD, Kenan S, Klein MJ. Case report 810. Skeletal Radiol 1993;22:543–5.
35. Baker JF, Perera A, Kiely PD, et al. Giant cell tumour in the foot of a skeletally immature girl: a case report. J Orthop Surg 2009;17(2):248–50.
36. Dridi M, Ben SS, M'Barek M, et al. Metatarsal giant cell tumour in a 7-year-old child: a case report. Acta Orthop Belg 2011;77(6):843–6.
37. Strom TMA, Skeie AT, Lobmaier IK, et al. Giant cell tumor: a rare condition in the immature skeleton—a retrospective study of symptoms, treatment, and outcome in 16 children. Sarcom 2016.
38. Campanacci M, Baldini N, Boriani S, et al. Giant- cell tumor of bone. J Bone Joint Surg Am 1987;69(1):106–14.
39. Hoch B, Inwards C, Sundaram M, et al. Multicentric giant cell tumor of bone. Clinicopathologic analysis of thirty cases. J Bone Joint Surg Am 2006;88:1998–2008.
40. Varshney A, Rao H, Sadh R. Multicentric GCT of tarsal bones in an immature skeleton: a case report with review of literature. J Foot Ankle Surg 2010;49:399e1–4.
41. Bickels j, Campanacci DA. Local adjuvant substances following curettage of bone tumors. J Bone Joint Am 2020;102(2):164–74.
42. Budny AM, Ismail A, Osher. Chondromyxoid fibroma. J Foot Ankle Surg 2008; 47(2):153–9.
43. Wu CT, Inwards CY, O'Laughlin S, et al. Chondromyxoid fibroma of bone: a clinicopathologic review of 278 cases. Hum Pathol 1998;29(5):438–44.
44. Lersundi A, Mankin H, Mourikis A, et al. Chondromyxoidfibroma:a rarely encountered and puzzling tumor. Clin Orthop Rel Res 2005;439:171–5.
45. Dahlin DC, Unni KK. Bone tumors: general aspects and data on 8542 cases. 4th edition. Springfield: Thomas; 1987. p. 88–101.
46. Jordan RW, Koc T, Chapman AW, et al. Osteoid osteoma of the foot and ankle–a systematic review. Foot Ankle Surg 2015;21:228–34.
47. Makley JT, Dunn MJ. Prostaglandin synthesis by osteoid osteoma. Lancet 1982; 2:42.
48. Donkol RH, Al-Nammi A, Moghazi K. Efficacy of percutaneous radiofrequency ablation of osteoid osteoma in children. Pediatr Radiol 2008;38:180–5.
49. Peyser A, Applbaum Y, Khoury A, et al. Osteoid osteoma: CT-guided radiofrequency ablation using a water-cooled probe. Ann Surg Oncol 2007;14:591–6.

50. Whitmore MJ, Hawkins CM, Prologo JD, et al. Cryoablation of osteoid osteoma in the pediatric and adolescent population. J Vasc Interv Radiol 2016;27:232–7.
51. Hage N, Beecham Chick JF, Gemmete JJ, et al. Percutaneous radiofrequency ablation for the treatment of osteoid osteoma in children and adults: a comparative analysis in 92 patients. Cardiovasc Intervent Radiol 2018;41(9):1384–90.
52. Resnick RB, Jarolem KL, Sheskier SC, et al. Arthroscopic removal of an osteoid osteoma of the talus: a case report. Foot Ankle Int 1995;16(4):212–5.
53. Temple HT, Mizel MS, Murphey MD, et al. Osteoblastoma of the foot and ankle. Foot Ankle Int 1998;19(10):698–704.
54. Cazzato RL, Auloge P, Dalili D, et al. Percutaneous image-guided cryoablation of osteoblastoma. Am J Roentgenol 2019;213(5):1157–62.
55. Bertoni F, Unni KK, McLeod RA, et al. Osteosarcoma resembling osteoblastoma. Cancer 1985;55(2):416–26.
56. Gambarotti M, Dei Tos AP, Vanel D, et al. Osteoblastoma-like osteosarcoma: high-grade or low-grade osteosarcoma? Histopathology 2019;74(3):494–503.
57. Wu W, Zhao G, Chen J, et al. Osteoblastoma-like osteosarcoma of the cuboid and skull: a case report and review of the literature. J Foot Ankle Surg 2020;59(1): 156–61.
58. Lau LMS, Stuurman K, Weitzman S. Skeletal langerhans cell histiocytosis in children: permanent consequences and health-related quality of life in long-term survivors. Pediatr Blood Cancer 2008;50:607–12.
59. Ghanem I, Tolo VT, D'Ambra P, et al. Langerhans cell histiocytosis of bone in children and adolescents. J Pediatr Orthop 2003;23(1):124–30.
60. Baptista AM, Camargo AF, de Camargo OP, et al. Does adjunctive chemotherapy reduce remission rates compared to cortisone alone in unifocal or multifocal histiocytosis of bone? Clin Orthop Relat Res 2012;470(3):663–9.
61. Choong PFM, Qureshi AA, Sim FH, et al. Osteosarcoma of the foot: a review of 52 patients at the Mayo Clinic. Acta Orthop Scand 1999;70(4):361–4.
62. Murai NO, Teniola O, Wang WL, et al. Bone and soft tissue tumors about the foot and ankle. Radiol Clin North Am 2018;56(6):917–34.
63. Adkins CD, Kitaoka HB, Seidl RK, et al. Ewing's sarcoma of the foot. Clin Orthop Relat Res 1997;343:173–82.
64. Casadei R, Magnani M, Biagini R, et al. Prognostic factors in Ewing's sarcoma of the foot. Clin Orthop Rel Res 2004;420:230–8.
65. Jamshidi K, Shiradi MR. Unusual form and location for a tumor: multiosseous Ewing sarcoma in the foot. Am J Orthop (Belle Mead NJ) 2015;44(1):E32–5.
66. Gerrand C, Athanasou N, Brennan B, et al, British Sarcoma Group. UK guidelines for the management of bone sarcomas. Clin Sarcoma Res 2016;6:7.
67. Thompson MJ, Shapton JC, Punt SE, et al. MRI Identification of the osseous extent of pediatric bone sarcomas. Clin Orthop Relat Res 2018;476:559–64.
68. Thévenin-Lemoine C, Destombes L, Vial J, et al. Planning for bone excision in ewing sarcoma: post-chemotherapy MRI more accurate than pre-chemotherapy MRI assessment. J Bone Joint Surg Am 2018;100(1):13–20.
69. La TH, Meyers PA, Wexler LH, et al. Radiation therapy for Ewing's sarcoma: results from Memorial Sloan-Kettering in the modern era. Int J Radiat Oncol Biol Phys 2006;64(2):544–50.
70. Albergo JI, Gaston CLL, Parry MC, et al. Risk analysis factors for local recurrence in Ewing's sarcoma: when should adjuvant radiotherapy be administered? Bone Joint J 2018;100-B(2):247–55.
71. Campanacci M. Bone and soft tissue tumors. 2nd edition. Padova – Wien New York: Piccin – Springer-Verlag; 1999. p. 213–28.

72. Thorkildsen J, Taksdal I, Bjerkehagen B, et al. Chondrosarcoma in Norway 1990-2013; an epidemiological and prognostic observational study of a complete national cohort. Acta Oncol 2019;58(3):273–82.
73. Wu AM, Li G, Zheng JW, et al. Chondrosarcoma in a paediatric population: a study of 247 cases. J Child Orthop 2019;13(1):89–99.
74. McCarville MB. The child with bone pain: malignancies and mimickers. Cancer Imaging 2009;9:S115–21.
75. Singer AD, Datir A, Tresley J, et al. Benign and malignant tumors of the foot and ankle. Skeletal Radiol 2016;45(3):287–330.
76. Ayerza MA, Piuzzi NS, Aponte-Tinao LA, et al. Structural allograft reconstruction of the foot and ankle after tumor resections. Musculoskelet Surg 2016;100(2): 149–56.
77. Weiland A, Daniel R. Microvascular anastomoses for bone grafts in treatment of massive defects in bone". J Bone Joint Surg Am 1979;61:98–104.
78. Ishida O, Tsai T. Free vascularized whole joint transfer in children. Microsurgery 1991;12:196–206.
79. Shenaq SM, Dinh TA. Heel reconstruction with an iliac osteocutaneous free flap in a child. Microsurgery 1989;10:93–6.

Surgical Treatment of Calcaneonavicular and Talocalcaneal Coalitions

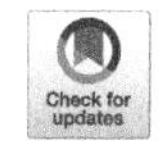

Désirée Moharamzadeh, MD[a], Maurizio De Pellegrin, MD[b,*]

KEYWORDS

- Tarsal coalition • Calcaneonavicular coalition • Talocalcaneal coalition
- Rigid flatfoot • Imaging • Alignement • Calcaneo-stop

KEY POINTS

- Calcaneonavicular (CNC) and talocalcaneal (TCC) coalitions are the most common causes of rigid flatfoot (RFF) in children. Resection with interposition of fat graft is the treatment of choice in symptomatic flatfeet.
- Plan radiographs are not always able to reveal the presence of CNC and TCC. Computed tomography (CT) is a useful tool for assessment, particularly of TCC, while MRI plays an important role in painful RFF with a suspected fibrous or cartilaginous CNC and/or TCC coalition; CT technique should be performed perpendicular to the subtalar joint ("coalition-specific axial plane") to permit a better visualization of the facets and with 1.0 × 1.0-mm slices. CT scan 3D reconstruction is useful for surgical planning.
- MRI can detect earlier the presence of a painful non-ossified coalition allowing an early resection of the fibrous or cartilaginous tissue before a complete osseous or rigid deformity develops.
- After resection, the correction of the most frequent hindfoot valgus deformity usually requires further surgery, such as lateral column lengthening. Arthrodesis is the most common surgical procedure for symptomatic flatfeet in adulthood.
- Adult patients with untreated coalitions or residual valgus deformity of the hindfoot often complain of anterolateral pain due to the calcaneofibular impingement and/or arthritis and medial pain around the osseous coalition. MRI can show bone marrow edema in the coalition area and in other areas of the affected foot, explaining symptoms and aiding in surgical indications, even in osseous coalitions.
- Subtalar arthroereisis for correction of residual hindfoot valgus can be performed after resection in one step.

[a] Orthopedic and Traumatology Unit, San Raffaele Hospital, Via Olgettina 60, Milan 20132, Italy; [b] Head Pediatric Orthopedic and Traumatology Unit, San Raffaele Hospital, Via Olgettina 60, Milan 20132, Italy
* Corresponding author.
E-mail address: depellegrin.maurizio@hsr.it

Foot Ankle Clin N Am 26 (2021) 873–901
https://doi.org/10.1016/j.fcl.2021.07.011

INTRODUCTION

Tarsal coalition is determined by an absence of segmentation between one or more foot bones, therefore, resulting in a failed joint cleft development. The first anatomic description of a coalition is around 1750 by Buffon[1]; Cruveilhier in 1829 described the anatomy of a calcaneonavicular coalition (CNC),[2] while in 1877, Zukerkandl described talocalcaneal coalition (TCC) and its anatomy.[3] Although the true incidence of tarsal coalitions is unknown, as many cases are not symptomatic, estimates are between 1% and 13%,[4,5] with a bilateral presentation in 50% of cases.[6] All tarsal joints may be involved; however, most coalitions (90%) involve the calcaneonavicular joint and the talocalcaneal joint.[7] The cited relative frequencies of coalitions are 53% for CNC, 37% for TCC, and infrequent appearances for the remaining talonavicular, calcaneocuboidal, and naviculocuneiform coalitions.[8]

As described in a study by Mosca,[9] in genetically programmed individuals, the coalition starts as a syndesmosis with fibrous tissue, which undergoes metaplasia to cartilage (synchondrosis) and subsequently to bone (synostosis). Therefore, although the coalition develops during embryogenesis, the synostosis forms only during growth. As a matter of fact, symptoms' onset occurs when the coalition ossifies; this generally is between 8 and 12 years for CNC and between 12 and 16 years for TCC.[10] In a large prospective MRI study,[4] tarsal coalitions were described precisely per type (osseous, cartilaginous, or fibrous) and location (calcaneonavicular and/or talocalcaneal/subtalar), confirming an underestimation of their prevalence.

As the subtalar motion is progressively limited, the foot becomes symptomatic and increasingly flat and rigid. The rotatory and gliding motion of the subtalar joint, if restricted, limits the physiologic compensatory external rotation of the foot during gait, forcing the calcaneus in a fixed valgus position, and the navicular overrides the talar head, with flattening of the arch.[10] Although valgus hindfoot has been addressed in many studies, it must be noted that it is not the only clinical presentation. In some patients, the arch develops, and the hindfoot may be in neutral or in varus position. If the posterior facet is involved, the clinical appearance may be of a pes cavus.[11–13] Clinical evaluation of patients with tarsal coalitions has been addressed in detail by Cass and Camasta.[14]

The main symptom is activity-related foot pain, usually dorsolateral for CNCs and medial for TCCs.[15] Pain is suggested to be caused by abnormal mechanical stresses due to the coalition.[16] Actually, although it has been postulated that an inflammatory process contributes to pain, Kumai and colleagues demonstrated in their histopathological study that no inflammatory cell infiltration or nerve elements are present at the coalition site or its boundaries.[17] In the untreated valgus deformity (before or after coalition resection), the main concerns are caused by the shear stresses due to the calcaneofibular impingement and the articular incongruity in weight-bearing, both of which may lead to degenerative changes of the articular surfaces in the subtalar joint and, therefore, pain.[18,19]

In this review, we will be addressing exclusively CNC and TCC.

IMAGING

Imaging has recently acquired an important role not only for the detailed analysis of the complex subtalar joint but also in detecting tarsal coalitions, their shape, and location and for surgical planning, particularly in TCC.[14] Many authors reported data of imaging mostly on TCC[20–25] and less on CNC.[14,26,27]

Radiological features for identifying TCC in lateral radiographs are indirect radiological signs of suspect. According to Phyo and colleagues,[22] the C-sign was recorded in

69%, the talar beaking sign in 29%, a dysmorphic sustentaculum in 74%, and the absence of the middle facet in 58% of TCC cases. According to Lee and colleagues[21] who reviewed radiological findings, CT and MRI images in 43 feet affected by TCC, the typical C-sign, which is generally present in middle facet coalitions, was present in only 32% of the TCC cases; in 68%, the posterior facet was involved, and a "deformed C-sign" was described. CT technique should be performed perpendicular to the subtalar joint ("coalition-specific axial plane") to permit a better visualization of the facets and with 1.0 × 1.0-mm slices.[14]

In a retrospective study, ultrasound appearance of TCC was studied. In 9 out of 11 patients (average age 35.3 years; range 17–58 years), a fibrous coalition was detected showing a reduced joint space of the medial aspect of the anterior talocalcaneal joint. Instead in the remaining 2 patients, an osseous coalition was detected; a smooth continuity of the bone surface was seen between the talus and the sustentaculum. Confirmation of the coalition was obtained by CT or MRI, which were suggested for preoperative assessment.[20]

An elongated anterior process of the calcaneus or irregular bony margins may hide a non-osseous CNC which can be visualized with a CT scan. Performing 26 CT scans and 40 MRI examinations in 65 TCCs did not only permit to visualize the anterior, middle, posterior facet TCC and extra-articular posteromedial (EA-PM) coalition with or without *os sustentaculum* but also allowed to identify cases (31.3%) where more than one facet was involved or a CNC was present, classifying these cases as "complex."[22]

Guignand and colleagues[26] report in a specific study the role of MRI in CNC in 24 children (34 feet; average age at surgery 12.9 years), determining that in the presence of a rigid and painful foot and a negative radiograph, MRI was the most effective examination for detecting CNC, replacing the previously used CT. Bone scintigraphy was also performed in this study in 7 cases; only 3 showed hyperfixation. The results of bone scan with single photon emission computed tomography/computed tomography (SPECT/CT) were recently reported in a study with 33 patients (mean age 13.4 years) with complex foot and ankle pain; in 8 of 9 tarsal coalitions, decisive clinical value added by SPECT/CT was reported.[28]

Hamel stated that an oblique view of a plain radiograph is sufficient for diagnosing CNC. Instead in TCC, CT and MRI should be performed to understand exactly the shape of the coalition (CT) and to evaluate the bone signal (edema) of the involved joints (MRI). Both are useful for preoperative planning.[27] CT was considered the gold standard of imaging in TCC because of its ability to show the osseous anatomy. Many authors underlined the role of MRI for detecting non-osseous coalitions and differentiating the fibrous from the cartilaginous coalition.[14,25–27] Cass and Camasta demonstrated in a review of tarsal coalitions the role of MRI which can show bony edema of the medial aspect of the subtalar joint also in complete osseous TCC, implying a mechanical stress of the bones and explaining the pain.[14] MRI findings include bone marrow edema in the coalition area and in other areas of the affected foot, such as in the calcaneofibular area.[22,25]

For a better understanding of the coalition and a correct preoperative planning, Upasani and colleagues analyzed 3D CT images of patients with CNC, further defining the variants, from type I (forme fruste variant), type II (fibrous coalition), type III (cartilaginous synchondrosis), and type IV (osseous coalition).[29] Similarly, Rozansky and colleagues described a 3D CT-based classification for TCC[30]: type I (linear), the commonest; type II (linear with posterior hook), similar to type I but with a hook on the posterior aspect of the sustentaculum tali; type III (shingled), hypoplastic sustentaculum tali; type IV (bone) is the most controversial regarding treatment (resection or realignment) (**Fig. 1**); type V (posterior) usually small and located in the posterior subtalar joint, close to the neurovascular bundle. Lim and colleagues[23] introduced a new radiological classification for TCC based on a multiplanar imaging study using CT and MRI in 70 feet: type I linear TCC (65%), type II talar overgrowth (14%) (see **Fig. 1**), type III calcaneal overgrowth (19%), type IV complete osseous (3%). The classification provides information regarding the surgical approach. Yun and colleagues[24] reported the necessity of a continuous revision of the classification, introducing after evaluation of CT and MRI images, the "extraarticular TCC with *os sustentaculum*" as a different type of coalition; it was demostrated in 13 of 81 foot coalitions (16%) and in 13 of 54 TCCs (24.1%). The patients with an *os sustentaculum* presented symptoms in the medial talocalcaneal region. Phyo and colleagues introduced later the EA-PM TCC which cannot be diagnosed with the classical indirect radiological signs; in patients with vague ankle symptoms and a prominence of the posterior facet of the subtalar joint, MRI and CT studies should be carefully assessed.[22]

Summarizing imaging roles, (1) CT is useful for assessment, particularly in TCC, while MRI plays a role in painful rigid feet with suspected fibrous and cartilaginous TCC and/or CNC coalition (**Fig. 2**); (2) the ability of MRI to detect at an earlier stage the presence of a painful non-ossified coalition allows an early resection of the fibrous or cartilaginous tissue before the development of a complete rigid deformity; resection at an early age yields better results and permits to later avoid invasive surgery due to

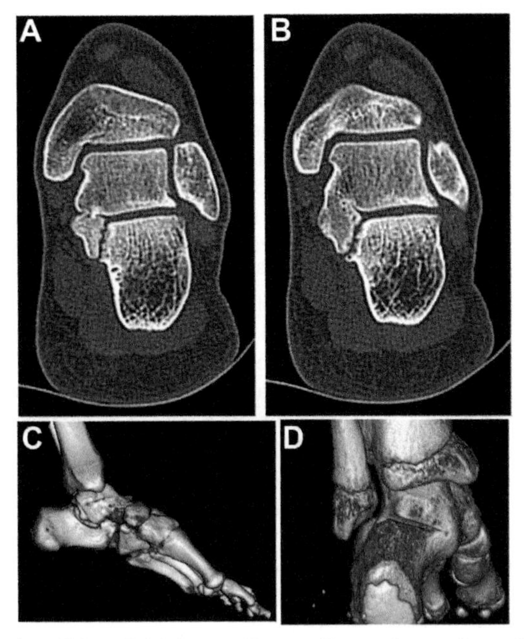

Fig. 1. Talocalcaneal coalitions (TCCs). Type III according to Rozansky and colleagues[30] (shingled shape) on CT scan (*A, B*) and on 3D reconstruction in a 14-year-old boy and type II (talar overgrowth) according to Lim and colleagues[23] (*C*). Type IV (complete osseous coalition) according to Rozansky and colleagues[30] and Lim and colleagues[23] on 3D reconstruction in a 13-year-old boy (*D*). (*From* Rozansky A, Varley E, Moor M, Wenger DR, Mubarak SJ. A radiologic classification of talocalcaneal coalitions based on 3D reconstruction. JCO 2010; 4: 129 – 35 and Lim S, Lee HK, Bae S, et al. A radiological classification system for talocalcaneal coalition based on a multi-planar imaging study using CT and MRI. Insights Imaging 2013 Oct; 4 (5): 563 – 67.)

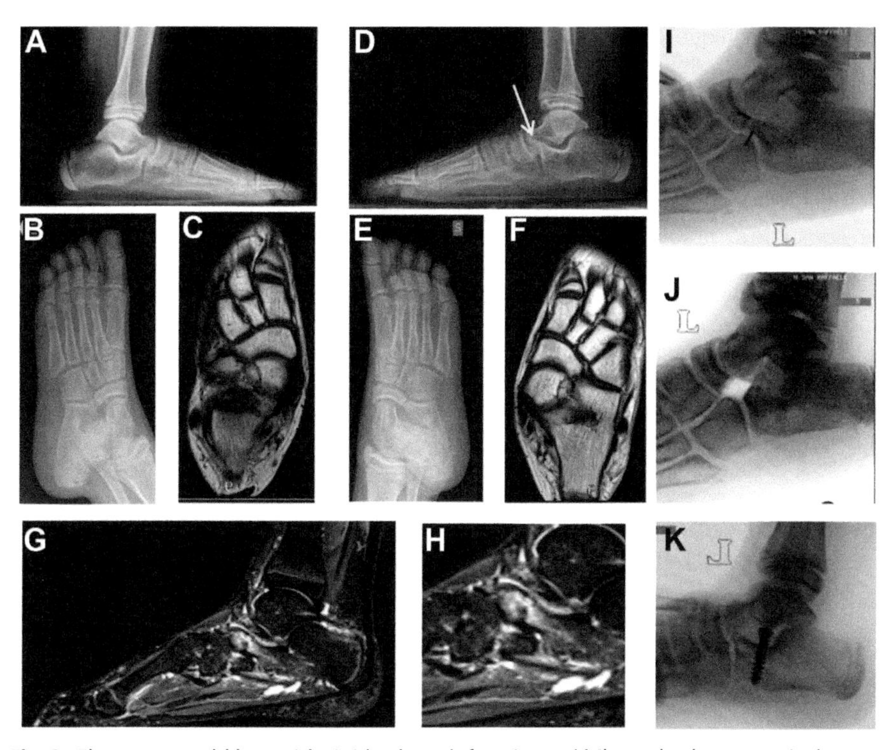

Fig. 2. Eleven years old boy with rigid valgus deformity and bilateral calcaneonavicular coalition (CNC) complaining of pain after sport activities. Weight-bearing lateral view radiograph (*A*) and oblique view (*B*) of the right and left foot (D-E, respectively). "Anteater–sign" (yellow *arrow*). MRI-T1 weighted showing fibrocartilaginous tissue between the calcaneal and navicular bony border (*C-F*) and MRI-dP (diffusion prepared) fat weighted showing perilesional signal alterations (*G*), magnification (*H*). Preoperative fluoroscopy check with two landmark needles (*I*). Intraoperative radiograph after bar resection (*J*). Calcaneo-stop procedure for residual valgus deformity (*K*).

pain in adulthood[27,31]; (3) bone marrow edema in the coalition area and in other areas of the affected foot such as the calcaneofibular area helps in explaining symptoms and determining surgical indications, even in osseous types.

SURGICAL TECHNIQUES

At presentation, a symptomatic tarsal coalition (CNC or TCC) must be treated conservatively for at least 6 months. If the conservative treatment fails after 6 months of trial[32–35] and the foot is still painful, provided it is a single coalition and no degenerative signs present, resection is the treatment of choice. Advantage of surgery is to restore mobility and reduce the risk of subsequent degenerative arthritis.[36] Aims of surgery are to relieve pain of the foot and ankle, to restore subtalar and midtarsal movement, and to correct deformity and have a well-aligned foot.[32] Resection surgery has some common pitfalls. First, in 4% of cases, there may be a failure to recognize associated coalitions. Second, the resection may be inadequate, with a nonresected medial plantar aspect. On the contrary, the resection may be too extensive determining an iatrogenic uncovering of the talus. Finally, adjoining bones may be injured during resection, such as the talar head or the cuboid.[32]

Surgical technique of excision and interposition of fat graft in CNC and TCC is described in the following paragraph.

CALCANEONAVICULAR COALITION

Surgical resection of calcaneonavicular bar (1927) was first described by Badgley[37] in a study in 1967 as a technique for resection (largest series at that time, n = 41 feet)[38] with complete symptom relief in 68% (n = 28 feet), thereby introducing it in the surgical practice (**Figs. 3–5**). To be successful, the operation had to be confined to the younger patient. Long-standing deformity or adaptive joint changes diminished the chances of success and were responsible for some of the poor results in this study. The ideal case for operation was described as "that of a young patient with symptoms of recent origin and no adaptive joint changes visible in the radiographs."[38] No interposition was performed, but the raw bone exposed was cauterized by diathermy to prevent regrowth. However, recurrence of the bar occurred to a large extent in one-third of the feet and to a slight extent in another third, so concern regarding ossification after resection of the coalition led to the addition of tissue interposition (muscle, tendon) or bone wax, after the removal of the bar. To avoid recurrence of the bone bar and improve long-term pain relief, the CNC resection was associated to the interposition of the extensor

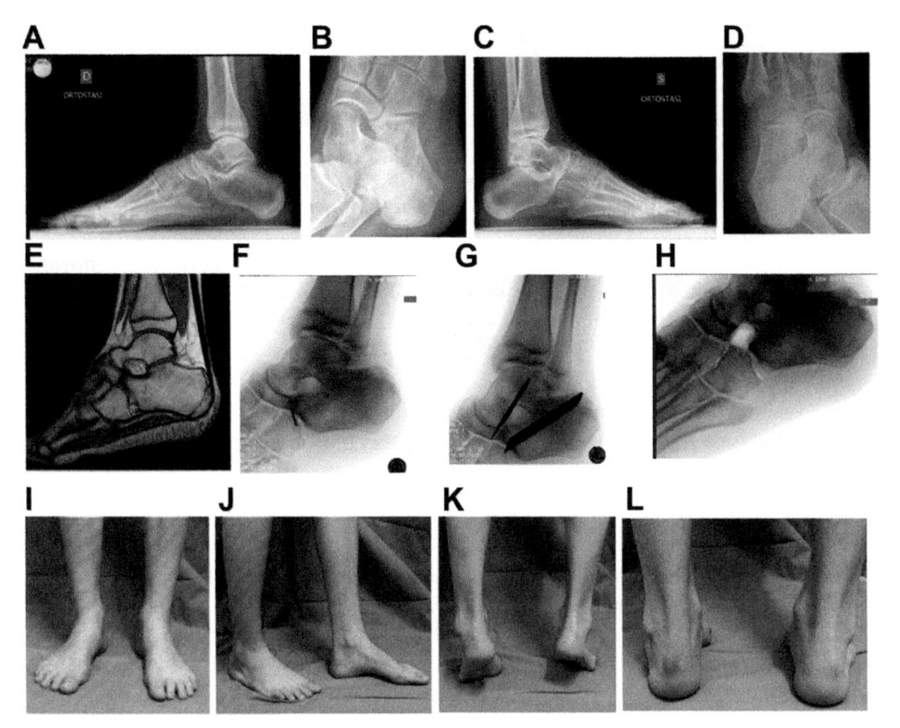

Fig. 3. Twelve-year-old girl with rigid symptomatic cavovarus deformity bilateral complaining of many ankle sprains on the left. Weight-bearing lateral view radiograph (*A*) and oblique view (*B*) of the right and left foot (*C, D*, respectively). "Anteater-sign". MRI of the left foot showing fibrocartilaginous coalition (*E*). Preoperative fluoroscopy check with landmark needle (*F*). Intraoperative radiograph for correct resection (*G*) and after bar resection left (*H*). Clinical aspect at follow-up with residual mild cavus and varus deformity of the left foot (*I–L*).

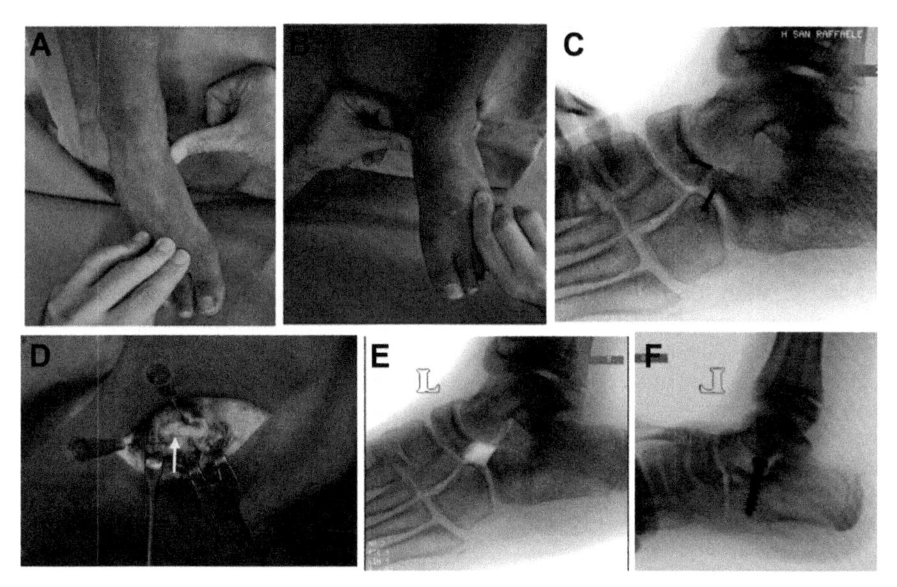

Fig. 4. Fourteen-year-old boy with calcaneonavicular coalition left (CNC). Clinical evaluation of the normal right foot with normal range of motion of supination and adduction (*A*). Limited painful supination and adduction motion of the left foot (*B*). Preoperative fluoroscopy check with two needles percutaneously inserted to identify the correct site of CNC (*C*). CNC exposition (yellow *arrow*) between the two landmark needles after dissection of the exstensor muscles (*D*). Intraoperative radiograph after correct osteotomy of the bar (*E*). A calcaneo-stop procedure is performed to correct the residual hind foot valgus (*F*).

digitorum brevis (EDB) muscle.[10,33,39] Relative contraindication to resection is complete ossification because degenerative changes may have occurred in other tarsal joints. As a matter of fact, in patients with large coalitions, failed resection or advanced degenerative changes, arthrodesis is recommended.[40] Triple arthrodesis in CNC is described by Mitchell and Gibson in 1967,[38] in the adult foot or in the adolescent

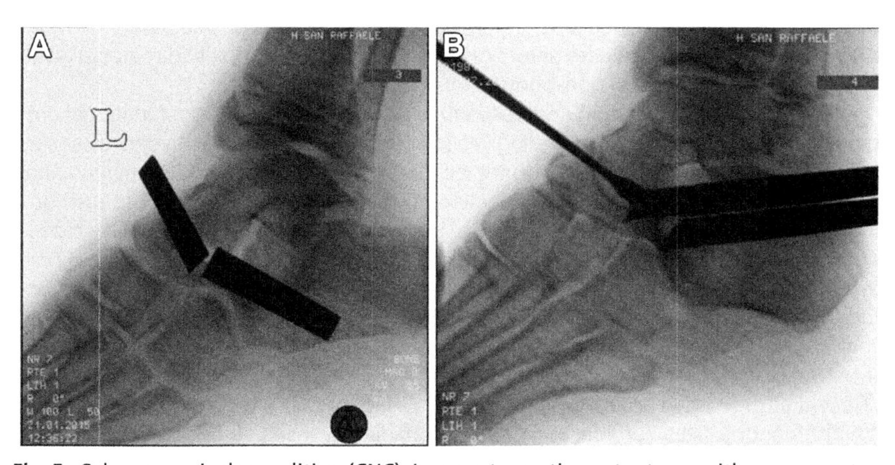

Fig. 5. Calcaneonavicular coalition (CNC). Incorrect resection osteotomy with convergent osteotomes (*A*) and correct 1-cm resection technique with parallel osteotomes (*B*).

foot which underwent adaptive joint changes. Andreasen in a study in 1968 confirmed his recommendation on triple arthrodesis instead of resection as he considered the former much safer with respect to secondary osteoarthritis.[41]

When resection is performed, all cartilage and bone from the bar must be excised completely from the calcaneus and the navicular ones (see **Fig. 5**). The surgeon should be cautious not to enter the talonavicular joint because cutting the talonavicular capsule will allow the navicular to ride up on the talus.[10] After the resection, the origin of the EDB (anterior part of the dorsal surface of the calcaneus) is interposed and held there by a catgut suture passed through the medial aspect of the foot and tied over a button. Between 1983 and 1993, other authors[42–46] described retrospectively their results with excision and EBD muscle interposition. Results were reported from good to excellent (88%–69%), and the technique has been the gold standard for many years. In 2009, a study describes open excision of the calcaneonavicular bar associated with fat grafting to achieve functional improvement and full recovery in sports activities, with a low reossification rate.[33] In this study, 69 feet with CNC underwent fat graft interposition to address patient and parents' complaints of a bony prominence on the lateral border of the foot resulting in difficulties while wearing shoes following the near-traditional method of EBD interposition after coalition resection (1990s). Postoperatively, 89% had pain improvement, and 87% were able to fully return to sport or past level of activity. Fat was grafted from the gluteal cleft or, in alternative form, the abdomen in obese children. Furthermore, they suspected that EDB muscle was not long enough to fill the gap. In fact, in their cadaveric study, Mubarak and colleagues[33] demonstrated that the EBD muscle was able to fill on average 64% of the gap. A previous CT analysis of CNC verified the depth of the coalition to be 25 mm,[29] supporting the data on EBD muscle's insufficient filling. This study was confirmed by Masquijo and colleagues in 2017.[47] In their study, where 3 groups of patients were compared (fat graft vs bone wax vs EBD muscle belly), autogenous fat graft and bone wax interposition techniques provided better pain relief, gave better functional scores, and avoided more effectively coalition reossification than EBD technique, in a statistically significant manner (4% wax, 6% fat, and 40% EBD). Interposition with bone wax has the advantage of avoiding an accessory incision, but once placed, it is not reabsorbed. It is very effective in reducing intraoperative bleeding and is known to interfere with bone healing and osteogenesis, which is useful for the treatment of coalitions. However, it also induces chronic inflammation and reduces bacterial clearance in cancellous bone, increasing the risk of infection.[48] Further studies are required to evaluate safety of bone wax as an interposition material given the potential to produce foreign-body reactions and infections.[48,49]

In a study in 2013, Khoshbin and colleagues analyzed the long-term functional outcomes of bar resection, demonstrating in a long follow-up period (14.4 years after surgery) that primary arthrodesis may not be necessary as initial treatment and that resection should be considered irrespective of coalition size.[50] Although, in previous studies, CNC resections are reported to have better outcomes than TCC resections,[18,51] Khoshbin and colleagues in their study reported similar function and pain for both CNC and TCC.[50] Mahan and colleagues describe similar findings in a recent study, where no significant difference is reported between CNC and TCC outcome groups, confirming the high rates of return to full activity (based on patient reports) after bar resection.[52]

Recent studies have addressed the topic of resection, via a less invasive approach, with arthroscopy. This surgical technique is a minimally invasive alternative which allows a quicker postoperative recovery, as weight-bearing is not always restricted, earlier hospital discharge, reduced levels of postoperative pain, lower rates of infections and wound complications, and better esthetic results.[36,53–55] These studies, although presenting a valid option, with referred excellent outcomes, require a longer follow-up and larger series to assess the long-term efficacy.

The main advantage of arthroscopic resection is to perfectly visualize the area and to completely remove the coalition and avoid the risk of a plantar residual bone bar. Another important advantage is the possibility to assess and treat in the same procedure associated pathologies such as degenerative changes in the lateral side of the talar head with debridement and resection.[56] One of the difficulties of arthroscopy is the location of the portals; both visualization and working portals must be identified accurately so to achieve a complete resection.[57] Another disadvantage is the obvious difficulty in positioning an interposition graft. However, in a review, Raikin and colleagues found no cases of recurrence after arthroscopic resection of tarsal coalitions, despite the absence of a tissue interposition[58]; this could be due to the early mobilization and weight-bearing, which may inhibit reossification of the coalition.[57]

TALOCALCANEAL COALITION

TCC is the most common cause of rigid flatfoot (RFF) (**Figs. 6–9**). In the past, it was mistakenly referred to as peroneal spastic flat foot, characterized by limited tarsal joint motion, a clonus response to evertors and a pes planus deformity[59]; however, it has since been recognized that the deformity is present despite the absence of spasticity.[60] The subsequent RFF associated to a TCC is often symptomatic (25% of cases).[8,10,14] Anatomy of a TCC must be considered in preoperative planning; the coalition may be either central (articular) or peripheral (extraarticular), as described in Downey classification.[61] In the central form, all 3 facets may be involved (in order of decreasing frequency: (1) middle facet, (2) posterior facet, (3) anterior facet). See imaging paragraph.

For many years, subtalar or triple arthrodesis was the treatment of choice for pain relief.[62–65] These are now limited to feet which have an extensive coalition, failed resection secondary to an unrecognized bar before surgery or radiographic evidence of osteoarthritis,[10,66] as otherwise, with a primary arthrodesis, one achieves pain relief

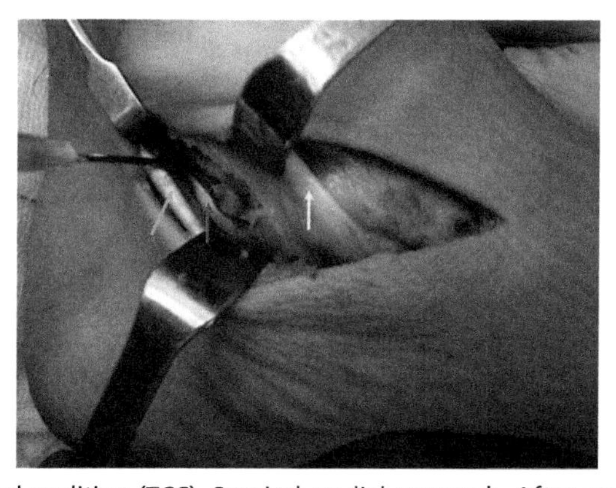

Fig. 6. Talocalcaneal coalition (TCC). Surgical medial approach. After opening sheaths, the tendon of the tibialis posterior muscle (TP) (*yellow arrow*) and of the flexor digitorum longus (FDL) (*blue arrow*) will appear. The flexor hallucis longus (FHL) tendon (*red arrow*) is located under the *sustentaculum tali* and represents a landmark for the above present coalition. The TP is retracted dorsally, and the FHL and FDL plantarly.

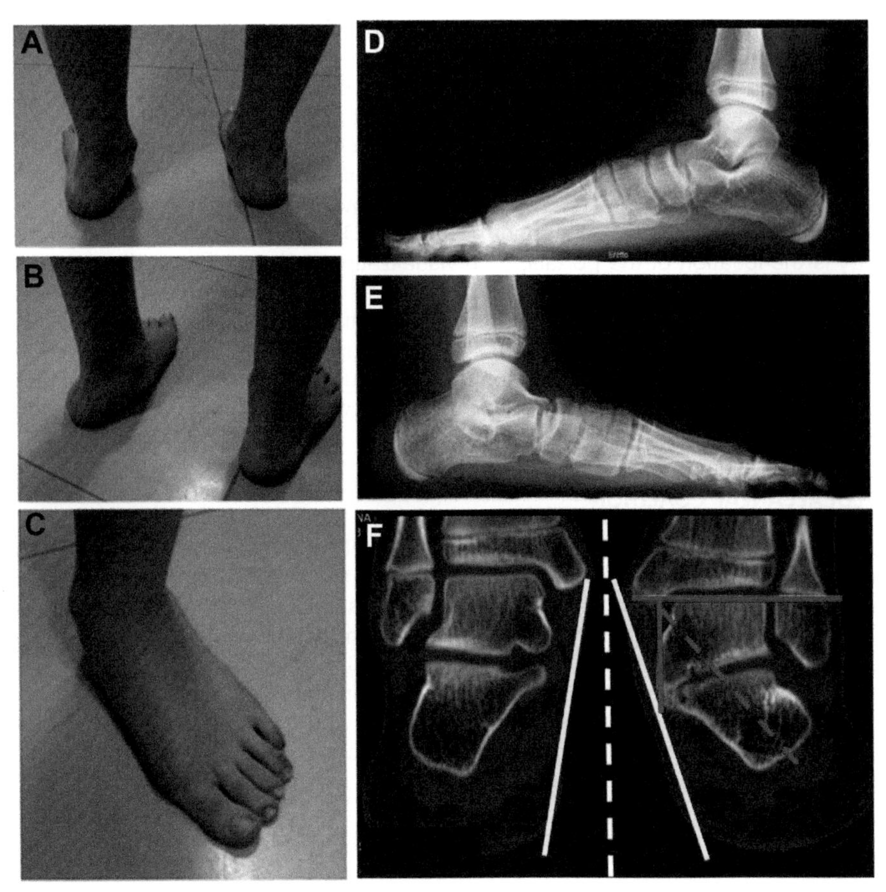

Fig. 7. Twelve-year-old girl with severe rigid symptomatic flat foot deformity left and asymptomatic flexible flat foot right. Upon weight-bearing, marked hindfoot valgus (*A*), collapse of the medial longitudinal arch (*B*), and supination of the forefoot (*C*) were observed. Lateral radiographic evaluation of the right (*D*) and left foot showing the "C-sign" left (*E*). Coronal slice CT scan image shows the angle measured between the axis of the calcaneus (dashed *line*) and the line perpendicular to the ankle joint (red *line*). Yellow lines show the valgus rearfoot profile (*F*).

with the sacrifice of the affected joint's motion and with the risk in the long term of tibio-talar arthritis after triple arthrodesis.[67] Early attempts of resection were limited to the young population, and arthrodesis/fusion were recommended to older patients; however, this was probably due to the delay in treatment and the onset of secondary changes in the subtalar joints.[34]

Now, many studies reported good results with resection and interposition of various tissues.[18,51,68–70] Commonly used materials are fat, bone wax, flexor hallucis longus tendon, pediculated tibialis posterior tendon sheath, fascia lata allograft, or cartilage allograft.[58,71–74] As reported, the three most important symptoms of a TCC are pain, valgus deformity of the hindfoot, and stiffness of the subtalar joint. According to Salomão and colleagues, the absence of heel varus when on tip toe was most helpful in identifying clinically a TCC, present in all cases. Similarly, as in other studies, in 1984, Salomão and colleagues also preferred to perform triple arthrodesis for the deformity.

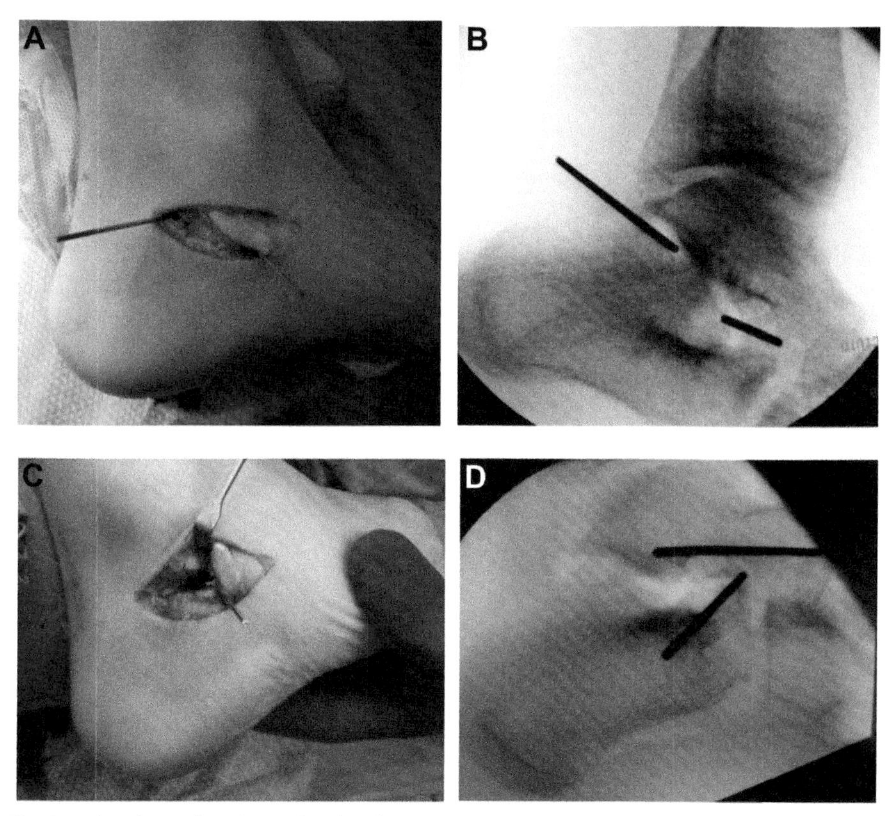

Fig. 8. Talocalcaneal coalition (TCC). After retraction of the TP tendon, the posterior limit of the coalition is identified with a K-wire (*A*). A fluoroscopy check is useful to show the exact positioning of the K-wires in the subtalar joint also of the anterior limit of the coalition (*B*). After resection of the coalition, the subtalar joint motion has to be checked clinically (*C*) and documented by X-ray (*D*).

However, in this study in 1992, the results reported on TC bar resection and fat graft interposition were gratifying with 78% of pain-free feet after surgery.[75]

Patients will often present with foot and/or ankle sprains, pain on the medial aspect of the foot, or flat feet.[35] Gantsoudes and colleagues report that excision of TC bar helps to prevent future pathology, such as sprains, fractures, and ankle arthritis.[76] In fact, according to Moraleda and colleagues,[77] all symptomatic TCC should undergo resection (unless there are other concomitant coalitions or the TCC are solid and large), as the underlying pathology will eventually lead to painful degenerative changes throughout the course of the patient's life. In their case study, the preferred surgical treatment was represented by resection and fat interposition,[76] harvested from the gluteus or the abdomen, as well as bone wax, with approximately 86% of good-excellent outcomes based on The American Orthopedic Foot and Ankle Score (AOFAS) score and an improvement of range of motion in 92% of cases. However, they did not assess preoperative hindfoot deformity when approaching surgery and concluded that excision with interposition was the best treatment for TCC to improve joint motion and relieve pain. Further surgery to correct realignment was to be taken into consideration as a secondary procedure. In a review in 2015, the authors[35]

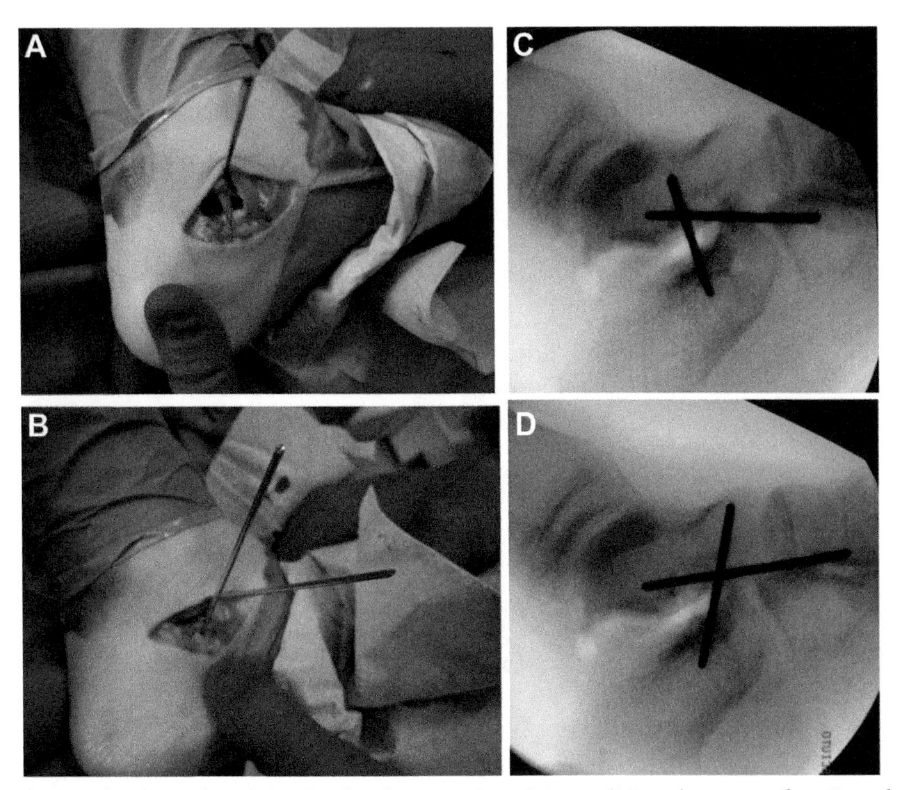

Fig. 9. Talocalcaneal coalition (TCC). After resection of the coalition, the range of motion of the subtalar joint is checked clinically in eversion (*A*) and inversion (*B*) and radiologically (*C*) and (*D*), respectively.

reported the same conclusions, as they believed that TCC and valgus hindfoot are two separate conditions and must be approached as such. First, resection must be performed to regain subtalar motion, then after 1 year at most, realignment surgery may be considered.

As seen, many different open techniques with or without tissue interposition for TCC resection have been described, and until 2011, arthroscopic resection was addressed only for CNC.[54,56] Introducing a new technique, Bonasia and colleagues in 2011[78] described the posterior arthroscopic resection of a TCC, with excellent results and low complication rates. They described an algorhythm for surgical approach to TCC, and their inclusion criteria for arthroscopy were very selective; posterior-facet TCC, after failure of adequate conservative management and no prior foot surgery. Contraindications to arthroscopy were if the coalition had an anterior, middle facet involvement and if the posterior facet's involvement was more than 50%. As most TCCs involve the middle facet,[24] their application of arthroscopic resection was further limited. Knörr and colleagues[79] extended the inclusion criteria of a posterior ankle arthroscopic approach to medial facet TCC (Rozansky types I to IV), although surgically more challenging. Fifteen patients with symptomatic TCC were treated with an arthroscopic resection, and 4 underwent simultaneously a calcaneo-stop technique to correct a hindfoot valgus greater than 20°, with postoperative improvement in motion and alignment.

Compared with the lateral approach described by Jagodzinski and colleagues,[13] the posterior portals allow to visualize the medial anatomic structures, avoiding the risk of their injury. However, similar to arthroscopic resection of CNC, ankle arthroscopy for TCC has a longer learning curve, increased duration of the procedure, posterior tibial neurovascular bundle damage, and difficulty in using interposition material. It remains nevertheless a valid alternative to open surgery.[78]

POSTOPERATIVE CARE

Postoperative care varies depending on the type of surgery performed.

After resection of any tarsal coalition, if open excision is performed, the consensus is to apply a short-leg cast and allow immediate weight-bearing, as tolerated. Different authors suggested 3 weeks of cast after excision and fat interposition of TCC; after 3 weeks, the patients transition to a sturdy athletic shoe and begin physical therapy.[35,51,76] In a large series of 96 feet with CNC, treated with resection and fat interposition, a short-leg walking cast was applied for 2 to 3 weeks, and at removal, subtalar motion and plantarflexion were encouraged with a home exercise regimen. At 6 weeks after surgery, patients returned to their activities.[33]

In cases where a different type of interposition graft was used, such as tibialis posterior tendon sheath, patients were kept in cast with no weight-bearing for 2 weeks to protect the graft. Then, partial weight-bearing was recommended for 4 weeks, combined with physical therapy; full weight-bearing was allowed at 6 weeks postoperatively.[69]

If open resection of the tarsal coalition and immediate foot realignment with an arthroereisis was performed, patients wore a cast for 2 to 4 weeks, and full weight-bearing was allowed as soon as pain was tolerable. If an Achilles' tendon lengthening was performed, the cast was removed after 4 weeks.[31,80]

In TCC, where patients are managed with calcaneal lengthening osteotomies, regardless of concomitant resection of the coalition, a short-leg non-weight-bearing cast is used for 8 weeks. At 6 weeks postoperatively, the cast is changed, and the lateral column Steinmann pin is removed. Weight-bearing is commenced after 8 weeks.[81]

In a bicentre case series on arthroscopic excision of TCC, Jagodzinski and colleagues encourage the subtalar movement from the immediate postoperative period.[13] No casting is applied, only a bandage for 48 hours and foot elevation is highly recommended. These 9 patients had a slightly different approach to weight-bearing: In the first institute, they were mobilized with no weight-bearing for 2 weeks; and in the second institute, they were allowed to mobilize with weight-bearing and crutches for comfort. All walked unaided by the 6th week postoperatively. All patients returned to good level of activity within 6 months to 1 year from surgery.[13] Similarly, in CNC, as described by Lui, the postoperative care of an arthroscopic resection is the active and passive mobilization of the foot, started on day 1. Weight-bearing was allowed, as tolerated.[54]

A literature review of the last 10 years (2010–2020) regarding tarsal coalition surgery techniques and results is reported in **Table 1**.

COMPLICATIONS

In a total of 18 articles selected from 2010 to 2020, 603 feet were included from the studies on coalitions' operative[13,16,47,50,52,64,68,73,76,79–86] and nonoperative treatment.[80,87] Among operative treatment with different surgical techniques, authors classified outcome data on 343 feet as excellent, good, fair, and poor. Out of these 343

Table 1
Literature review of the last 10-year period (2010–2020) regarding tarsal coalition surgery techniques and results

Author, Year	Title	N° Patients (N° Feet)	Mean Age at Treatment	Type of Treatment	Follow-up (y)	Results	Complications/ Recurrence
Sperl et al,[16] 2010	Preliminary report: resection and interposition of a deepithelialized skin flap graft in tarsal coalition in children	3 (3)	13.4 (10–15)	Resection + deepithelialized skin flap interposition.	3.3 (0.5–8)	Good/excellent 3/3 (100%)	none
Lisella et al,[83] 2011	Tarsal coalition resection with pes planovalgus hindfoot reconstruction	7 (8)	15 (12–18)	Resection + reconstruction	3 (2–5)	Good/excellent 8/8 (100%)	1 infection 1 deep vein thrombosis
Mosca and Bevan,[81] 2012	Talocalcaneal tarsal coalitions and the calcaneal lengthening osteotomy: the role of deformity correction	8 (13)	13 (10–18)	a. 5 patients (9 ft) with RFF and TCC (coalition area >50%): CLO + strayer or TAL + medial plication.	2–15	Good/excellent: Group 1: 9/9 (100%) Group 2: 2/2 (100%) Group 3: 1/2 (50%)	Group 1: 1 patient developed pain under the fourth and fifth metatarsal heads on

				b. 1 patient (2 ft) with RFF and TCC (coalition area >50%): simultaneous CLO + resection of the middle facet coalition + strayer. c. 2 patients (2 ft) with residual RFF after the resection of a middle facet tarsal coalition: CLO + TAL + talonavicular arthrodesis (1 ft)			both feet. Grouo 2: None. Group 3: 1 patient underwent talonavicular arthrodesis for symptomatic arthritis
Gantsoudes et al,[76] 2012	Treatment of talocalcaneal coalitions	32 (49)	13	TCC resection + fat graft interposition	3.5	Poor (1) 2% Fair (6) 12% Good (10) 20% Excellent (32) 64%	11 ft (22%) underwent a total of 12 secondary procedures involving the lower extremity, including 2 revisions (4%)
Khoshbin et al,[50] 2013	Long-term functional outcomes of resected tarsal coalitions	24 (32) TCC: 11 (13) CNC: 13 (19)	TCC: 11.9 (8–16) CNC: 11.8 (10–13)	TCC: Resection alone (1) or with interposition of fat/wax graft (7), flexor digitorum longus (4) or flexor hallucis longus (1)	TCC: 13.1 CNC: 15.3	13/13 (100%) TCC with hindfoot valgus less or equal to 16° had comparable outcomes to those >16°	TCC: Wound infection (1)

(*continued on next page*)

Table 1
(continued)

Author, Year	Title	N° Patients (N° Feet)	Mean Age at Treatment	Type of Treatment	Follow-up (y)	Results	Complications/ Recurrence
				CNC: resection alone (1) or with interposition extensor digitorum brevis (18), Achilles tendon lengthening (1)		Subtalar inversion/ eversion TCC < CNC Questionnaire/ scores no differences between TCC & CNC	
Jagodzinski et al,[13] 2013	Arthroscopic resection of talocalcaneal coalitions—a bicentre case series of a new technique	8 (9)	15 (11–20)	Arthroscopic resection.	1–5.5	Good/excellent 7/9 (78%)	1 patient developed scar sensitivity at one of the portal sites. 1 patient had posterior tibial nerve damage. 1 patient (2 ft) required further surgery (fusion)
de Wouters et al,[73] 2014	Patient-specific instruments for surgical resection of painful tarsal coalition in adolescents	9 TCC (7) CNC (2)	14 (11–16)	CNC: Resection TCC: Resection using 3D printed cutting guides + fascia lata allograft interposition.	1.5	Excellent (5) 55.5% Satisfactory (4) 44.5%	None

Kemppainen et al,[84] 2014	The use of a portable CT scanner for the intraoperative assessment of talocalcaneal coalition resections	19 (26)	13.5 (9–17)	Resection with (14) or without (12) intraoperative assessment through a portable CT scanner	2 (0.5–4)	Intraop group • Excellent 57% • Fair 21% • Poor 21% Control group 25% • Excellent 25% • Fair 42% • Poor 33% Intraoperative CT scan changed surgical decision making in 21% (3) Pain improvement: 75% (9/12) of patients in the control group and 79% (11/14) in the intraoperative CT group reported	1 case required further surgery Intraop group: • 3 persistent pain • 2/3 correction of flat foot Control group: • 5 feet (4 pts) flat foot correction • (2) 16% persistent pain
Krief et al,[68] 2016	Tarsal coalitions: preliminary results after operative excision and silicone sheet interposition in children	3 (3)	10 (8–12)	Resection + interposition of a sterile silicone sheet	3.3 (1–6.7)	3/3 (100%)	none
Knörr et al,[79] 2015	Arthroscopic talocalcaneal coalition resection in children	15 (16)	11.8 (8–15)	Arthroscopic resection	2.3 (1–3.7)	Mean AOFAS 90.9 Excellent 67% Fair 27% Poor (1) 7%	Complex regional pain syndrome in 1 patient. No recurrences.

(*continued on next page*)

Table 1
(continued)

Author, Year	Title	N° Patients (N° Feet)	Mean Age at Treatment	Type of Treatment	Follow-up (y)	Results	Complications/ Recurrence
Mahan et al,[52] 2015	Patient-reported outcomes of tarsal coalitions treated with surgical excision	63 (87) CNC (43) 68% TCC (20) 32%	4.62	Resection	4.62 (1.8–10.6)	Overall: AOFAS mean 88.3 UCLA mean 8.33 73% (32 CNC, 14 TCC): • Activity levels not limited by foot pain • AOFAS 93.9 • UCLA 8.9 27% (11 CNC, 6 TCC): • Activity levels limited • AOFAS 72.9 • UCLA 6.9 TCC: AOFAS 88.4 UCLA 8.4 CNC: AOFAS 88 UCLA 8.3 Type of coalition not indicative factor in determining the outcome	Unilateral surgery: worse outcome

Hamel et al,[85] 2016	Surgical treatment of talocalcaneal coalition: experience with 80 cases of pediatric or adolescent patients	(80)	8–17	1. Resection + fat interposition (31) 2. Resection + fat interposition + tarsal osteotomy (26) 3. Fusion (20) 4. Fusion + tarsal osteotomy (3)	3	Group 1: 27/31 (87%) Group 2: 20/26 (77%) Group 3: 18/20 (90%) Group 4: 3/3 (100%)	Group 1: • Persistent pain after 15 mo (2) • Further surgery (1) Group 2: • Further surgery (2) Group 3: • Moderate tarsal pain (2)
Mahan et al,[86] 2017	Subtalar coalitions: Does the morphology of the subtalar joint involvement influence outcomes after coalition excision?	36 (51)	13.1	Resection	2.7	41/51 (80%)	2 patients developed superficial wound infection
Masquijo et al,[82] 2017	Surgical reconstruction for talocalcaneal coalitions with severe hindfoot valgus deformity	13 (14)	14 (11–16)	7 patients (8 ft): simultaneous TCC resection and reconstruction (CSO, CNL MCO) 6 patients (6 ft): isolated reconstruction	3.7	14/14 (100%) significative improvement of AOFAS scores	Hardware prominence (1) Superficial infection (1)

(continued on next page)

Table 1
(continued)

Author, Year	Title	N° Patients (N° Feet)	Mean Age at Treatment	Type of Treatment	Follow-up (y)	Results	Complications/ Recurrence
Masquijo et al,[47] 2017	Fat graft and bone wax interposition provides better functional outcomes and lower reossification rates than extensor digitorum brevis after calcaneonavicular coalition resection	48 (56)	Group 1: 12 (10–17) Group 2: 12.5 (11–15) Group 3: 12 (11–14)	July 2008-July 2015 CNC resection-interposition Group 1: Fat graft (23) Group 2: Bone graft (18) Group 3: Extensor digitorum brevis (15)	2.91 (1–6.5) Group 1: 2 (1–6.5) Group 2: 3.2 (2–4.5) Group 3: 3.1 (2.1–4.3)	Preoperative AOFAS Group 1: 59 (33–71) Group 2: 50 (34–62) Group 3: 48 (30–60) Postoperative AOFAS Group 1: 98 (62–100) Group 2: 98 (88–100) Group 3: 75 (70–95)	Regrowth: Group 1: 4% Group 2: 6% Group 3: 40% Progressive symptoms: Group 3: 5 feet
Hubert et al,[69] 2018	Resection of medial talocalcaneal coalition with interposition of a pediculated flap of tibialis posterior tendon sheath	10 (12)	12.2 (10–18)	TCC resection and interposition of pediculated flap of the tibialis posterior tendon sheath	4.8	12/12 (100%) • Pain reduction • Activity improvement • Subtalar joint motion improvement • AOFAS score improvement	None
Shirley et al,[87] 2018	Results of nonoperative treatment for symptomatic tarsal coalitions	49 (50) CNC (33) TCC (16) TNC (1)	11.4 (8.1–17.9)	Conservative treatment	1.7 (0.2–7.4)	Pain relief 53% of 81 nonoperative treatment trials	Cases required surgery: • CNC 21% • TCC 38%

Di Gennaro et al,[80] 2020	Operative vs nonoperative treatment in children with painful rigid flatfoot and talocalcaneal coalition	55 (81)	11.8 (9–17)	Group 1: nonoperative treatment (47); Group 2: coalition resection, graft interposition and subtalar arthroereisis (34)	6.6 (3–12)	26/47 (55%) 26/34 (76%)	No complications, but 6 patients (7) in group 1 were unsatisfied and required surgery

Abbreviations: AOFAS, The American Orthopedic Foot and Ankle Score; CNC, calcaneonavicular coalition; CNL, calcaneal neck lengthening; CLO, calcaneal lengthening osteotomy; CSO, calcaneal sliding osteotomy; MCO, medial cuneiform osteotomy; RFF, rigid flatfoot; TAL, tendon Achilles lengthening; TCC, talocalcaneal coalition; TNC, talonavicular coalition; UCLA, University of California and Los Angeles Activity Score.

feet, 291 were excellent, and 18 were good (90.08%). In the remaining 54 cases, data were incomplete, reporting 19 fair results and 11 poor results. The most frequent complication is foot pain (persistent pain, pain limiting activity) described in 26 patients.[16,79,83–86] In 21 cases, further surgery to solve unsatisfactory outcome was necessary.[13,47,76,81,84,85] In 7 cases, flatfoot correction was needed.[84] Surgical site infections were reported in 6 cases.[47,50,82,83,86] Moreover, in 2 cases, surgical scar dehiscence occurred.[47] Other complications reported were deep vein thrombosis (1),[83] posterior tibial nerve damage (1),[13] hardware prominence (1),[82] which needed further surgery to remove it, and development scar sensitivity at one of the portal sites (1).[13]

DEFORMITY CORRECTION

Mosca and Bevan defined pain as a consensual indication for treatment.[81] Pain may be located at the site of a fibrocartilaginous coalition; pain in the ankle joint or Chopart joint implies transferred stress in those joints; pain under the head of a plantar-flexed talus or in the sinus tarsi is characteristic of a flatfoot in a patient with a tight Achilles tendon.[81]

The goal of treatment is to relieve pain and not to simply eliminate the coalition, and the management of the symptomatic flatfoot associated to TCC is still controversial. However, in a recent study, 47 feet (non-operative) versus 34 feet (op) were compared, and the postoperative AOFAS-Ankle Hindfoot Scale scores were significantly better with respect to conservative treatment.[80]

General consensus considers resection and fat interposition a gold standard for persistently painful middle facet TCC.[32,62] However, when hindfoot deformity is considered, the outcomes are not always good. In a study, resection of coalitions with an area at CT greater than 50% and heel valgus greater than 16°, narrowing of the posterior talocalcaneal joint, and impingement of the lateral talar process on the calcaneus showed unsatisfactory results.[18] Differently, in another study, although the indication for resection and interposition was still a symptomatic TCC with failed conservative treatment, patients with a coalition greater than 50% or a heel valgus greater than 21° had still a very satisfactory outcome.[19] However, these patients had to correct the hindfoot deformity, either conservatively with orthoses or surgically with osteotomies or lateral column-lengthening. Arthrodesis was used as a salvage procedure.[19] In another study, only the degenerative changes were taken into consideration, recommending resection in a painful coalition, regardless of the dimension of TCC.[72]

In recent years, the approach to TCC coalition with or without hindfoot deformity has required the development of treatment algorhythms as it is quite controversial. In fact, Hamel in 2013[27] suggested a treatment algorhythm taking into consideration the size of coalition, age, and other involved joints. However, in a painful coalition with a hindfoot deformity, the surgical options suggested were resection with or without immediate realignment surgery. Pain is not only referred around the coalition site but may also be at sinus tarsi level or anterolateral region (impingement).

Recently an algorithm was proposed for treatment of TCC[32,82] where the main criteria are area (on CT scan) of the subtalar posterior facet, hindfoot valgus, and degenerative signs in the subtalar joint. If the area of coalition is less than 50%, with a valgus less than 16° and no degenerative signs, the pain is due to the coalition, so resection is recommended. If the area is less than 50%, without degenerative signs, but the hindfoot valgus greater than 16°, resection and realignment surgery is recommended. These data are in accordance with the study by Mosca and Bevan.[81] If instead the area is greater than 50%, hindfoot valgus is >16°, and initial degenerative signs are present, the pain is mainly caused by the deformity. The marked valgus of the hindfoot bar acts as a tether, so its removal allows a collapse of the hindfoot, increasing the deformity.[5] Therefore, in severe valgus of the hindfoot, realignment surgery is recommended, without necessarily the resection of the bar. This permits to reserve arthrodesis in case of failure, as a salvage surgery.

When surgery is recommended, the criteria proposed included a middle facet coalition which involves 30% to 50% of the surface area of the posterior facet (on CT scan), with a 16° – 21° of hindfoot valgus, measured on coronal image, and with minimal or no narrowing or degeneration of the posterior facet of the subtalar joint[18,19,71] (**Fig. 10**).

The hindfoot valgus deformity has been addressed in the surgical strategy,[81] as it is considered fundamental for pain relief, before the onset of degenerative changes of the subtalar joint. Its alignment is as important as the size of the coalition. In fact, they conclude that if there is excessive hindfoot valgus deformity, with or without a resectable coalition (and regardless of a resection), a valgus correction (calcaneal lengthening osteotomy) is necessary for pain relief. Also considering CNC, if a valgus deformity is present, an Evans osteotomy or medializing calcaneal osteotomy is suggested in association to the bar resection.[14]

Arthroereisis is a valid, alternative procedure to calcaneal osteotomy, to realign the hindfoot (**Fig. 11**). Three authors confirmed the less invasiveness, describing a decreased period of immobilization in cast and a low complication rate. Giannini and colleagues reported the use of a bioabsorbable screw (intra-articular) with good

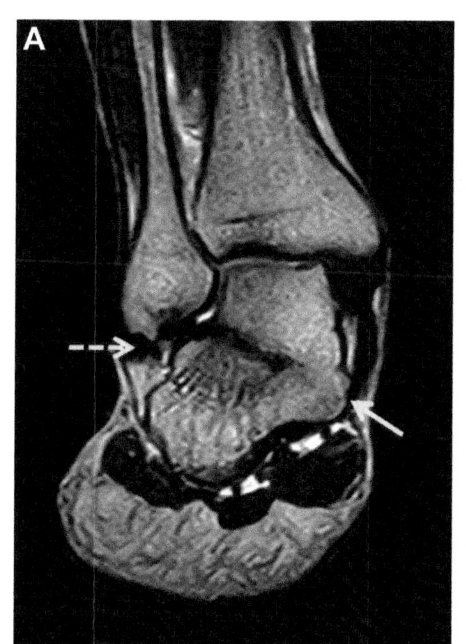

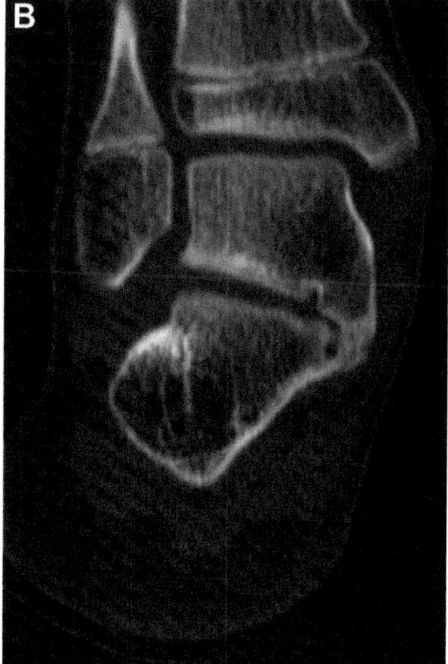

Fig. 10. MRI slice of an untreated talocalcaneal coalition (TCC) of a 32-year-old patient with a rigid valgus deformity of the hindfoot complaining of pain laterally for the calcaneofibular impingement and arthritis (*yellow dashed arrow*) and medially on the osseous coalition (*yellow arrow*) (*A*). Coronal slice CT scan of the same region in a 12-year-old patient with similar type of TCC and valgus deformity (*B*) for comparison (same patient of **Fig.7**).

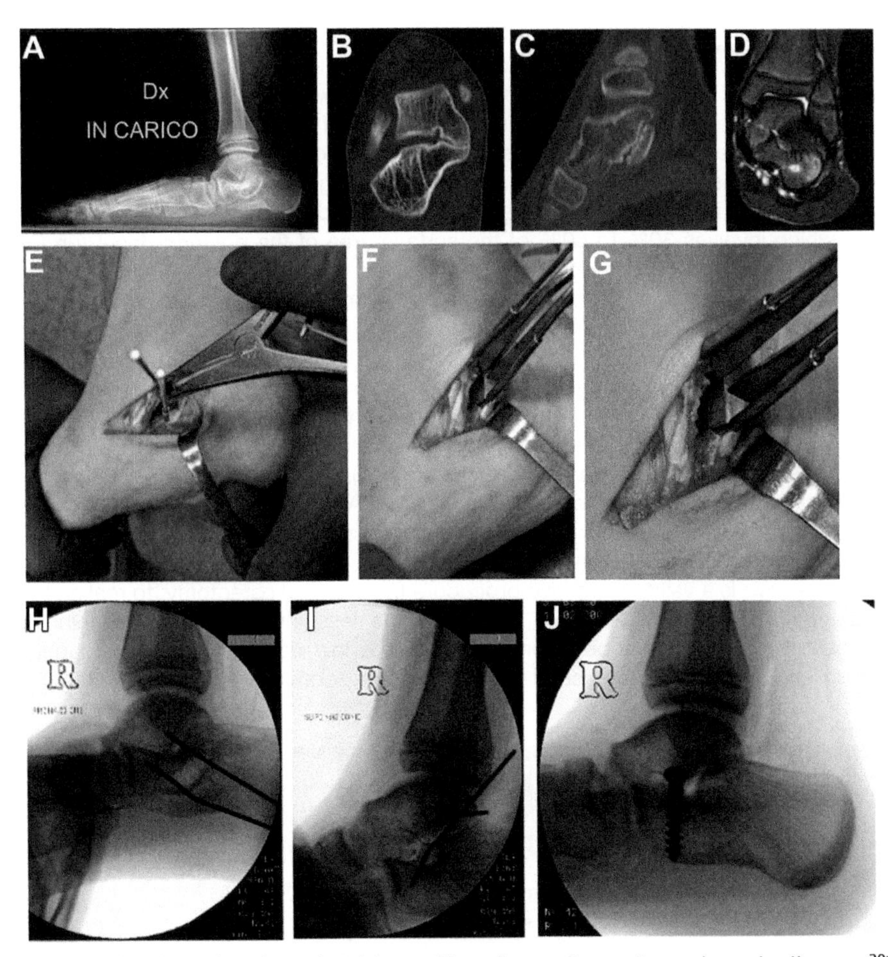

Fig. 11. Talocalcaneal coalition (TCC) (type I [linear] according to Rozansky and colleagues[30]) (type I [linear] according to Lim and colleagues[23]) with severe rigid flat foot deformity. Weight-bearing lateral view radiograph (*A*), coronal (*B*) and sagittal CT slice (*C*). MRI showing associated perilesional signal alterations and calcaneo-fibular impingement (*D*). Positioning of two 1.8-K wires (in the talus and in the calcaneus) (*E*). Positioning of the Kirschner pin open distractor (*F*). Opening of the distractor for checking the achieved motion of subtalar joint (*G*). Intraoperative fluoroscopy check before resection (corresponding to the position in *A*) (*H*) and after resection of the coalition showing divergent K-wires in supination (*I*). A calcaneo-stop procedure is performed to maintain the correction of the hind foot at the level of the subtalar joint (*J*). (*From* Rozansky A, Varley E, Moor M, Wenger DR, Mubarak SJ. A radiologic classification of talocalcaneal coalitions based on 3D reconstruction. JCO 2010; 4: 129 – 35 and Lim S, Lee HK, Bae S, et al. A radiological classification system for talocalcaneal coalition based on a multi-planar imaging study using CT and MRI. Insights Imaging 2013 Oct; 4 (5): 563 – 67.)

results, after resection of a TCC.[31] The results considered the postoperative realignment of the hindfoot, subtalar motion, and the absence of pain.[31] Differently, a non-bioabsorbable screw can be used with the aim of obtaining a “calcaneo-stop” effect[80] in association to the TCC resection, as described recently, although taking into consideration a different position of the screw (in the talus, not in the calcaneus).

Knörr and colleagues[79] reported 4 calcaneo-stop procedures simultaneously performed in 15 patients with symptomatic TCC and a hindfoot valgus greater than 20°, after arthroscopic resection.

In our unpublished data, 17 patients (20 feet) affected by CNC (13) and TCC (7) underwent a one-step procedure, combining open resection, fat graft interposition, and subtalar extraarticular screw arthroereisis. The average postoperative AOFAS Ankle-Hindfoot score was 94.46, and no patient had recurrency or secondary realignment surgery. This validates the mini-invasiveness of the calcaneo-stop technique associated to coalition resection, for the correction of the hindfoot valgus deformity, which otherwise may lead to poor results and further surgery for pain and secondary degenerative changes.[88]

SUMMARY

CNCs and TCCs are the most common cause of RFF in children. Resection with interposition of fat graft is still the treatment of choice in symptomatic flatfeet. Imaging has an important role not only for the detailed analysis of the pathologic anatomy of the tarsal coalitions but also for surgical planning, particularly in TCC. MRI can detect earlier the presence of a painful non-ossified coalition, allowing an early resection of the fibrous or cartilaginous tissue before the development of a complete rigid deformity; resection at an early age yields better results and permits to later avoid invasive surgery due to pain in adulthood. Bone marrow edema in the coalition area and in other areas of the affected foot, such as the calcaneo-fibular area, helps in explaining symptoms and determining surgical indications, even in osseous types.

The hindfoot valgus deformity has been addressed in the surgical strategy as its correction is considered fundamental for pain relief, before the onset of degenerative changes. The hindfoot alignment is considered to be important; as a matter of fact, valgus correction techniques such a calcaneal lengthening osteotomy are necessary for pain relief. Arthroereisis is an alternative procedure to realign the hindfoot after coalition resection.

CLINICS CARE POINTS

- Clinical examination and history are important for diagnosis of tarsal coalitions; however, imaging has a fundamental role for surgical planning, espacially in TCC.
- Hindfoot alignment must be addressed correctly and is the main goal in surgery.
- Recent minimally invasive techniques for valgus realignment after coalition resection show interesting results, with good outcomes and low complication rates.

DISCLOSURE

The authors have nothing to disclose.

REFERENCES

1. Compte de Buffon GLL. Histoire naturelle avec la description du cabinet du Roy. Tome 1975;3:47.
2. Cruveilhier J. Anatomie pathologique du corps humain. In: Tome I, editor. Paris: Bailliere JB; 1829.

3. Zukerkandl E. Ueber einen Fall von Synostose zwischen Talus und Calcaneus. Allg Wein Med Zeitung 1877;22:293.
4. Nalaboff KM, Schweitzer ME. MRI of tarsal coalition. Frequency, distribution and innovative signs. Bull NYU Hosp Jt Dis 2008;66(1):14–21.
5. Rühli FJ, Solomon LB, Henneberg M. High prevalence of tarsal coalitions and tarsal joint variants in a recent cadaver sample and its possible significance. Clin Anat 2003;16:411–5.
6. Leonard MA. The inheritance of tarsal coalition and its relationship to spastic flat foot. J Bone Joint Surg Br 1974;56B:520–6.
7. Kawashima T, Uhthoff HK. The development of the ankle and foot. In: Uhthoff HK, editor. The embryology of the human locomotor system. Berlin: Heidelberg Springer; 1990.
8. Stormont DM, Peterson HA. The relative incidence of tarsal coalition. Clin Orthop Relat Res 1983;181:28–36.
9. Mosca VS. Subtalar coalition in pediatrics. Foot Ankle Clin Am 2015;20:265–81.
10. Jayakumar S, Cowell HR. Rigid flatfoot. Clin Orthop Relat Res 1977;(122):77–84.
11. Docquier PL, Maldaque P, Bouchard M. Tarsal coalition in paediatric patients. Orthop Traum Surg Res 2019;105:S123–31.
12. Van Rysselberghe NL, Souder CD, Mubarak SJ. Unsuspected tarsal coalitions in equinus and varus foot deformities. J Pediatr Orthop B 2020;29(4):370–4.
13. Jagodzinski NA, Hughes A, Davis NP, et al. Arthroscopic resection of talocalcaneal coalitions – a bicentre case series of a new technique. Foot Ankle Surg 2013; 19:125–30.
14. Cass AD, Camasta CA. A review of tarsal coalition and pes planovalgus: clinical examination, diagnostic imaging, and surgical planning. J Foot Ankle Surg 2010; 49(3):274–93.
15. Zhou B, Tang K, Hardy M. Talocalcaneal coalition combined with flatfoot in children: diagnosis and treatment: a review. J Orthop Surg Res 2014;9:129.
16. Sperl M, Saraph V, Zwick EB, et al. Preliminary report: resection and interposition of a deepithelialized skin flap graft in tarsal coalition in children. J Ped Orthop B 2010;19:171–6.
17. Kumai T, Takakura Y, Akiyama K, et al. Histopathological study of nonosseos tarsal coalition. Foot Ankle Int 1998;19:525–31.
18. Wilde PH, Torode IP, Dickens DR, et al. resection for symptomatic talocalcaneal coalition. J Bone Joint Surg Br 1994;76:797–801.
19. Luhmann SJ, Schoenecker PL. Symptomatic talocalcaneal coalition resection: indications and results. J Pediatr Orthop 1998;18:748–54.
20. Bianchi S, Hoffman D. Ultrasound of talocalcaneal coalition: retrospective study of 11 patients. Skeletal Radiol 2013;42(9):1209–14.
21. Lee SH, Park HJ, Yeo ED, et al. Talocalcaneal coalition: a focus on radiographic findings and sites of bridging. Indian J Orthop 2016;50(6):661–8.
22. Phyo N, Pressnet I, Khoo M, et al. The radiological diagnosis of extra-articular posteromedial talocalcaneal coalition. Skeletal Radiol 2020;49(9):1413–22.
23. Lim S, Lee HK, Bae S, et al. A radiological classification system for talocalcaneal coalition based on a multi-planar imaging study using CT and MRI. Insights Imaging 2013;4(5):563–7.
24. Yun SJ, Jin W, Kim GY, et al. A different type of talocalcaneal coalition with Os sustentaculum: the continued necessity of revision of classification. AJR Am J Roentgenol 2015;205(6):W612–8.
25. Umul A. MRI findings of talocalcaneal coalition: two case reports. Acta Inform Med 2015;23(4):248–9.

26. Guignand D, Journeau P, Mainard-Simard L, et al. Child calcaneonavicular coalitions: MRI diagnostic value in a 19-case series. Orthop Traumatol Surg Res 2011;97(1):67–72.
27. Hamel J. Diagnosis and treatment of tarsal coalitions and synostoses in children and adolescents. Orthopade 2013;42(6):442–8.
28. Yeats JC, Rahbek O, Griffith N, et al. Bone scan with SPECT/CT in children with complex foot and ankle pain: initial experience of a paediatric tertiary referral centre. J Child Orthop 2020;14(5):433–9.
29. Upasani VV, Chambers RC, Mubarak SJ. Analysis of calcaneonavicular coalitions using multi-planar three-dimensional computed tomography. J Child Orthop 2008;2:301–7.
30. Rozansky A, Varley E, Moor M, et al. A radiologic classification of talocalcaneal coalitions based on 3D reconstruction. J Child Orthop 2010;4:129–35.
31. Giannini S, Ceccarelli F, Vannini F, et al. Operative treatment of flatfoot with talocalcaneal coalition. Clin Orthop Relat Res 2003;411:178–87.
32. Kothari A, Masquijo J. Surgical treatment of tarsal coalitions in children and adolescents. EFORT Open Rev 2020;5:80–9.
33. Mubarak SJ, Patel PN, Upasani VV, et al. Calcaneonavicular coalition: treatment by excision and fat graft. J Pediatr Orthop 2009;29:418–26.
34. Cowell HR. Talocalcaneal coalition and new causes of peroneal spastic foot. Clin Orthop Relat Res 1972;85:16–22.
35. Murphy JS, Mubarak SJ. Talocalcaneal coalitions. Foot Ankle Clin 2015;20:681–91.
36. Nehme AH, Bou Monsef J, Bou Ghannam AG, et al. Arthroscopic resection of a bilateral calcaneonavicular coalition in a child. J Foot Ankle Surg 2016;55:1079–82.
37. Badgley CE. Coalition of the calcaneus and the navicular. Arch Surg 1927;15:75–88.
38. Mitchell GP, Gibson JMC. Excision of calcaneo-navicular bar for painful spasmodic flat foot. J Bone Joint Surg Br 1967;49 B(2):281–7.
39. Cohen BE, Davis WH, Anderson RB. Success of calcaneonavicular coalition resection in the adult population. Foot Ankle Int 1996;17:569–72.
40. Bohne WH. Tarsal coalition. Curr Opin Pediatr 2001;13:29–35.
41. Andreasen E. Calcaneo-navicular coalition. Late results of resection. Acta Orthop Scand 1968;39(3):424–32.
42. Inglis G, Buxton RA, Macnicol MF. Symptomatic calcaneonavicular bars. The results 20 years after surgical excision. J Bone Joint Surg Br 1986;68(1):128–31.
43. Gonzalez P, Kumar SJ. Calcaneonavicular coalition treated by resection and interposition of the extensor digitorum brevis muscle. J Bone Joint Surg Am 1990;72(1):71–7.
44. Swiontkowski MF, Scranton PE, Hansen S. Tarsal coalitions: long-term results of surgical treatment. J Pediatr Orthop 1983;3(3):287–92.
45. Alter SA, McCarthy BE, Mendicino S, et al. Calcaneonavicular bar resection: a retrospective study. J Foot Surg 1991;30(4):383–9.
46. Cohen AH, Laughner TE, Pupp GR. Calcaneonavicular bar resection. A retrospective review. J Am Podiatr Med Assoc 1993;83(1):10–7.
47. Masquijo J, Allende V, Torres-Gomez A, et al. Fat graft and bone wax interposition provides better functional outcomes and lower reossification rates than extensor digitorum brevis after calcaneonavicular coalition resection. J Pediatr Orthop 2017;37:e427–31.

48. Vestergaard RF, Jensen H, Vind-Kezunovic S, et al. Bone healing after median sternotomy: a comparison of two hemostatic devices. J Cardiothorac Surg 2010;5:117.
49. Qayum A, Koka AH. Foreign body reaction to bone wax an unusual cause of persistent serous discharge from iliac crest graft donor site and the possible means to avoid such complication - a case report. Cases J 2009;2:9097.
50. Khoshbin A, Law PW, Caspi L, et al. Long-term functional outcomes of resected tarsal coalitions. Foot Ankle Int 2013;34(10):1370–5.
51. Kitaoka HB, Wikenheiser MA, Shaughnessy WJ, et al. Gait abnormalities following resection of talocalcaneal coalition. J Bone Joint Surg Am 1997;79:369–74.
52. Mahan ST, Spencer SA, Vezeridis PS, et al. Patient-reported outcomes of tarsal coalitions treated with surgical excision. J Pediatr Orthop 2015;35(6):583–8.
53. Knörr J, Accadbled F, Abid A, et al. Arthroscopic treatment of calcaneonavicular coalition in children. Orthop Traumatol Surg Res 2011;97(5):565–8.
54. Lui TH. Arthroscopic resection of the calcaneonavicular coalition or the "too long" anterior process of the calcaneus. Arthroscopy 2006;22(8):903.e1–4.
55. Zekry M, Shahban SA, El Gamal T, et al. A literature review of the complications following anterior and posterior ankle arthroscopy. Foot Ankle Surg 2019;25(5): 553–8.
56. Bauer T, Golano P, Hardy P. Endoscopic resection of a calcaneonavicular coalition. Knee Surg Sports Traumatol Arthrosc 2010;18(5):669–72.
57. Malik-Tabassum K, Wahed K, To C, et al. Post-operative outcomes of arthroscopic tarsal coalition resection: a systematic review. J Orthop 2020;21:537–43.
58. Raikin S, Cooperman DR, Thompson GH. Interposition of the split flexor hallucis longus tendon after resection of a coalition of the middle facet of the talocalcaneal joint. J Bone Joint Surg Am 1999;81:11–9.
59. Kelo MJ, Riddle DL. Examination and management of a patient with tarsal coalition. Phys Ther 1998;78:518–25.
60. Harris RI, Beath T. Etiology of peroneal spastic flat foot. J Bone Joint Surg Am 1948;30B:624–34.
61. Downey M. Tarsal coalitions. A surgical classification. J Am Podiatr Med Assoc 1991;81:187–97.
62. Takakura Y, Sugimoto K, Tanaka Y, et al. Symptomatic talocalcaneal coalition: its clinical significance and treatment. Clin Orthop Relat Res 1991;269:249–56.
63. Cowell HR, Elener V. Rigid painful flatfoot secondary to tarsal coalition. Clin Orthop Relat Res 1983;177:54–60.
64. Mann RA, Baumgarten M. Subtalar fusion for isolated subtalar disorders. Preliminary report. Clin Orthop Relat Res 1988;226:260–5.
65. Mann RA, Beaman DN, Horton GA. Isolated subtalar arthrodesis. Foot Ankle Int 1998;19:511–9.
66. Greer E. Tarsal coalition. In: Myerson MS, editor. Foot and ankle disorders, vol. 1. Philadelphia: Saunders WB; 2000. p. 729–48.
67. Pell RF, Myerson MS, Schon LC. Clinical outcome after primary triple arthrodesis. J Bone Joint Surg Am 2000;82:47–57.
68. Krief E, Ferraz L, Appy-Fedida B, et al. Tarsal coalitions: preliminary results after operative excision and silicone sheet interposition in children. J Foot Ankle Surg 2016;55(6):1264–70.
69. Hubert J, Hawellek T, Beil FT, et al. Resection of medial talocalcaneal coalition with interposition of a pediculated flap of tibialis posterior tendon sheath. Foot Ankle Int 2018;39(8):935–41.
70. Dutoit M. Talocalcaneal bar resection. J Foot Ankle Surg 1998;37:199–203.

71. Comfort TK, Johnson LO. Resection for symptomatic talocalcaneal coalition. J Pediatr Orthop 1998;18:283–8.
72. McCormack TJ, Olney B, Asher M. Talocalcaneal coalition resection: a 10-year follow-up. J Pediatr Orthop 1997;17:13–5.
73. de Wouters S, Tran Duy K, Docquier PL. Patient-specific instruments for surgical resection of painful tarsal coalition in adolescents. Orthop Traumatol Surg Res 2014;100:423–7.
74. Tower DE, Wood RW, Vaardahl MD. Talocalcaneal joint middle facet coalition resection with interposition of a juvenile hyaline cartilage graft. J Foot Ankle Surg 2015;54:1178–82.
75. Salomão O, Napoli MMM, de Carvalho AE Jr, et al. Talocalcaneal coalition: diagnosis and surgical management. Foot and Ankle 1992;13(5):251–6.
76. Gantsoudes GD, Roocroft JH, Mubarak SJ. Treatment of talocalcaneal coalitions. J Pediatr Orthop 2012;32(3):301–7.
77. Moraleda L, Gantsoudes GD, Mubarak SJ. C Sign: talocalcaneal coalition or flat foot deformity? J Pediatr Orthop 2014;34:814–9.
78. Bonasia DE, Phisitkul P, Saltzman CL, et al. Arthroscopic resection of talocalcaneal coalitions. Arthroscopy 2011;27(3):430–5.
79. Knörr J, Soldado F, Menendez ME, et al. Arthroscopic talocalcaneal coalition resection in children. Arthroscopy 2015;31(12):2417–23.
80. Di Gennaro GL, Stallone S, Olivotto E, et al. Operative versus nonoperative treatment in children with painful rigid flatfoot and talocalcaneal coalition. BMC Musculoskelet Disord 2020;21:185.
81. Mosca VS, Bevan WP. Talocalcaneal tarsal coalitions and the calcaneal lengthening osteotomy: the role of deformity correction. J Bone Joint Surg Am 2012;94:1584–94.
82. Masquijo J, Vazquez I, Allende V, et al. Surgical reconstruction for talocalcaneal coalitions with severe hindfoot valgus deformity. J Pediatr Orthop 2017;37:293–7.
83. Lisella JM, Bellapianta JM, Manoli A 2nd. Tarsal coalition resection with pes planovalgus hindfoot reconstruction. J Surg Orthop Adv 2011;20(2):102–5.
84. Kemppainen J, Pennock AT, Roocroft JH, et al. The use of a portable CT scanner for the intraoperative assessment of talocalcaneal coalition resections. J Pediatr Orthop 2014;34(5):559–64.
85. Hamel J, Nell M, Rist C. Surgical treatment of talocalcaneal coalition: experience with 80 cases of pediatric or adolescent patients. Orthopade 2016;45(12):1058–65.
86. Mahan ST, Prete VI, Spencer SA, et al. Subtalar coalitions: does the morphology of the subtalar joint involvement influence outcomes after coalition excision? J Foot Ankle Surg 2017;56(4):797–801.
87. Shirley E, Gheorghe R, Neal KM. Results of nonoperative treatment for symptomatic tarsal coalitions. Cureus 2018;10(7):e2944.
88. Fracassetti D, Moharamzadeh D, De Pellegrin M. Resection of tarsal coalition and surgical correction of the hindfoot deformity in one step. J Child Orthop 2017;10(Suppl 1):S159–60.

Congenital Vertical Talus

Thomas Wirth, MD, PhD

KEYWORDS

- Congenital vertical talus • Reverse ponseti method • Percutaneous achillotenotomy
- Peritalar release

KEY POINTS

- The main feature of congenital vertical talus (CVT) is a dislocation of the talonavicular joint in combination with contractures of the dorsolateral tendons of the foot and tendo Achilles.
- Functional results of the miniinvasive method are superior to those of the former more extensive surgical releases.
- Syndromic or neurmuscular CVT often require extensive surgical release to correct the deformity.

INTRODUCTION

Congenital vertical talus (CVT; synonyms: congenital convex pes valgus, congenital flat foot) describes a distinct structural foot deformity present at birth, 10 times rarer than congenital clubfoot. The frequency is 1:10.000 live births, and the main feature is a fixed dorsal dislocation of the navicular bone in the talonavicular joint.[1] There is a very characteristic postpartum appearance of CVT with the typical rocker bottom deformity, forefoot abduction, midfoot dorsiflexion, and hindfoot equinus. The head of the talus can be palpated on the plantar and medial aspect of the foot.[1–3] Typically this deformity is rigid and hence discriminates CVT clinically from talus obliquus and pes calcaneus, both entirely flexible foot deformities, which need to be considered as differential diagnoses. Talus obliquus is charaterised by a fully reducible talo-navicular joint both manually and confirmed by a lateral plantarflexion radiograph. In CVT the talus is in a vertical position on the radiograph and the os calcis remains in an equinus position with the forefoot elevated and abducted. Functional lateral radiographs in maximum dorsiflexion fail to align the forefoot bones with the talus, which is possible in all functional flatfoot deformities. In roughly 50% of cases bilateral deformity is present (**Fig. 1**).

About one-half of the vertical talus cases are known to be idiopathic because of lacking association with other underlying diseases and also referred to as isolated pathology. The true causes here remain unclear despite some familial predispositions and associations with HOXD10, 5′HOXC, and GDF5 gene mutations pointing out a possible genetic background.[4–8] The other half of CVT deformities, the so-called

Department of Orthopaedics, Klinikum Stuttgart, Olgahospital, Kriegsbergstraße 62, D-70174 Stuttgart, Germany
E-mail address: t.wirth@klinikum-stuttgart.de

Foot Ankle Clin N Am 26 (2021) 903–913
https://doi.org/10.1016/j.fcl.2021.08.002

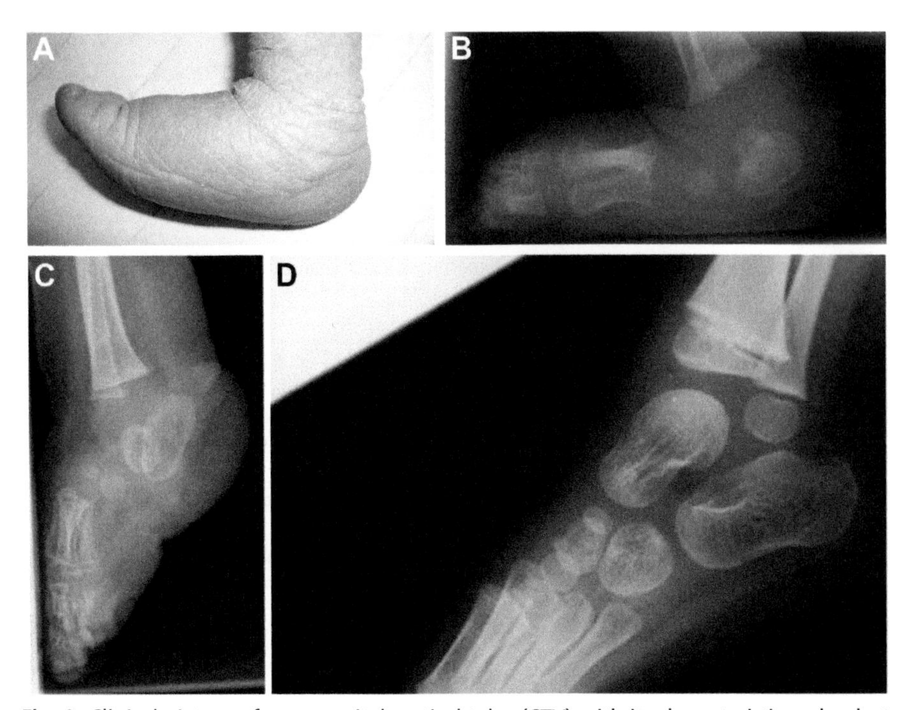

Fig. 1. Clinical picture of a congenital vertical talus (CTV) with its characteristic rocker bottom deformity (*A*). Radiographic appearance of CVT in a true lateral foot radiograph (*B*). Lateral radiograph in maximum plantar flexion: discrimination between CVT with lacking realignment of the first metatarsal and talus in CVT (*C*) and perfectly aligned first ray and reduced talonavicular joint in oblique talus (*D*).

unisolated pathology, is associated with syndromal or neuromuscular conditions, such as arthrogryposis multiplex congenita, and myelomeningocele (**Table 1**). Unisolated CVT are regarded as being more severe with greater rigidity and posing bigger treatment challenges with a larger rate of recurrences.[9–11]

CLINICAL AND RADIOGRAPHIC PATHOANATOMY

In CVT the principal pathology is dislocation of the subtalar complex along with its rotation into a plantar and medial direction; this leaves the forefoot abducted, the midfoot dorsiflexed, and the hindfoot in an equinus position. The key anatomic feature is a dislocation of the talonavicular joint with the navicular sitting irreducibly dorsally on the talar neck (**Fig. 2**). Both navicular and talus are abnormal in shape with the navicular

Table 1
Underlying conditions and possible associations of unisolated congenital vertical talus[12]

Underlying Condition	Association with
Neuromuscular	Myelomeningocele
Congenital contractures	Distal arthrogryposis multiplex congenital
Syndromal	Aneuploidy (chromosomes 1, 8, 13, 15, 18)
Syndromal	ie, De Barsy, Costello, and Rasmussen syndromes
Limb malformation	Split hand and foot

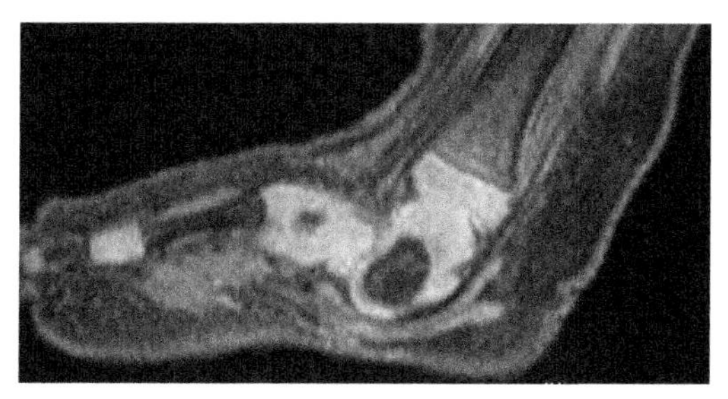

Fig. 2. MRI of a foot with congenital vertical talus, sagittal plane. The navicular is sitting dorsally on the talar neck.

bone frequently being triangular and the talus exhibiting a deeper talar neck. In addition, the calcaneocuboid joint may be subluxed or even dislocated.[11,12] Tendo Achilles, the peroneal and extensor tendons, as well as the tibialis anterior muscle are contracted and short. The posterior capsule of the subtalar and talonavicular joint demonstrates a significant contracture as well.

Anteroposterior and lateral radiographs of the foot are being used for assessment. In addition, 2 lateral functional radiographs in maximum plantar and dorsiflexion are necessary to discriminate between structural and positional deformities. The severity of the deformity can be evaluated by measuring a variety of angles (**Fig. 3**).[1] More recently the talar and calcaneal axis, first metatarsal base angles (TAMBA and CAMBA, respectively), first described by Hamanishi, have been used for classification of severity and for reference to select the best treatment modalities (see **Fig. 3**C).[13,14] The functional radiographs help distinguishing vertical talus from the flexible flatfoot entities, such as oblique talus and flexible pes calcaneovalgus (see **Fig. 1**). Other differential diagnoses like pes calcaneus and posteromedial tibial bowing should be identified clinically. In vertical talus the radiograph in maximum plantar flexion fails to demonstrate alignment of the first metatarsal and the talus, which typically occurs in the talus obliquus and all flexible deformities. The position of the calcaneus and its relation to the cuboid needs to be assessed carefully as well. In vertical talus there is considerable equinus of the calcaneus. In severe cases a posterior displacement or even dislocation of the cuboid can be seen as well. Positional deformities do not show both these features. There are borderline cases, which are more difficult to differentiate between oblique and vertical talus, if just mild calcaneal equinus is

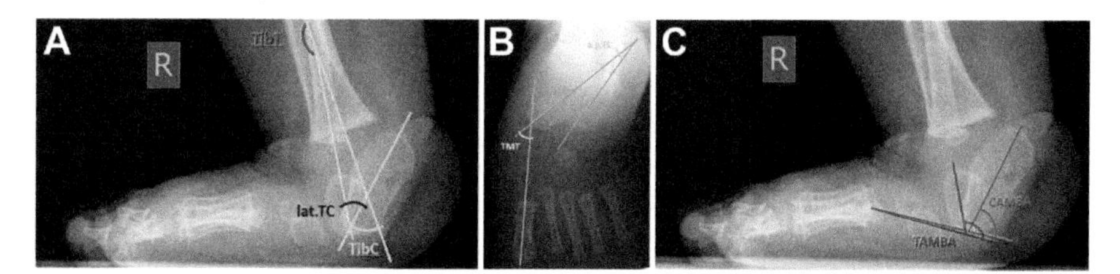

Fig. 3. Lateral radiograph of the foot showing typical angle measurements. (*A*) Lateral talocalcaneal angle (TC, *dark blue*), tibiocalcaneal angle (TibC, *dark yellow*), and tibiotalar angle (TibT, *red*). Anteroposterior radiograph of a foot with CVT demonstrating typical angles. (*B*) Talocalcaneal angle (TC, *light green*) and tarso-first-metatarsal angle (TMT, *yellow*). (*C*) Lateral radiograph of a foot with CVT, demonstrating the talar and calcaneal axis, first metatarsal base angles (TAMBA, *red*; CAMBA, *blue*).

present on the lateral radiograph but complete reduction of the talonavicular joint is present on the lateral plantar flexion film; they represent mild vertical talus cases, which are best treated according to the vertical talus treatment protocol.[12]

CLINICAL EXAMINATION

The clinical appearance of talus verticalis is very characteristic and must not be missed after birth. There is the typical convex sole of the foot, fore- and midfoot dorsiflexion and abduction, and significant equinus of the hindfoot with a skin crease just above the palpable upper end of the heel bone giving the foot the well-known rocker bottom shape (see **Fig. 1**A). Forced dorsiflexion cannot bring the heel down, and forced plantar flexion will not overcome the midfoot break. The head of the talus can be palpated on the plantar medial aspect of the foot. In positional flatfoot conditions, the posterior skin crease and the hindfoot equinus are lacking. The medioplantarily positioned talar head can easily be reduced, which leads to normalization of the fore- and hindfoot alignment. If possible, a limited functional assessment of the feet should be attempted even in the little newborns. The passive range of motion of the ankle and subtalar joints as well as of the toes should be recorded, and the active mobility of the toes can be evaluated by touching the sole and the dorsum of the foot. Functional toes indicate a higher probability of a good response to treatment.[12] It is very important to search for other associated deformities and conditions to discriminate between isolated and nonisolated CVT and to thoroughly explore the family history.

CLASSIFICATION

The mainly used classifications refer to the pathoanatomy detected. Coleman differentiates between type I with an irreducible talonavicular joint and a type II with additional subluxation or dislocation of the calcaneocuboid joint.[15] Several investigators have tried to classify CVT according to its cause (**Table 2**)[8,14]. Ogata and colleagues[8] classified the patients into 3 groups: (1) primary isolated form, (2) associated form without neurologic deficit, and (3) associated form with neurologic deficit. Hamanishi[14] has used the TAMBA and CAMBA to find guidelines for grading severity and selecting treatment strategies. He stated that the cutoff between true CVT and oblique talus is TAMBA of greater than 60° and CAMBA greater than 20°.[14] In our experience the rigidity of the feet during manipulation characterizes their severity. In a less severe deformity manual reduction of the talonavicular joint in plantar flexion is possible with the heel staying in equinus. Rigid feet do not respond to this maneuver in the first instance and need persistent stretching of soft tissue before a reduction may occur. Active toe movement seems to play a role as well with no movement detectable in the most severely affected feet.

Table 2
Classification of congenital vertical talus according to cause

Grade	Ogata et al,[8] 1979	Hamanishi,[14] 1984
I	Idiopathic	Neural tube defects
II	Associated without neurologic deficit	Neuromuscular disorders
III	Associated with neurologic deficit	Malformation syndromes
IV		Chromosomal aberrations
V		Idiopathic

EVOLUTION OF TREATMENT

Treatment of CVT always consisted of a combination of serial manipulative casting followed by limited or extensive surgical releases, because purely conservative management has been proved to be unsuccessful in most cases.[16] In the 1960s and the 1970s reports on staged procedures initially were more common. Following the plaster cast treatment persistent tight structures of the dorsum of the foot such as extensors and contracted joints were released to allow reduction of the talonavicular joint followed by a limited posterior release including lengthening of tendo Achilles and the posterior capsular structures of the ankle and subtalar joints.[3,17] Badelon and colleagues[18] have reported the results of their staged approach by reducing the talonavicular joint surgically in the first step and correcting the hindfoot equinus next 6 weeks later. More and more it was found that combining the 2 interventions to a single-stage surgical correction was superior to the staged procedures and gained wide acceptance.[19–22] With the introduction of the peritalar release for surgical clubfoot correction, the same incision was being used to correct CVT (**Fig. 4**)[23]. More detailed analysis of the pathoanatomy of CVT found that the key anatomic changes were seen in the bones forming the talonavicular joint and in the hindfoot but not in the subtalar joint itself.[24] Therefore surgical approaches were limited to address only the most relevant pathologic conditions[25] and an à la carte treatment was recommended.[1,26] Similar to the results in extensive clubfoot surgeries, several stiff and less functional feet were recognized after complete peritalar releases.[12] As a consequence a minimally invasive treatment method was developed,[27] and it has been made state-of-the-art treatment at present.

The timing of initiating surgical procedures varies a lot. Most investigators have described their surgical methods for children younger than 2 years. Increasingly it was pointed out that a beginning of casting shortly after birth and early surgical interventions were yielding better results with less extensive releases.[1,22,25,26] It is consensus today that treatment of CVT should be commenced within the first 2 weeks after birth or immediately after confirming the diagnosis.

CURRENT TREATMENT

Minimally invasive treatment of clubfoot has led the way since Ponseti and Campos'[28] treatment method gained worldwide acceptance more than 20 years ago (**Fig. 5**). For CVT a minimally invasive treatment method, which was also addressed as reverse Ponseti method, was reported in 2006.[27] This method consisted of manual manipulation of the deformed foot before serial casting into a progressive clubfoot position,

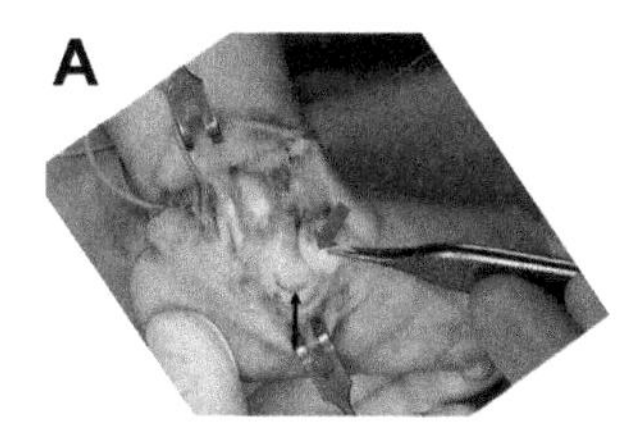

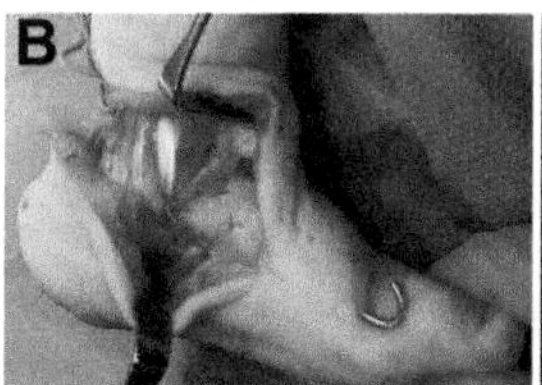

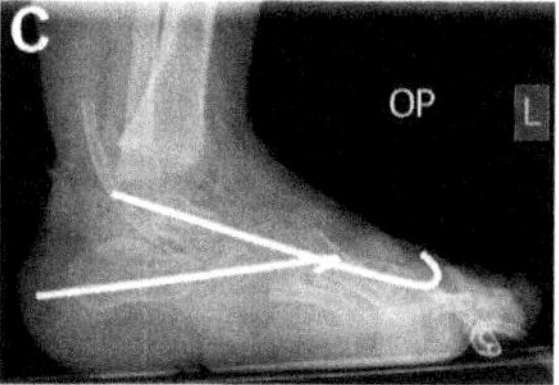

Fig. 4. Intraoperative picture of a severe arthrogrypotic CVT, operated by peritalar release through a Cincinnati incision, before talonavicular joint reduction (*A*), (talar head, *black arrow*; navicular bone, *red arrow*), tibialis posterior tendon detached. After reduction the position of the talonacvicular joint is secured by a K-wire, tibialis posterior tendon reinserted (*B*), position of navicular bone indicated by red arrow; corresponding postoperative lateral radiograph (*C*).

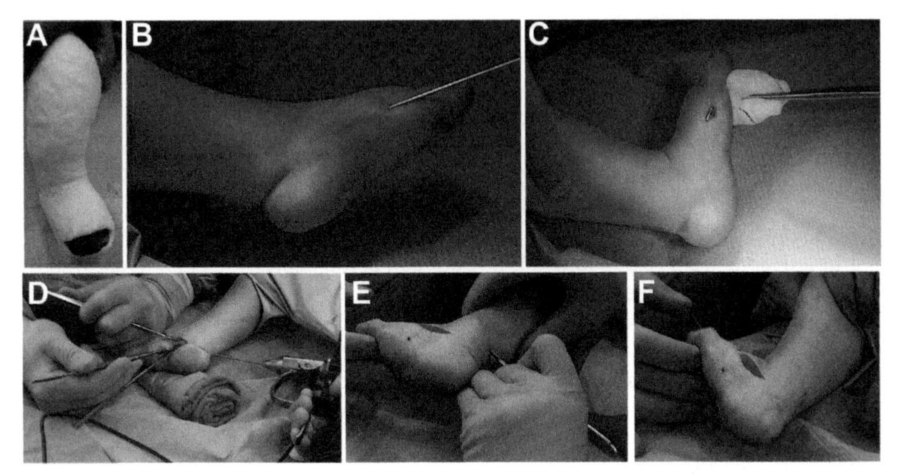

Fig. 5. Syndromic patient with bilateral CVT. Serial above-knee plaster casts in progressive forefoot supination and plantar flexion preoperatively (*A*); closed reduction and percutaneous K-wire fixation of the talonavicular joint performed (*B*); satisfactory ankle dorsiflexion after tendo Achilles tenotomy (*C*). Miniopen reduction and retrograde K-wire fixation of the talonavicular joint on the left side (*D*). The K-wire is first inserted in the talus under direct vision in an antegrade fashion. Very good ankle dorsiflexion following percutaneous tendo Achilles tenotomy (*E, F*).

followed by closed or miniopen reduction of the talonavicular joint and K-wire fixation and percutaneous achillotenotomy. The treatment ideally commences in the first weeks of life but can also be used in older children.[12] The session starts by manipulative correction of the fore- and midfoot deformity by stretching the short extensors and dorsolateral soft tissues followed by a corrective above-knee plaster with the knee in 90° flexion. Week by week, the foot is gradually brought into plantar flexion and supination, increasing this clubfootlike position with every subsequent plaster change. During the manipulation process it becomes increasingly possible to reduce the talonavicular joint. It is absolutely crucial to just put the pressure on the talar head and not on the anterior part of the calcaneus to allow reduction. After completing the plaster cast series by using 5 casts in average in a weekly sequence a limited surgical intervention under general anesthesia is performed. The talonavicular joint is reduced by closed means, or its reduction confirmed, and is then fixed by a K-wire along the first ray into the talus. To prevent early dislocation of the K-wire it is preferably buried under the skin. In more severe cases a closed reduction of the talonavcular joint may not be possible. In those cases an open reduction through a small incision is needed to align the talus and navicular under direct vision. Then a percutaneous tenotomy of tendo Achilles is added. The procedure is concluded by application of an above-knee plaster, the knee placed in 90° flexion.

Postoperatively the foot is kept in plaster for 6 weeks. The plaster and the K-wire are removed under a short general anesthesia, and an ankle foot orthosis with an elevated longitudinal arch is applied; this represents a modification to the original Dobbs method, which uses an abduction brace in neutral foot position for 2 years of age. In our protocol an insole with an elevated medial arch is used from walking age onward. When the foot seems to be stable, any orthotic support is discontinued.[29]

RESULTS

The treatment of vertical talus bears the risk of undercorrection, overcorrection, and relapse, regardless of which method has been used for correction. The key issue remains the accurate reduction of the talonavicular joint. Most undercorrected feet are the result of an incomplete realignment of the talus and navicular bones in this joint. In some cases the contracture of the tendons and joints may have been underestimated and additional tendon lengthenings have been omitted to allow joint reduction. This is the reason why we advocate the miniopen procedure whenever there is doubt of perfect alignment of talus and navicular bones.[12] Generally, unisolated feet demonstrate a higher risk of unsatisfactory results in the longer term.[11] Arthrogrypotic and syndromic feet are known to be stiffer and often more severe in the first instance and apparently more difficult to correct. The underlying condition may be responsible for muscular imbalance and dysfunction, leading to less functional feet with greater risks of overcorrection or relapse.[30] If we respect the treatment principles outlined earlier, both isolated and unisolated CVT can be equally well corrected initially with any treatment modality, but in particular with the minimally invasive reverse Ponseti technique.[11,13,26,27] Mid- and long-term results are promising (**Fig. 6**). However, stiff feet, identified by measuring the talar axis, first metatarsal base angle difference in the neutral and plantar-flexed lateral radiograph, may exhibit a higher risk of being undercorrected.[13]

Going into a more detailed analysis of mid- and long-term results, there is proof that the isolated or idiopathic CVT performs better.[13] By using the minimally invasive method, Chan and colleagues[30] reported the recurrence rate being twice as high in unisolated CVT. Wright and colleagues[31] found a recurrence rate of 33% in isolated (idiopathic) and 67% in unisolated (teratological) vertical tali with the Dobbs method. More recent publications used the talar axis, the first metatarsal base angle (TAMBA), for the radiographic analysis of surgical outcomes with the Dobbs method.[14] TAMBA

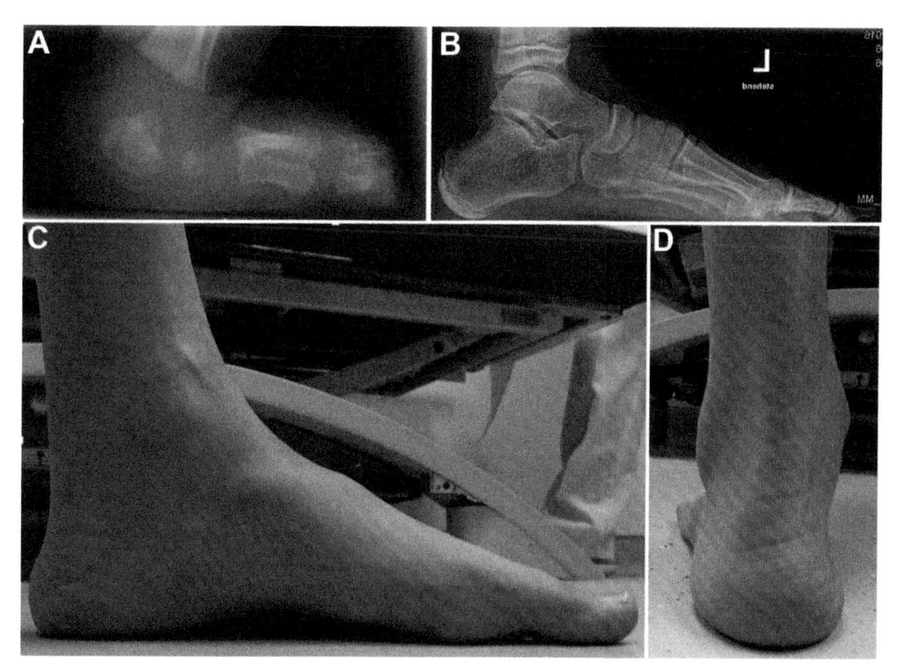

Fig. 6. Radiograph of a left isolated idiopathic CVT (*A*). Eleven years follow-up radiograph following the Dobbs protocol at age 3 months (*B*). The clinical appearance is very satisfactory 11 years after the correction, no functional deficits (*C, D*).

was reduced by average to values between 8° and 15°,[27,29] which are close to normal (3.3° ± 6.4°). These findings are well known from the era of more extensive surgical interventions as primary treatment. Series with more or less extensive soft tissue release report a better functionality and range of motion in idiopathic CVT.[11,32] Fair and bad results are predominantly related to relapses. Overcorrection and partial talar head necrosis are rarely reported.[1,32] The relapse rate varies between studies, but it does not seem to be related to the ratio between isolated and unisolated feet. The recurrence rate in studies reporting soft tissue releases through the Cincinnati approach range from 18% to 23%.[21,23] Studies that report the results of limited soft tissue releases mention a relapse rate between 15% and 33%.[1,11,26,32] The Dobbs method creates similar recurrence rates, 15% to 33%,[11,27,29,30] with one study reporting 10 relapses of 21 treated CVT (47%).[31] Eberhardt and colleagues[13] found the preoperative TAMBA of greater than 120° and the TAMBA difference of less than 25° predictive for the success of a minimally invasive treatment. Similar to the results in clubfoot treatment less extensive surgical interventions produce significantly better functional outcomes. Yang and Dobbs[11] compared soft tissue releases with the Dobbs method and found a much better functional outcome measured by the Pediatric Outcomes Data Collection Instrument and range of ankle movement in the minimal invasively treated patients (42.4° in the Dobbs and 12.7° in the soft tissue release group). In addition, idiopathic feet show the greater range of motion of the ankle joint.[11,32]

TREATMENT OF RECURRENCE

The treatment modality in relapsed cases is related to the flexibility or rigidity of the deformity. Like in clubfoot treatment, there is an option of repeating the Dobbs protocol for CVT recurrences as well. Serial casting is followed by preferably miniopen reduction of the talonavicular joint and K-wire fixation and percutaneous tenotomy of tendo Achilles.[11] Most relapsed CVT, however, are stiff and unsuitable to the minimally invasive approach. For correction they require an à la carte peritalar and soft tissue release including complete reduction of the talonavicular and calcaneocuboid joints. Short tendons have to be lengthened, and capsular contractures of the ankle and posterior subtalar joints need to be released. K-wire stabilization may be not only needed for maintaining the reduction of the talonavicular joint but also to fix the reduction of the calcaneocuboid joint. Every case and every foot is different and has to be treated on an individual basis and by a specifically adapted approach.

The older the child at the time of revision, the more likely extensive or more radical operations may be required. In very rigid feet talonavicular joint reduction may not be achievable. Alignment of the medial structures of the foot can be obtained by naviculectomy and direct articulation between the talar head and the first cuneiform bone.[33] In arthrogrypotic feet of older children naviculectomy may not be sufficient and a formal talectomy may be required instead.[34] Those radical procedures are clearly limited to the very particular case and patient and not part of the routine program.

Partially relapsed feet may only require limited local surgical corrections such as mid- and forefoot alignment osteotomies (**Fig. 7**) or limited posterior releases for persistent or recurrent pes equinus.

Untreated CVT or severely deformed feet following failed initial treatment may need bony surgical interventions such as subtalar extra-articular stabilization according to Grice in younger children and corrective pretalar arthrodeses or corrective triple arthrodeses in adolescents or young adults. By these means the goal of plantigrade and stable feet can be achieved. Despite sacrificing subtalar joint motion those

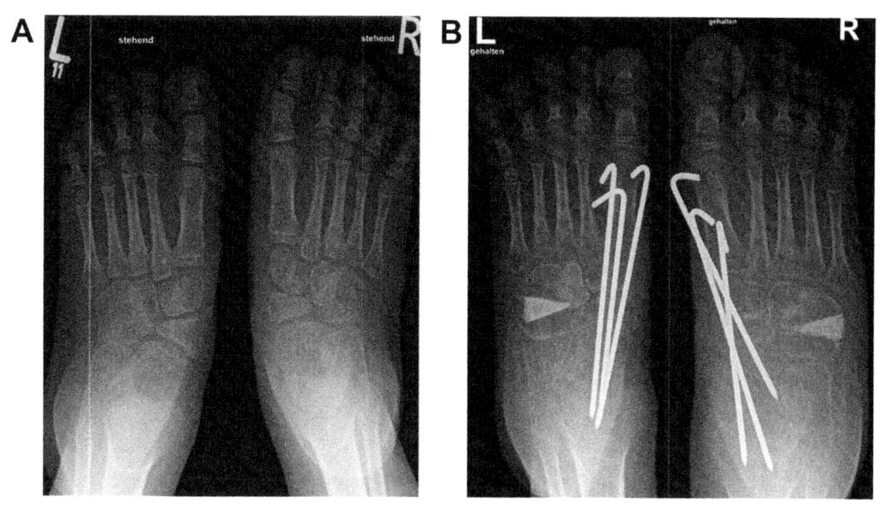

Fig. 7. Partial recurrence of CVT in a child with distal arthrogryposis. Bilateral persistent forefoot abduction (*A*). Treatment by a combination of open wedge osteotomy of the cuboid and closing wedge osteotomy of the first cuneiform (*B*).

patients may benefit from pain-free and more functional feet compared with the preoperative situation.

CLINICS CARE POINTS

- Early diagnosis allows early and successful minimal invasive treatment.
- Open reduction of the talo-navicular joint required , if closed reduction fails.
- Syndromic and neuromuscular CVT are much more difficult to treat.
- Peritalar release only necessary in very severely deformed and rigid feet.

DISCLOSURE

The author states that there is no conflict of interest related to this work.

REFERENCES

1. Wirth T, Schuler P, Griss P. Early surgical treatment for congenital vertical talus. Arch Orthop Trauma Surg 1994;113:248–53.
2. Giannestras NJ. Recognition and treatment of flatfeet in infancy. Clin Orthop Relat Res 1970;70:10–29.
3. Silk FF, Wainwright D. The recognition and treatment of congenital flatfeet in infancy. J Bone Joint Surg Br 1967;49-B:628–33.
4. Alvarado DM, McCall K, Hecht JT, et al. Deletions of 5' HOXC genes are associated with lower extremity malformations including clubfoot and vertical talus. J Med Genet 2016;53:250–5.
5. Dobbs MB, Schoenecker PL, Gordon JE. Autosomal dominant transmission of isolated congenital vertical talus. Iowa Orthop J 2002;22:25–7.

6. Dobbs MB, Gurnett CA, Robarge J, et al. Variable hand and foot abnormalities in family with congenital vertical talus and CDMP-1 gene mutation. J Orthop Res 2005;23:1490–4.
7. Dobbs MB, Gurnett CA, Pierce B, et al. HOXD10 M319K mutation in a family with isolated congenital vertical talus. J Orthop Res 2006;24:448–53.
8. Ogata K, Schoenecker PL, Sheridan J. Congenital vertical talus and its familial occurrence: an analysis of 36 patients. Clin Orthop Relat Res 1979;139:128–32.
9. Sharrard WJ, Grosfield I. The management of deformity and paralysis of the foot in myelomeningocele. J Bone Joint Surg Br 1968;50-B:456–65.
10. Townes PL, Dehart GK Jr, Hecht F, et al. Trisomy 13-15 in a male infant. J Pediatr 1962;60:528–32.
11. Yang JS, Dobbs MB. Treatment of congenital vertical talus: comparison of minimally invasive and extensive soft-tissue release procedures at minimum five-year follow-up. J Bone Joint Surg Am 2015;97-A:1354–65.
12. Miller M, Dobbs MB. Congenital vertical talus: etiology and management. J Am Acad Orthop Surg 2015;23:604–11.
13. Eberhardt O, Fernandez FF, Wirth T. The talar axis-first metatarsal base angle in CVT treatment: a comparison of idiopathic and non-idiopathic cases treated with the Dobbs method. J Child Orthop 2012;6:491–6.
14. Hamanishi C. Congenital vertical talus: classification with 69 cases and new measurement system. J Pediatr Orthop 1984;4:318–26.
15. Coleman SS, Stelling FH III, Jarrett J. Pathomechanics and treatment of congenital vertical talus. Clin Orthop Relat Res 1970;70:62–72.
16. Becker-Andersen H, Reimann I. Congenital vertical talus. Reevaluation of early manipulative treatment. Acta Orthop Scand 1974;45:130–44.
17. Walker AP, Ghali NN, Silk FF. Congenital vertical talus. The results of staged operative reduction. J Bone Joint Surg Br 1985;67-B:117–21.
18. Badelon O, Rigault P, Pouliquen JC, et al. Congenital convex clubfoot: a diagnostic and therapeutic study of 71 cases. Int Orthop 1984;8:211–21.
19. Duncan RD, Fixsen JA. Congenital convex pes valgus. J Bone Joint Surg Br 1999;81-B:250–4.
20. Fitton JM, Nevelös AB. The treatment of congenital vertical talus. J Bone Joint Surg Br 1979;61-B:481–3.
21. Kodros SA, Dias LS. Single-stage surgical correction of congenital vertical talus. J Pediatr Orthop 1999;19:42–8.
22. Tachdjian MO. Congenital convex pes valgus. Orthop Clin North Am 1972;3:131–48.
23. Zorer G, Bagatur AE, Dogan A. Single stage surgical correction of congenital vertical talus by complete subtalar release and peritalar reduction by using the Cincinnati incision. J Pediatr Orthop B 2002;11:60–7.
24. Séringe R, Martin G, Katti E, et al. Le pied convexe congénital. Etude anatomique et déductions pratiques. Rev Chir Orthop 1990;76:234–44.
25. Seimon LP. Surgical correction of congenital vertical talus under the age of 2 years. J Pediatr Orthop 1987;7:405–11.
26. Daumas L, Filipe G, Carlioz H. Congenital convex talus. Methods and results of a single-stage surgical correction. Rev Chir Orthop Reparatrice Appar Mot 1995;81:527–37.
27. Dobbs MB, Purcell DB, Nunley R, et al. Early results of a new method of treatment for idiopathic congenital vertical talus. J Bone Joint Surg Am 2006;88-A:1192–200.

28. Ponseti IV, Campos J. Observations on pathogenesis and treatment of congenital clubfoot. Clin Orthop Relat Res 1972;84:50–60.
29. Eberhardt O, Fernandez FF, Wirth T. Treatment of vertical talus with the Dobbs method. Z Orthop Unfall 2011;149:219–24.
30. Chan Y, Selvaratnam V, Garg N. A comparison of the Dobbs method for correction of idiopathic and teratological congenital vertical talus. J Child Orthop 2016; 10:93–9.
31. Wright J, Coggings D, Maizen C, et al. Reverse Ponseti-type treatment for children with congenital vertical talus. Comparison between idiopathic and teratological patients. Bone Joint J 2014;96-B:274–8.
32. Malhotra M, Shah H. Comparison of outcome between idiopathic and non-idiopathic congenital vertical talus treated with soft tissue release. J Pediatr Orthop B 2020. https://doi.org/10.1097/BPB.0000000000000815.
33. Clark MW, D'Ambrosia RD, Ferguson AB. Congenital vertical talus. Treatment by open reduction and navicular excision. J Bone Joint Surg Am 1977;59-A:816–24.
34. Abraham E, Quan Soon CH, Murphy A, et al. Talectomy by medial surgical approach for congenital vertical talus in arthrogryposis multiplex congenita. Orthopedics 2020;43:e623–6.

Bony Procedures for Correction of the Flexible Pediatric Flatfoot Deformity

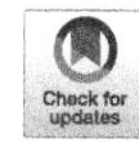

Maryse Bouchard, MD, MSc[a,b,c,*], Tayler Declan Ross, MB BCh BAO[d]

KEYWORDS

- Pediatric flatfoot • Flexible flatfoot • Osteotomy • Calcaneal lengthening

KEY POINTS

- Most pediatric flexible flatfeet are asymptomatic and do not require surgery.
- The calcaneal lengthening osteotomy is a powerful corrective procedure for symptomatic flexible pediatric flatfoot.
- Assess intraoperatively for residual forefoot supination after hindfoot correction.
- Evaluate for a concurrent gastrocnemius or tendoAchilles contracture.
- Choose osteotomies for flatfoot correction based on the flexibility, location, and severity of deformity.

INTRODUCTION

The pediatric flexible flatfoot is a common foot shape that is most often asymptomatic and may be a physiologic variant of normal.[1–3] A flexible flatfoot may become symptomatic if there is a concurrent equinus contracture or excessive deformity.[4] Surgery is only indicated when nonoperative interventions have failed to resolve symptoms.[5] The goal of surgery is to alleviate symptoms by improving hindfoot alignment and restoring the medial arch while preserving joint mobility.[6]

It is important to distinguish the flexible from a rigid flatfoot. Rigid flatfeet have restricted subtalar motion typically resulting from structural causes, such as tarsal coalitions or congenital vertical talus, or neuromuscular diseases such as cerebral palsy.[1,7–9] Treatment of the rigid flatfoot is more often surgical, and reconstruction may require procedures other than, or in addition to, the typical extra-articular osteotomies used for flexible flatfeet, such as arthrodesis or coalition resection.[6]

[a] Division of Orthopaedic Surgery, The Hospital for Sick Children, Toronto, Canada; [b] Department of Surgery, University of Toronto, Toronto, Canada; [c] Division of Orthopaedic Surgery, The University of Toronto, Toronto, Canada; [d] Division of Orthopaedic Surgery, The University of Toronto, 500 University Avenue #602, Toronto, Ontario M5G 1V7, Canada
* Corresponding author. 555 University Avenue, S107, Toronto, Ontario M5G 1X8, Canada.
E-mail address: Maryse.bouchard@sickkids.ca

Foot Ankle Clin N Am 26 (2021) 915–939
https://doi.org/10.1016/j.fcl.2021.09.001
1083-7515/21/

This article focuses on the common bony techniques for surgical correction of the pediatric flexible flatfoot that has failed nonoperative management, including calcaneal, midfoot, and supramalleolar osteotomies and distal tibial hemiepiphyseodesis.

PATHOANATOMY

Clinically, the flatfoot is described as loss of the medial arch, abduction of the forefoot relative to the hindfoot, and valgus hindfoot alignment.[10] There is no strict definition, although most investigators agree the flatfoot is a combination of dorsiflexion and external rotation of the subtalar joint, midfoot abduction, and forefoot supination.[10,11] When a flatfoot deformity is present, subtalar joint inversion is restricted causing inefficiency in gait and eventual fatigue and/or pain.[10] It remains unclear if the tendoAchilles contracture associated with some flatfeet is a secondary deformity or a primary pathology.[4,10]

EPIDEMIOLOGY AND CLINICAL FEATURES

The true incidence of flatfoot is unknown. Flatfoot is present in all infants.[3] By school age, approximately 50% of children have flatfeet.[12,13] Harris and Beath[4] noted flatfeet in 23% of adult army recruits. One-quarter had concurrent contractures of the tendoAchilles, and these recruits more often reported pain or disability.[4] Rigid flatfoot deformity occurred in less than 10% of the cohort.[4] It has been estimated that 95% of flatfeet are flexible and asymptomatic.[14]

Flatfoot deformity has been related to specific patient factors, including obesity and generalized ligamentous laxity.[13,15] Pfeiffer and colleagues[15] studied 835 Austrian schoolchildren and noted male children were twice as likely to have flatfeet and overweight children were 3 times more likely than normal weight children to have flatfeet. Ethnicity has also been related to flatfeet with multiple studies reporting a higher prevalence in Black individuals and Chinese populations.[16–19]

Assessment of the child with flatfoot requires a complete history with focus on pain location, aggravating factors, shoe wear difficulty, and functional disability.[1,5] Manual examination should be performed for restriction of subtalar motion. Subtalar motion should also be evaluated by having the patient rise on their toes. This position inverts the subtalar joint, and the arch reconstitutes when the flatfoot is flexible (**Fig. 1**).

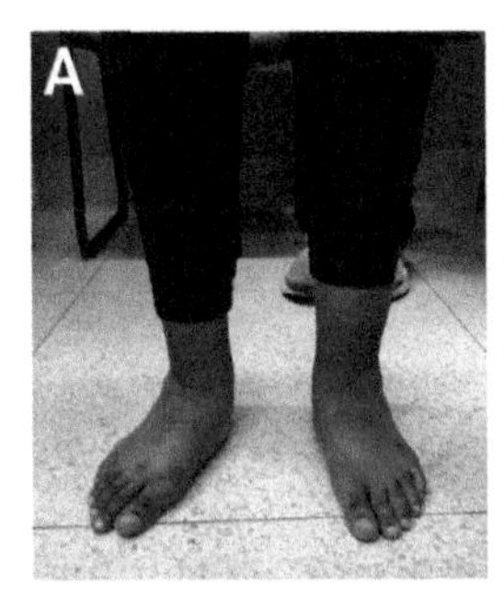

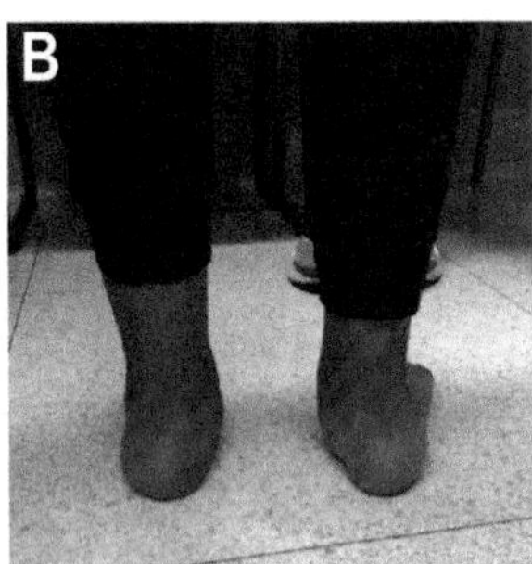

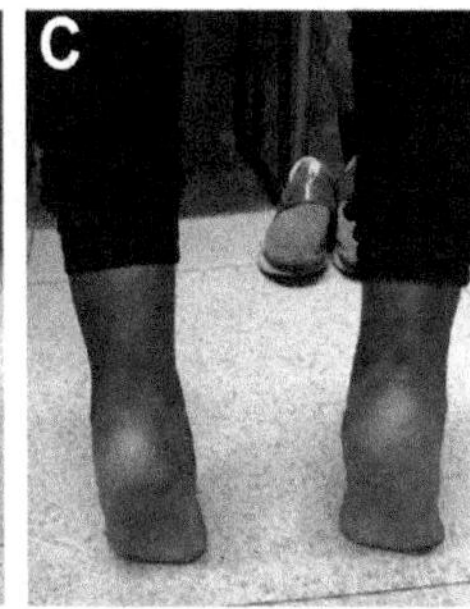

Fig. 1. (*A*) Clinical photograph of a 15-year-old girl with flexible flatfeet, most pronounced on the right. On this anterior view, note the collapsed medial longitudinal arch and forefoot abductus. (*B*) In this clinical photograph of the same patient, note on this posterior view the increased hindfoot valgus alignment on the right, collapsed medial arch, and too-many-toes sign representing forefoot abductus. (*C*) In this clinical photograph of the same patient, note how on toe-rise her medial arch is now present and the hindfeet are inverted, confirming a supple subtalar joint complex and flexible flatfoot deformities. (*Courtesy of* the private collection of Dr. M. Bouchard.)

Contracture of the tendoAchilles complex should be assessed with the Silfverskiold test[1,6] (**Fig. 2**). Calluses on the plantar aspect of the feet should be noted and a detailed neurologic examination performed.[20] Areas of pain and/or tenderness are classically located at the plantarmedial aspect of the arch under the talar head, in the sinus tarsi, and in the subfibular region in severe deformities causing impingement.[1,5]

RADIOGRAPHIC EVALUATION

Diagnosis of flatfoot is made by clinical examination, but radiographs are indicated for deformity assessment and surgical planning.[1,5,20,21] Weight-bearing anteroposterior (AP) and lateral radiographs of the feet and ankles are required. Ankle radiographs should be assessed to rule out concurrent distal tibial deformity and degenerative changes and instability within the ankle joint (**Fig. 3**).[6] Advanced imaging such as

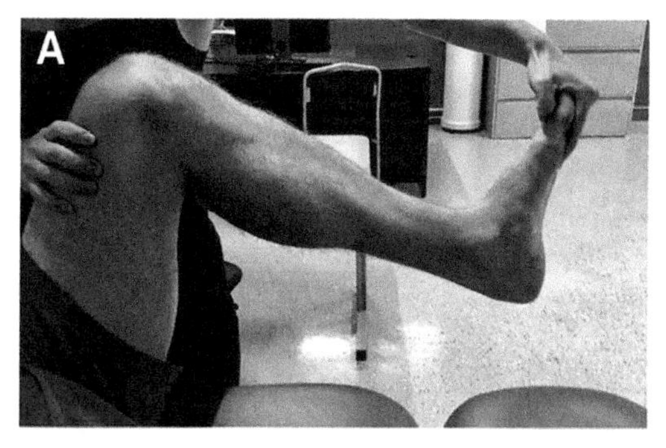

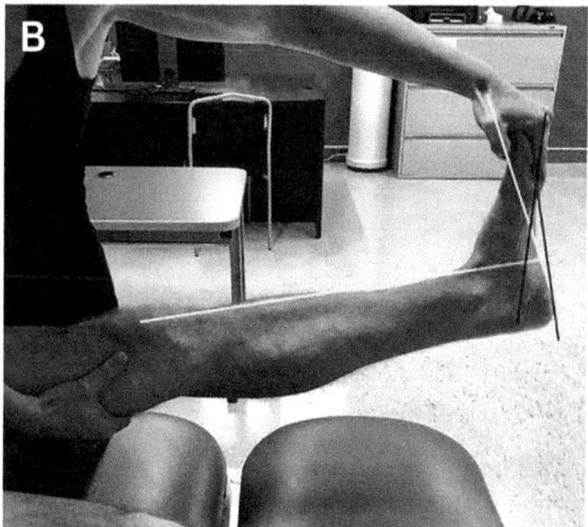

Fig. 2. Clinical photographs demonstrating the Silfverskiold test. (*A*) With the knee flexed to relax the gastrocnemius, the ankle is passively dorsiflexed. (*B*) Ankle dorsiflexion range is also assessed with the knee extended, now putting the gastrocnemius on stretch. The range of motion is assessed by comparing the axis of the anterior tibia to the lateral plantar border of the foot (*yellow lines*). Note the decrease in ankle dorsiflexion in this position (*B* vs *A*), confirming that there is an isolated gastrocnemius contracture. Also note that in feet with cavus, the amount of equinus is often overestimated because the first ray is excessively plantarflexed (*blue line*). If one judges the ankle range by a line subtending the heel to the first metatarsal head in a foot with cavus (*red line*), it falsely suggests more equinus than using the lateral border of the foot/heel (*yellow line*) that represents ankle motion. (*Courtesy of* the private collection of Dr. M. Bouchard.)

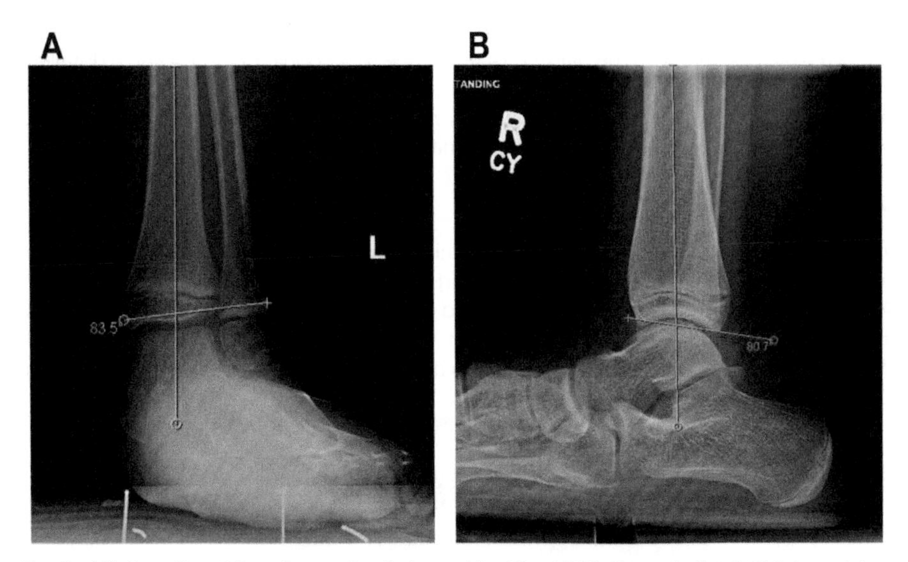

Fig. 3. (*A*) Standing AP radiograph of the ankle. The LDTA (lateral distal tibial angle) as measured by the tibial axis relative to the articular distal tibial surface is decreased suggesting a valgus deformity (normal 86°–92°). (*B*) Standing lateral radiograph of the ankle. The ADTA (anterior distal tibial angle) as measured by the tibial axis relative to the articular distal tibial surface is normal suggesting at 80°. (*Courtesy of* the private collection of Dr. M. Bouchard.)

computed tomography or MRI can be helpful for planning correction of severe deformities.[1,20]

Many angles and anatomic relationships have been described to characterize the flatfoot. Most important is the angle between the first metatarsal and talar axes (Meary angle) on the AP and lateral views because it confirms the flatfoot diagnosis and identifies the apex of the deformity. Normally, these should be collinear.[22] Deviations of up to 13° on the lateral/sagittal plane and 10° in the AP/axial plane are considered within normal limits.[22] On the lateral foot radiograph, a flatfoot deformity will therefore show increased angulation of Meary angle with the apex plantar.[6] If tendoAchilles contracture is present, the calcaneal pitch will be decreased.[5,22] On the AP view, Meary angle typically denotes abduction with the apex of the first metatarsal and talar axes being medial.[20] Talonavicular uncoverage may be noted but can be difficult to quantify before the navicular is fully ossified[10] (**Fig. 4**A, B). The surgeon should also take care to identify if a skewfoot variant is present.[21] In skewfoot, the first metatarsal and talar axes are parallel but translated[21] (**Fig. 4**C).

SURGICAL INDICATIONS

The literature is devoid of natural history, long-term, or prospective studies on pediatric flexible flatfeet. There is no evidence supporting operative treatment of the painless, asymptomatic flexible flatfoot.[1,5,13,20] Nonoperative management can include off-the-shelf and custom foot orthoses, and if a contracture is present, tendoAchilles stretching programs.[5,13] To date, there is no evidence to support any one nonoperative modality over another.[1,5,13,23]

When pain and/or functional disability persist despite nonoperative treatment for greater than 6 months, surgery may be indicated.[5,6,13,21] Surgery for the pediatric

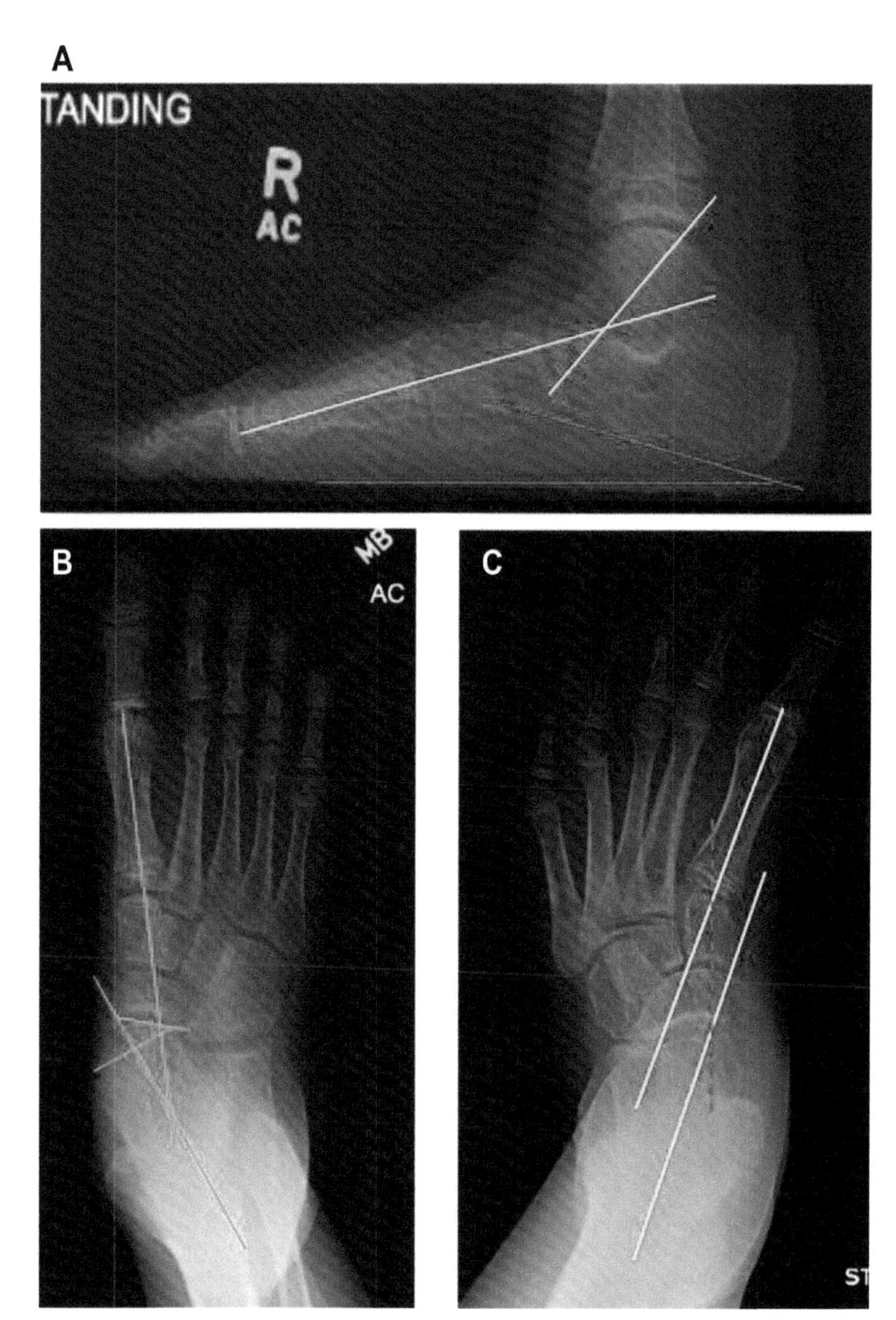

Fig. 4. (*A*) Standing lateral radiograph of the foot. The yellow lines denote Meary (first metatarsal-talar) angle with the intersection in the talar head and the apex plantar suggesting a flatfoot. The orange lines represent the calcaneal pitch. When decreased, equinus is typically present. On the lateral foot radiograph, a flatfoot deformity will therefore show increased angulation of Meary angle with the apex plantar. (*B*) Standing AP radiograph

flexible flatfoot generally consists of a combination of soft tissue and bony procedures to restore normal alignment of the midfoot and hindfoot while maintaining joint mobility.[5,24] Soft tissue procedures can include one or a combination of gastrocnemius recession, tendoAchilles lengthening, peroneus brevis lengthening, and medial plication of the spring ligament, talonavicular joint capsule, and/or tibialis posterior tendon.[24] Depending on deformity location and severity as determined on clinical and radiographic examination, bony procedures can include osteotomies of the midfoot, calcaneus, or distal tibia. Indications and techniques for arthroereisis and arthrodesis are described separately in other articles in this issue. When pathologic conditions such as skewfoot, tarsal coalition, accessory navicular, and hallux valgus are also present, the surgeon should consider additional procedures as indicated.

OUTCOMES OF BONY PROCEDURES

Generally, bony procedures for correction of the pediatric flexible foot have good outcomes and low complication rates.[24–27] Most studies comparing joint-sparing osteotomies to arthrodesis show improved mobility and equivalent or better pain and functional outcomes with osteotomies.[28,29] There is no literature comparing bony procedures to nonoperative management. Articles on outcomes of osteotomies for the pediatric flatfoot mostly report on small numbers of children, but the outcomes for flexible flatfeet are generally good.[21,29,30] Natural history studies of the untreated flexible flatfoot report long-term issues from tissue strain and poor propulsion strength including plantar fasciitis, posterior tibial tendon insufficiency, first-ray deformities such as hallux rigidus, and malalignment through the hip, knee, and pelvis.[31–37] A systematic review by Suh and colleagues[29] showed that calcaneal lengthening osteotomy (CLO) better radiographic outcome and American Orthopedic Foot and Ankle Society score improvement than subtalar arthroereisis for pediatric flatfoot correction. Independently, CLO had a reported success rate of 69% to 89%. Reoperation rates between the groups were similar. Marengo and colleagues[38] in a 2017 prospective study showed that symptomatic flatfeet treated with CLO had satisfactory outcomes in 89% of patients. Those with poor results were feet flattened secondary to neuromuscular conditions and therefore had rigid deformities, suggesting that CLO is an effective treatment in the flexible flatfoot.[38]

PATIENT POSITIONING AND PREPARATION

Most pediatric flatfoot reconstructions can be performed with the child supine on a radiolucent operating table with a bump under the ipsilateral hip and a nonsterile tourniquet on the ipsilateral thigh.[6] It is important to include the knee in the sterile field to more easily position the limb and assess limb alignment. A mini- or standard C-arm

of the foot. The green lines denote Meary (first metatarsal-talar) angle with apex medial suggesting abduction. The blue lines represent the articular surfaces of the talar head and navicular. Talar head uncoverage as a percentage or angle can be measured. Normally, these should be collinear. Deviations of up to 13° on the lateral/sagittal plane and 10° in the AP/axial plane are considered within normal limits. On the AP view, Meary angle typically denotes abduction with the apex of the first metatarsal and talar axes being medial. (*C*) AP lateral standing radiograph of a skewfoot. Note that the first metatarsal and talar axes are medially directed and parallel but translated (*yellow lines*). The midfoot aims slightly lateral (*dashed orange line*) giving the skewfoot its "s" shape. (*Courtesy of* the private collection of Dr. M. Bouchard.)

can be used for intraoperative fluoroscopy. If available, regional anesthesia with sciatic and/or saphenous nerve block, with or without an indwelling catheter, is an ideal technique for intraoperative and postoperative pain control and to minimize opiate use.[39]

SURGICAL TECHNIQUES

Calcaneal Lengthening Osteotomy

The foot is composed of a medial (first ray, medial cuneiform, navicular, and talus) and lateral column (fourth and fifth rays as they align with cuboid and calcaneus). As a flatfoot has an abduction deformity of the forefoot relative to the hindfoot, it therefore has a relatively long medial and short lateral column[22] (**Fig. 5**). The lateral column CLO was

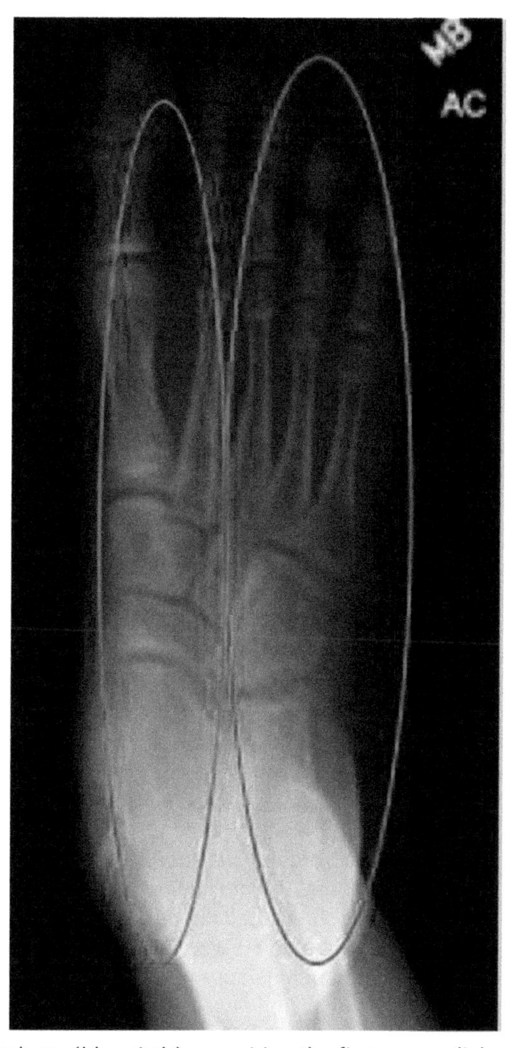

Fig. 5. The medial column (*blue circle*) comprising the first ray, medial cuneiform, and talus, and the lateral column (*green circle*), comprising the fourth and fifth rays, as they align with the cuboid and calcaneus are grossly identified on this standing AP radiograph of the foot. (*Courtesy of* the private collection of Dr. M. Bouchard.)

originally described by Evans[40] then modified by Mosca.[21] It enables simultaneous correction of hindfoot valgus, sag through the talonavicular joint, and navicular lateralization on the talar head by inserting a tricortical bone graft into an osteotomy in the anterior process of the calcaneus.[21,41,42] When the subtalar joint is supple, the corrective power of the CLO is significant and reliable, although good correction has also been reported in rigid flatfeet with tarsal coalitions.[7,38] CLO alone will not correct all components of the flatfoot deformity.[6] If significant hindfoot valgus persists after CLO, a medializing posterior displacement calcaneal osteotomy (PDCO) (section Posterior Calcaneal Displacement Osteotomy) can be added.[6] Residual supination of the forefoot will require a plantarflexion osteotomy (section Medial Cuneiform Osteotomy), and the appropriate soft tissue procedures such as Achilles lengthening, gastrocnemius recession, and medial plication.[6] Outcomes of the CLO, performed as described originally by Evans[40] and with the modified technique described by Mosca,[21] are favorable with good radiological deformity correction and pain reduction.[24,25,29,38,43–45]

Technique

A lateral longitudinal incision over the anterior process of the calcaneus or a modified Ollier incision is made.[21] It should be ensured that the sural and superficial peroneal nerves are protected.[21] The peroneus brevis is lengthened in a Z-fashion to accommodate the eventual CLO.[6] It should be ensured that all soft tissues are elevated off the anterior process of the calcaneus at the level of the osteotomy using a freer, Joker, and/or Crego retractors[21] (**Fig. 6**A, B).

To prevent subluxation of the calcaneocuboid joint (CCJ) with distraction of the CLO, a smooth 2- or 2.4-mm Steinman pin is placed across the joint in a retrograde fashion.[21] Fluoroscopy should be used to ensure that the wire crosses the center of the CCJ on both the AP and lateral radiographs[6] (**Fig. 6**B, C).

As described by Mosca,[21] the osteotomy for the modified CLO begins 1.5 to 2 cm behind the CCJ at the lowest point of the anterior process, generally within the sinus tarsi. The osteotomy should exit medially between the anterior and middle facets, aiming slightly distal, converging with the plane of the CCJ[21] (**Fig. 6**D). An oscillating sagittal saw or osteotome is used to divide the bone.[6]

A lamina spreader is inserted to distract the osteotomy.[21] Clinically, medial arch restoration and correction of hindfoot valgus should be confirmed (**Fig. 7**A, B). On fluoroscopy, it should be ensured that the AP first metatarsal-talar angle is restored and talonavicular coverage is improved[6] (**Fig. 7**C). The forefoot supination is now evident.[6] Generally, distraction of 8 to 12 mm is required to correct the alignment[6] (see **Fig. 7**A). As this is a lengthening osteotomy, and not a pure opening wedge, the graft should be cut as a trapezoid versus a triangle enabling distraction of the osteotomy to be greater from lateral to medial[21] (**Fig. 8**). Tricortical autograft from the iliac crest or fibula or allograft can be used. Union and complication rates are similar between graft types, although the latter saves morbidity from the graft donor site[21,45,46] (**Fig. 9**A). The graft is inherently stable, because it is press-fit into the osteotomy. The wire is advanced across the osteotomy into the posterior calcaneus (**Fig. 9**B). The wire is cut and bent at the skin and removed in clinic at the 6-week postoperative visit.[21] Other investigators have used internal fixation such as screws or plate and screw constructs.[47]

Posterior Calcaneal Displacement Osteotomy

The PDCO aligns the hindfoot by reapproximating the axes of the calcaneus and tibia.[48] PDCO neither alters the subtalar alignment nor will it address the midfoot deformities or talar head uncoverage.[5] This technique, originally described by Dwyer,

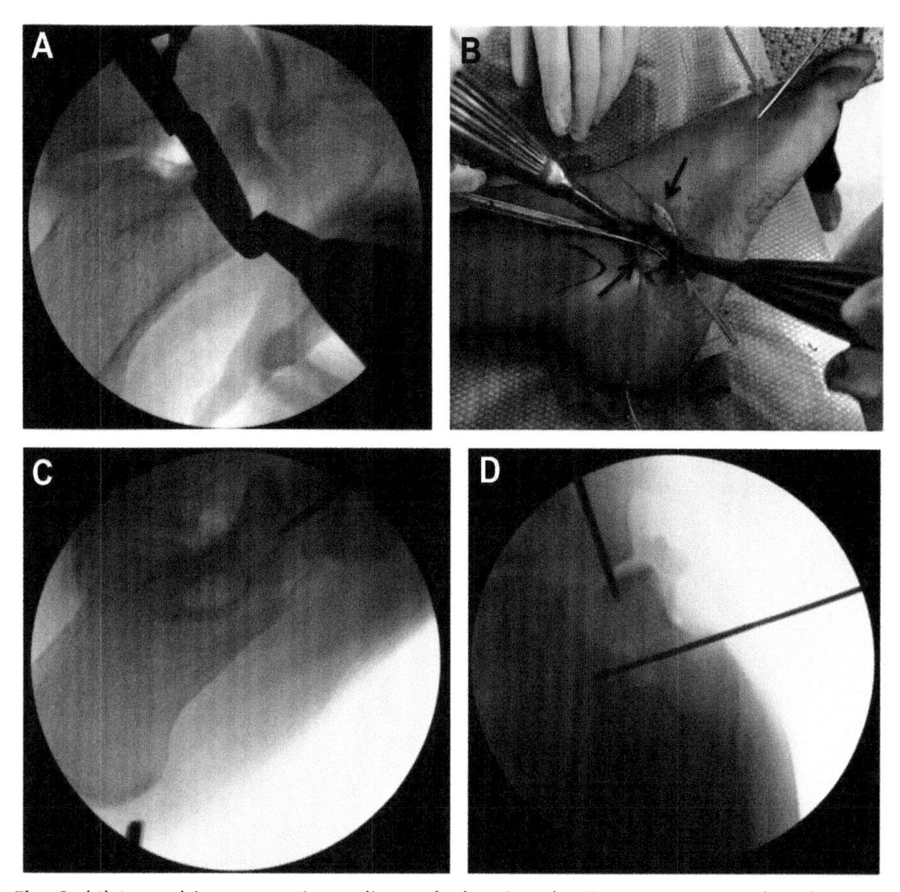

Fig. 6. (*A*) Lateral intraoperative radiograph showing the Crego retractors placed around the calcaneal anterior process at the site of the osteotomy. (*B*) Clinical intraoperative photograph with Crego retractors in place around the calcaneus through a modified Ollier incision. The z-lengthened ends of the peroneus brevis are denoted by the black arrows. The freer denotes the location of the osteotomy. The red arrows show the two smooth Steinman pins, one for fixation of the CCJ and the other to show the plane of the calcaneal osteotomy. (*C*) Lateral intraoperative radiograph showing the CCJ fixation wire in the center of the joint and stopping before the osteotomy. (*D*) AP intraoperative radiograph showing the same CCJ fixation wire in the center of the joint and stopping before the osteotomy and the second Steinman pin in the anterior process of the calcaneus aiming slightly distally as it exits medially between the anterior and middle facets, approximately 2 cm proximal to the CCJ. (*Courtesy of* the private collection of Dr. M. Bouchard.)

was a lateral opening wedge osteotomy, but owing to frequent wound issues it is most often modified to a medial displacement for flatfoot with reliable deformity correction and improves function postoperatively.[48,49]

A medial PDCO can improve hindfoot valgus in cases in which there is residual deformity after CLO or subtalar or triple arthrodesis or when CLO is contraindicated such as in severe rigid flatfoot.[48] Medial PDCO is commonly used in the adult acquired flatfoot.[50] A lateral PDCO is commonly used for correction of the cavovarus foot.[51] Recent advances in instrumentation have enabled for safe minimally invasive osteotomies.[52] These osteotomies are made through small percutaneous incisions with

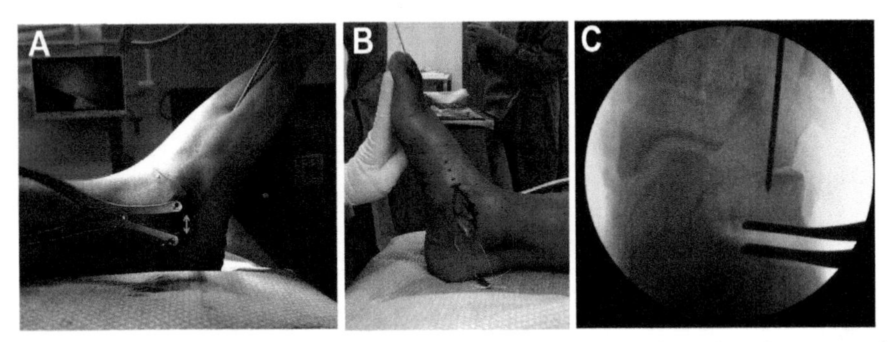

Fig. 7. (*A*) Clinical lateral-facing intraoperative photograph of the foot after distraction of the CLO with a Hintermann distractor in place. Note the arch has reconstituted. (*B*) Clinical medial-facing intraoperative photograph of the foot after distraction of the CLO with a Hintermann distractor in place. Note the arch has reconstituted. (*C*) AP intraoperative radiograph showing the lamina spreader in the CLO distracting to restore the arch clinically and talar head coverage radiographically. (*Courtesy of* the private collection of Dr. M. Bouchard.)

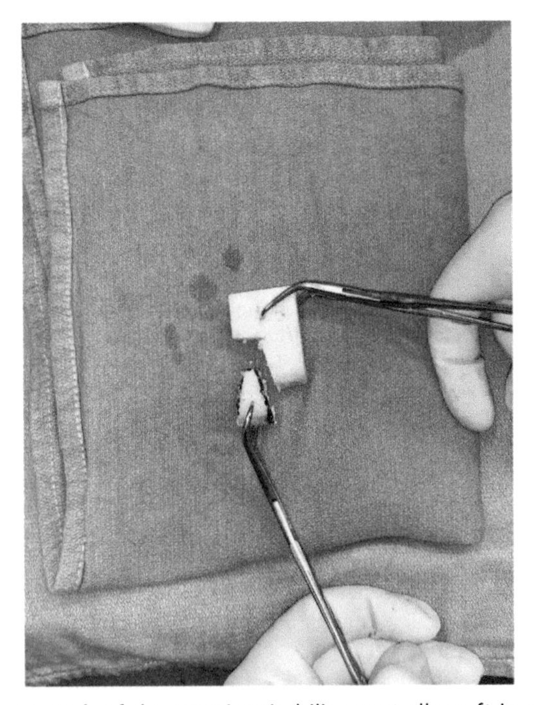

Fig. 8. Clinical photograph of the cut tricortical iliac crest allograft in a trapezoid with a 1 cm base. (*Courtesy of* the private collection of Dr. M. Bouchard.)

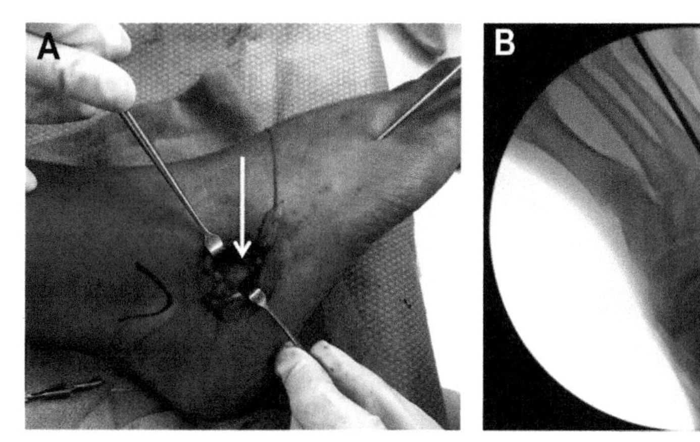

Fig. 9. (*A*) Clinical intraoperative photograph of the tricortical graft wedged into the CLO. (*B*) AP intraoperative radiograph showing the interposed tricortical allograft in the CLO with restored alignment. (*Courtesy of* the private collection of Dr. M. Bouchard.)

cooled high-torque low-speed burrs.[53] Although there are limited studies on its use in pediatrics, the adult literature growingly supports minimally invasive osteotomy techniques. There is less postoperative swelling and pain, without increased bone healing, wound complication, or neurovascular injury risks.[52–55] Both the open and minimally invasive techniques are described.

Open technique

An oblique incision is made laterally over the posterior calcaneus.[48] The sural nerve and peroneal tendons are protected.[48] Soft tissues should be bluntly elevated dorsally off the calcaneal tuberosity laterally, plantarly, and dorsally in the plane of the osteotomy to the medial side of the calcaneus remaining deep to the posterior tibial neurovascular bundle to ensure its protection during the osteotomy.[6,10] The periosteum should be incised and elevated in line with retractors along the lateral wall of the calcaneus.[48]

To avoid calcaneal shortening or lengthening or altering the vertical height of the bone, a wire can be placed in the plantar posterior aspect of the tuberosity from medial to lateral in the transverse plane of the metatarsal heads[10] (**Fig. 10**). The saw blade or osteotome should follow this plane and angle at approximately 45° from the plane of the foot from anterior-plantar to dorsal-posterior.[10] Care must be taken not to protrude excessively on the medial side to avoid injury of the neurovascular bundle.[6] As shown in cadaveric studies, performing the PDCO in the anterior or posterior third versus the middle third of the tuberosity carries the least risk of neurovascular injury.[56] A broad osteotome or blunt instrument like a Willegger elevator can be used from within the osteotomy to displace the tuberosity.[6] The long plantar ligament and/or periosteum may inhibit adequate displacement and can be released with scissors on the plantar aspect of the osteotomy.[48] Generally, 8 to 10 mm of medial displacement is sufficient. If more correction is required but not achieved with pure displacement, a medially based wedge of bone can be excised to further increase the varus alignment of the heel.[6]

Minimally invasive technique

The patient should be positioned in a sloppy lateral position, or supine with a bump under the knee to allow it to flex and the leg to lie in a more lateral position.[53,55] A mini c-arm with a flat panel is preferred because it can be used as the operating table and produces lower radiation.[57] Otherwise, a large c-arm over a radiolucent operating

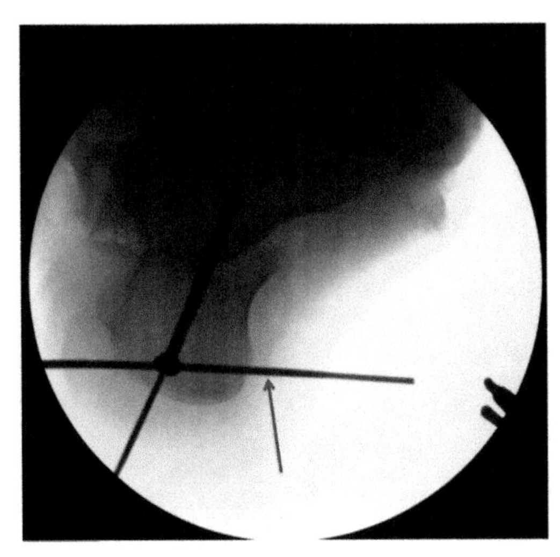

Fig. 10. Intraoperative Harris view radiograph. Note the wire in the posterior aspect of the tuberosity; this has been placed in the plane of the cascading metatarsal heads. Red arrow identifies the wire in the calcaneal tuberosity in line the with plane of the metatarsal heads. (*Courtesy of* the private collection of Dr. M. Bouchard.)

table can be used; it is, however, more cumbersome. The tourniquet is deflated for this procedure because the bleeding further cools the burr, preventing skin, tissue, and bone necrosis.[58]

The plane of the osteotomy is the same as described in the open technique. The orientation and start point are identified with fluoroscopy and marked on the lateral heel skin surface.[53–55] A knife is used to incise skin approximately 5 mm; then blunt dissection with a snap or artery clamp is made to the bone to displace the sural nerve and peroneal tendons. A small, curved instrument or rasp is used to elevate the soft tissues around the tuberosity from dorsomedial to plantarmedial.[52]

For pure displacement osteotomies, a Shannon burr is used.[54] The author (M.B.) prefers a 2 mm × 20-mm burr, although others may use 3 mm × 20-mm burr[52–54] (**Fig. 11**). The burr is powered on and penetrates the near lateral cortex, and the tuberostity is cut in 4 quadrants: the dorsal half of the near lateral cortex, the plantar half of the near lateral cortex, the dorsal half of the far medial cortex, and the plantar half of the far medial cortex. The lateral cortex cuts should be completed before the medial cuts.[52–54] Intermittent fluoroscopy is used to ensure the cuts remain in the desired plane.[53,55] Care should be taken not to plunge the burr medially beyond the cortex.[53,55] The surgeon can place their opposite hand on the medial cortex for sensory feedback.[54] The tuberosity should be displaced with a small instrument as described earlier[54] (**Fig. 12**).

Fixation is required and should be done with ankle in dorsiflexion, compressing the osteotomy.[53] For younger children when the apophysis is not yet fused, the author prefers to use a 2- or 2.4-mm smooth Steinman pin placed antegrade from the tuberosity, exiting on the dorsolateral foot. It is advanced until the wire is no longer felt at the heel, then cut and bent on the skin, and removed at the 6-week postoperative visit.[53] For older children, 1 or 2 percutaneous cannulated screws (4.5 mm preferred) can be placed in a retrograde fashion from the heel[59] (**Fig. 13**).

Step-Cut Calcaneal Osteotomy

The step-cut osteotomy of the calcaneal tuberosity (SCCO), originally described by Malerba and De Marchi,[60] was a lateral opening wedge in the sagittal plane.

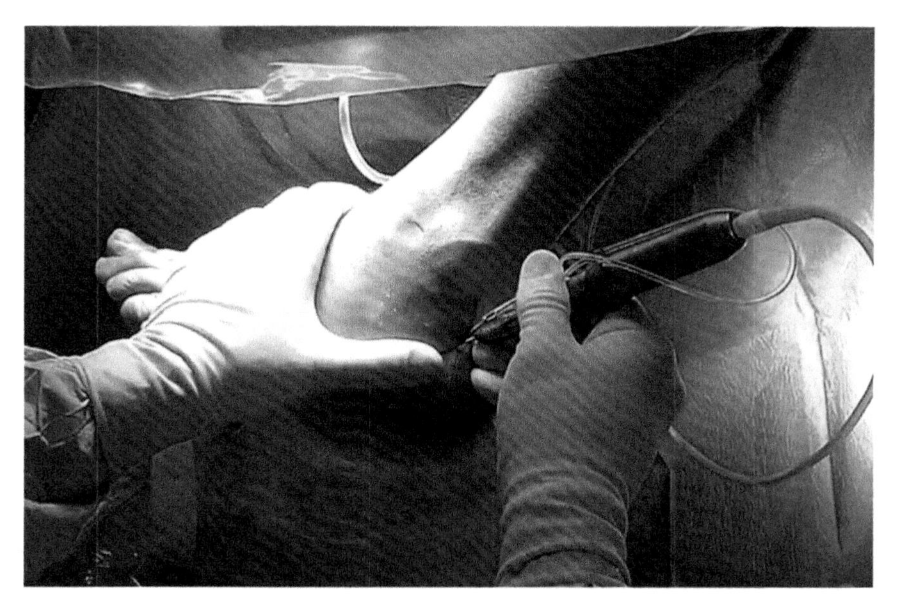

Fig. 11. Clinical intraoperative photograph of the burr introduced into the calcaneus though a keyhole incision on the lateral heel. Note the marking pen on the skin denoting the plane of the osteotomy. (*Courtesy of* the private collection of Dr. M. Bouchard.)

Modifications to the cuts and distraction techniques by multiple surgeons allow the SCCO to create triplanar deformity correction, including lateral lengthening, axial rotation, and sagittal plane correction[61]; it has been used for both flatfoot and cavus foot correction and deemed a more powerful correction than the CLO or PDCO.[62,63] When compared with the traditional Evans procedure, SCCO was found to have similar patient outcomes, but significantly faster healing times and lower nonunion rates.[63]

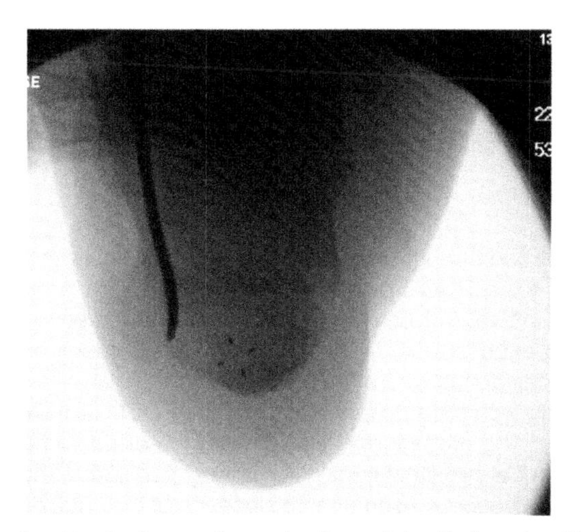

Fig. 12. Intraoperative Harris view radiograph after minimally invasive PDCO. A Willegger elevator is introduced into the tuberosity to help slide the posterior fragment. (*Courtesy of* the private collection of Dr. M. Bouchard.)

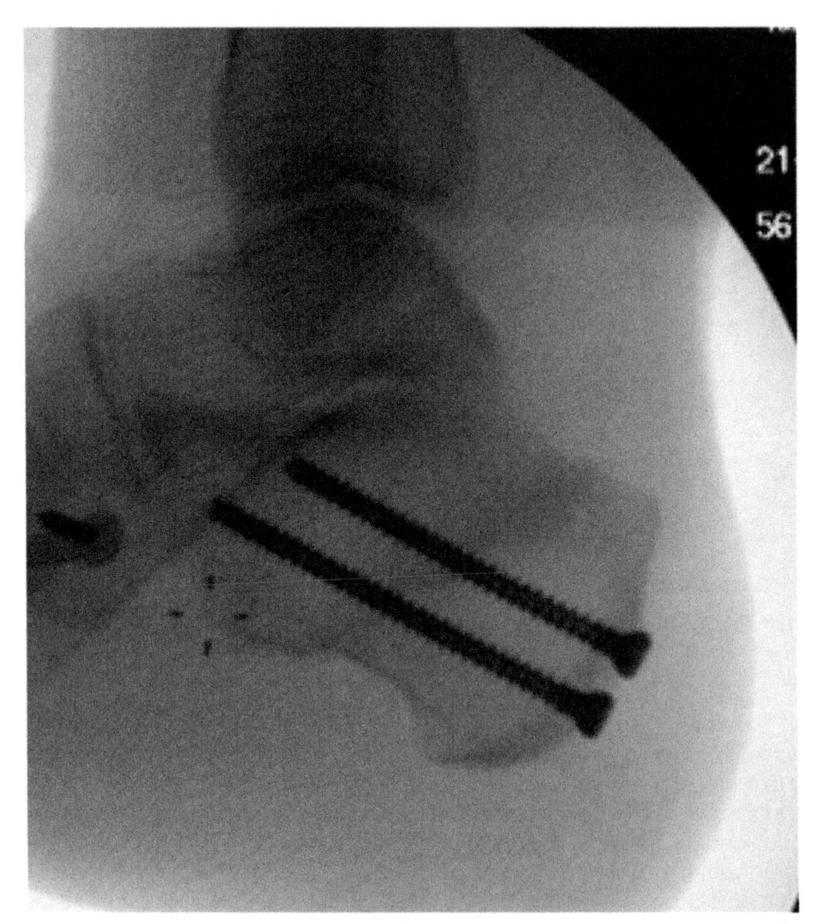

Fig. 13. Lateral intraoperative radiograph after minimally invasive PDCO showing fixation with 2 fully threaded 4.5-mm cannulated screws. Please note, the age of the patient in this radiograph is 16 years. (*Courtesy of* the private collection of Dr. M. Bouchard.)

Demetracopoulos and colleagues[61] found that patients treated for flatfoot deformity with an SCCO had significant improvement in pain and quality of life and no reported nonunions.

Technique

SCCO can be performed through 1 or 2 incisions, either a single oblique posterior incision as performed for a PDCO or this in combination with a modified Ollier incision.[61,63] The sural nerve and peroneal tendons are protected, and the lateral wall of the calcaneus is exposed extraperiosteally.[60,63] Soft tissues are elevated off the dorsal and plantar calcaneus where the osteotomies will exit.

The cuts are made with retractors in place per the PDCO and CLO using a sagittal saw or osteotome.[62] The procedure is started with the distal vertical limb, the transverse limb, and then the proximal limb.[61] A marking pen with a metal flat instrument can be used under fluoroscopy to confirm the location of the cuts, or smooth Steinman pins can be placed in the bone as "cut guides" (**Fig. 14**A, B).

A broad osteotome and/or lamina spreader should be used to distract the fragments[61] (**Fig. 14**C). Temporary smooth Steinman pins can be placed to hold the

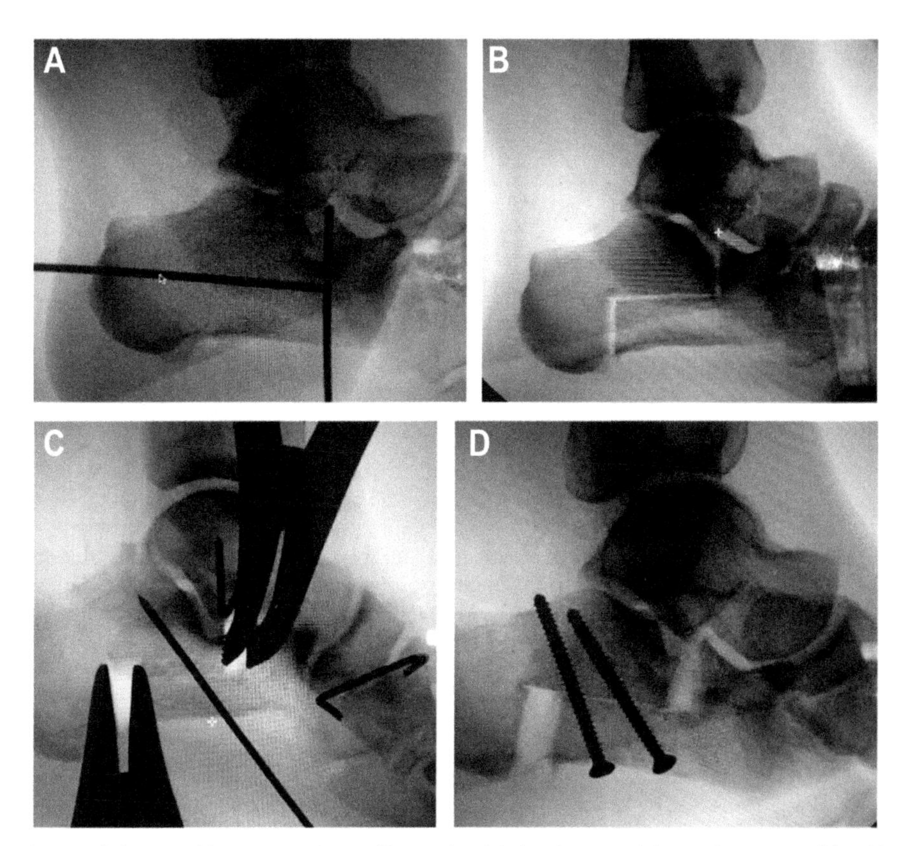

Fig. 14. (*A*) Lateral intraoperative radiograph with k-wires overlying calcaneus to identify planes of cuts. (*B*) Lateral intraoperative radiograph after completion the 3 limbs of the step cut. (*C*) Lateral intraoperative radiograph demonstrating lengthening distraction of the step cut osteotomy. (*D*) Final fixation of the step-cut osteotomy with two 4.5-mm fully threaded screws. Please note, the age of the patient in these radiographs is 19 or 20 years.

corrected position. If more hindfoot varus is needed, the osteotomy can be additionally opened laterally through the axial cut or rotated such that the posterior fragment moves further medially. If more talar coverage is desired, the distal anterior vertical cut can be additionally distracted. Once satisfied with the correction, fixation is placed. Options include screws, plate, and screw construct and staples[60–63] (**Fig. 14**D). No interpositional bone graft is required because this osteotomy has a large surface area of bony contact.[61–63]

Supramalleolar Tibial Osteotomy and Distal Tibial Hemiepiphyseodesis

The most common distal tibial deformity associated with a flatfoot is valgus, although the surgeon should evaluate for sagittal plane and rotational tibial deformities. Distal tibial valgus may result from sequelae of distal tibial growth arrest, fracture malunion, skeletal dysplasias, metabolic bone disease, and benign tumor conditions such as multiple hereditary exostoses.[6,64] A normal lateral distal tibial angle (LDTA) is between 86° and 92°.[65] There is no reported threshold at which distal tibial valgus must be treated; however, most surgeons consider correction when valgus is greater than

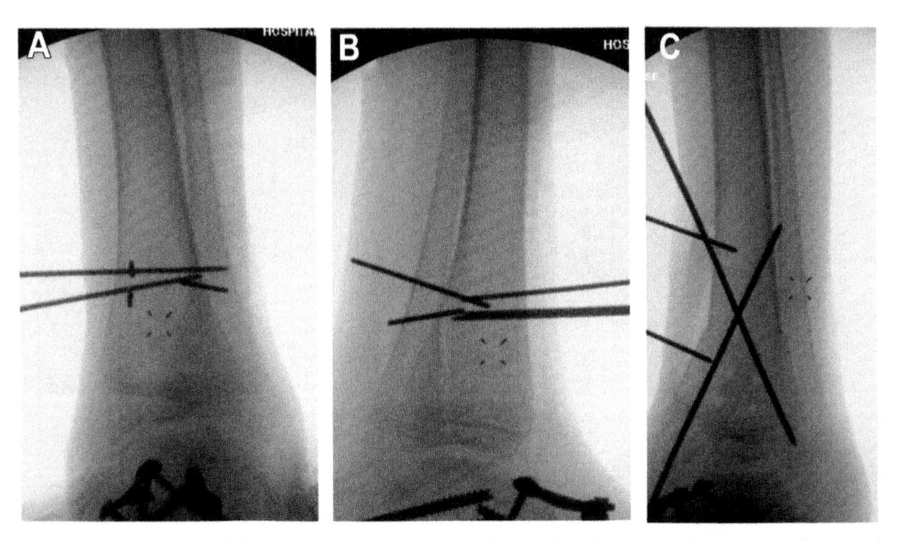

Fig. 15. (*A, B*) AP and lateral intraoperative radiographs showing placement of smooth Steinman pins to denote the plane of the medial closing wedge osteotomy. (*C*) AP intraoperative radiograph showing reduction of osteotomy after medial closing wedge has been resected with temporary fixation of 2 smooth Steinman pins running from proximal medial and distal medial across the osteotomy. (*Courtesy of* the private collection of Dr. M. Bouchard.)

10° or LDTA is less than 80° (**Fig. 15**A, B). Failure to address the supramalleolar deformity will leave residual hindfoot valgus alignment that can cause subfibular impingement, stress on the medial ankle ligaments, and pain at the plantar talar head from overload of the medial foot. When there is deformity at multiple levels in a limb, it is generally recommended to start with the proximal corrections and proceed distally.[6] Therefore in patients with concurrent distal tibial valgus and a flatfoot, the supramalleolar osteotomy (SMO) should in most cases be performed before the flatfoot reconstruction.

In children with open distal tibial physes and at least 2 years of growth remaining, guided growth can be considered.[66] A single cannulated 3.5- to 4.5-mm fully threaded cannulated screw is placed from the medial malleolus in the midcoronal plane hugging the medial cortex of the tibia[66]; this serves to slow the growth medially allowing for more lateral-based growth and gradual correction of the valgus alignment.[66] Alternatively, a 2-hole tension band plate and screw construct or staple spanning the medial physis can be used.[67] Deformity correction is reported in the range of 9.7° to 12°.[66,68] A rebound effect has been noted after screw removal, and therefore for younger children overcorrection is recommended.[69]

Acute correction of distal tibial valgus is preferred if the physes are closed or if the deformity in a younger child is severe or significantly symptomatic. Valgus correction is preferentially achieved with a medial closing wedge SMO over a lateral opening wedge to avoid distracting the fibula and the lateral soft tissues.[70] Healing and stability are also improved with a closing wedge osteotomy.[70] For optimal mobility of the fragments, an ipsilateral fibular osteotomy is recommended.[71] Literature on the outcomes of SMO specifically for flatfoot deformity and in pediatrics is limited; however, SMOs for valgus in the posttraumatic arthritic ankle effectively correct deformity and reduce pain.[70,72,73]

Technique

The fibular osteotomy is performed first through a 3- to 4-cm posterolateral incision at the level of the metadiaphysis and proposed tibial osteotomy.[6] The plane of the osteotomy is in an oblique coronal plane, that is, posterior proximal to anterior distal, to enable the fibula to swivel easily when the tibial valgus correction is performed.[6]

For a pure medial-closing/valgus-correcting SMO, a medial incision 5 to 7 cm long from the medial malleolus proximally is made.[6] Alternatively an anterior incision can be used.[6] The osteotomy should be at least 1 cm above the distal tibial physis if still open.[6] The author prefers to mark the osteotomy using smooth 1.6-mm Steinman pins as "cut guides." The first wire pin is placed under fluoroscopy from medial to lateral, remaining at least 1 cm above the physis, parallel to the joint. The second more proximal pin is placed medial to lateral remaining perpendicular to the shaft, meeting the first pin at the lateral cortex to enable removal of a triangular wedge that will restore the mechanical alignment of the tibia. Placing these 2 wires in the same coronal plane allows the surgeon to use them as a guide for assessing alignment and rotation (see **Fig. 15**A, B).

To enable immediate temporary fixation following wedge removal, smooth Steinman pins (1.6 to 2 mm) are advanced just shy of the osteotomy.[6] The wire beginning at the medial malleolus can also be the guide wire for a 3.5- or 4.5-mm cannulated screw that can be used as additional permanent fixation.[6]

The osteotomy is performed.[6] The triangular medially based wedge is resected and the cut surfaces of the tibia are opposed to correct the valgus.[6] Lateral translation of the distal fragment is required to maintain the mechanical axis of the tibia.[6] The provisional fixation wires are advanced (**Fig. 15**C). The coronal plane alignment and tibial rotation are assessed.[6] If satisfied, the final fixation is placed (**Fig. 16**).

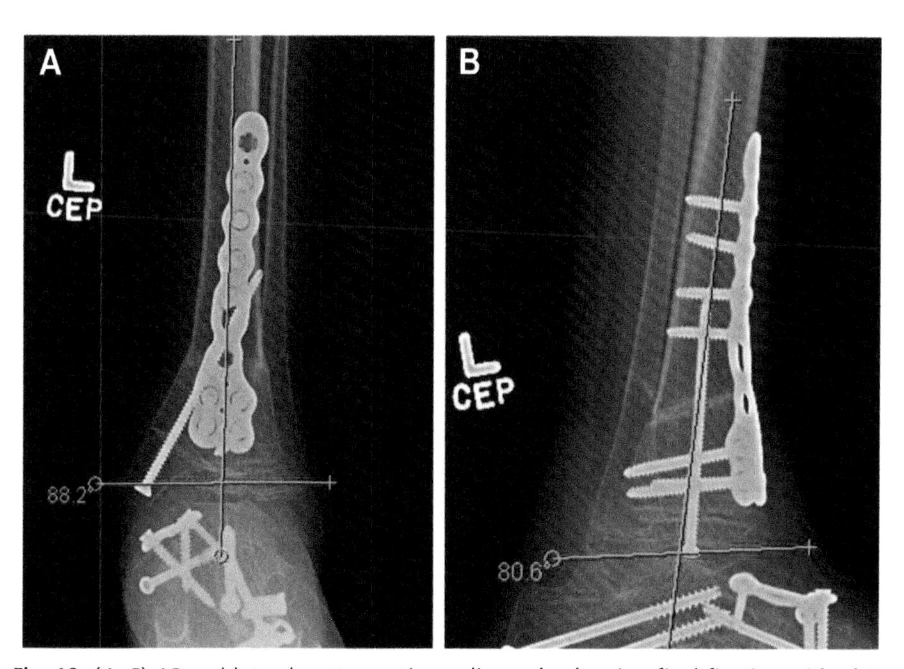

Fig. 16. (*A, B*) AP and lateral postoperative radiographs showing final fixation with plate and screw construct of a medial closing wedge SMO including medial malleolar lag screw. LDTA and ADTA have been restored. (*Courtesy of* the private collection of Dr. M. Bouchard.)

Medial Cuneiform Osteotomy

Once hindfoot alignment is restored, the forefoot supination becomes more obvious; this should be assessed intraoperatively after the calcaneal osteotomy.[6] Ideally, a firm platform is used to mimic weight-bearing.[6] Otherwise, the author keeps the ankle at neutral dorsiflexion and place her thumbs under the first and fifth metatarsal heads to simulate weight-bearing. Decreased pressure under the first metatarsal head or elevation of the first ray are noted when supination is present, indicating that a plantarflexion osteotomy of first ray is required.

In adults, this is traditionally done at the base of the first metatarsal as either a dorsal opening wedge or plantar closing wedge osteotomy.[6,10,11] In children, however, the medial cuneiform is preferred. Foremost, the physis of the first metatarsal is proximal and located at or adjacent to the site of a first metatarsal plantarflexion osteotomy. Second, when the lateral first metatarsal-talar axes are drawn, the apex of the deformity is in the medial cuneiform. Following deformity correction principles, osteotomies should be performed at the site of deformity when possible.[74] For these reasons, only the medial cuneiform osteotomy (MCO) is described in this article.

Both dorsal opening and plantar closing osteotomy techniques can be performed in the medial cuneiform to create plantarflexion. Since its description by Cotton in 1936,[75] the dorsal opening wedge MCO has been used to correct dorsiflexion of the first ray; it has been modified to correct other deformities such as forefoot adduction and forefoot supination. Outcomes of MCO are good with significant resolution of pain and significant improvement in radiographic angles.[76,77]

Selection of a dorsal opening or plantar closing wedge MCO is important. Mortimer and colleagues[78] described an unintentional biplanar effect that occurs during a sagittal plane MCO due to the tethering of soft tissues on the lateral aspect of the medial cuneiform, such as the intercuneiform joint capsule. Therefore, an intended purely dorsal opening wedge osteotomy will also distract slightly more medially than laterally, whereas a purely plantar closing wedge osteotomy will unintentionally close more medially than laterally,[78] and this means that a dorsal opening wedge osteotomy will create some forefoot abduction, whereas a plantar closing wedge will cause concurrent forefoot adduction.[78] Therefore, when correcting a flatfoot with already increased forefoot abduction, the author prefers a plantar closing MCO to simultaneously correct the supinated/dorsiflexed first ray with the residual forefoot abduction.

Technique

A longitudinal incision is made centered on the medial cuneiform.[6] The tibialis anterior is identified and retracted dorsally and distally.[6] The medial cuneiform is exposed extraperiosteally.[6] The plane of the first cut begins at the midpoint of the medial cuneiform from proximal to distal on the medial side and exits laterally aiming distally to the second tarsometatarsal joint.[6] This will enable the best mobility of the fragments[6] (**Fig. 17**). The first cut is made remaining perpendicular to the long axis of the first ray.[6] A second cut is made in the same medial to lateral direction, however, removing a 5- to 8-mm plantar wedge leaving the dorsal cortex intact to prevent translation of the fragments.[6] The correction is assessed. More bone is taken if supination persists.[6] Once adequate correction is achieved, fixation is placed. A smooth Steinman pin may be sufficient but is not compressive. The author prefers use of a nitinol staple. Plate and screw constructs are also available (**Fig. 18**).

Calcaneo-Cuboid-Cuneiform Osteotomies (Triple C Osteotomy)

The combination of a medial posterior calcaneal displacement, cuboid opening wedge, and medial cuneiform medial closing wedge osteotomies was originally

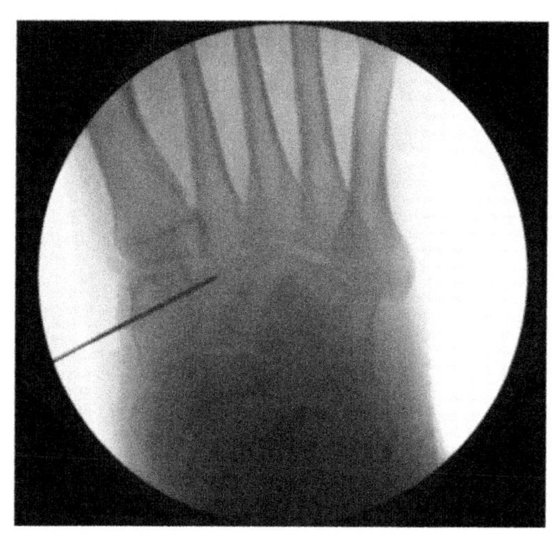

Fig. 17. AP intraoperative radiograph showing placement of Steinman pin to denote the plane of the osteotomy, aiming to the second tarsometatarsal joint and beginning in the midpoint on the medial surface of the medial cuneiform. (*Courtesy of* the private collection of Dr. M. Bouchard.)

described by Rathjen and Mubarak[79] and dubbed the triple C osteotomy for correction of the pediatric flatfoot. The triple C osteotomy has been shown to have good patient-reported, clinical, and radiological outcomes.[26,79–81] Compared with arthrodesis, outcomes are similar with the advantage of preserved joint mobility.[79] However, this procedure does not correct the subtalar joint orientation or talonavicular coverage because it does not correct the flatfoot at the site of the deformity, but proximal and distal to it.[26,65] The surgeon must not forget to include the necessary soft tissue procedures, such as gastrocnemius recession in case of contracture.

Technique

The PDCO is performed first and with an open technique as described earlier, followed by the medial cuneiform osteotomy removing a 5- to 8-mm wedge from the plantar or plantarmedial aspect.[6] The resected wedge is saved for insertion in the cuboid.[26,79] A

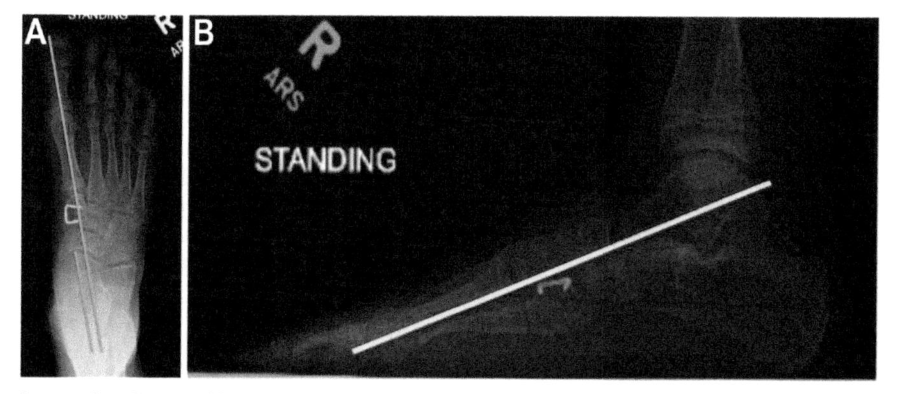

Fig. 18. (*A, B*) AP and lateral postoperative radiographs showing final fixation with staple of a plantar closing wedge medial cuneiform osteotomy. Meary angle on the AP and lateral radiographs are restored. (*Courtesy of* the private collection of Dr. M. Bouchard.)

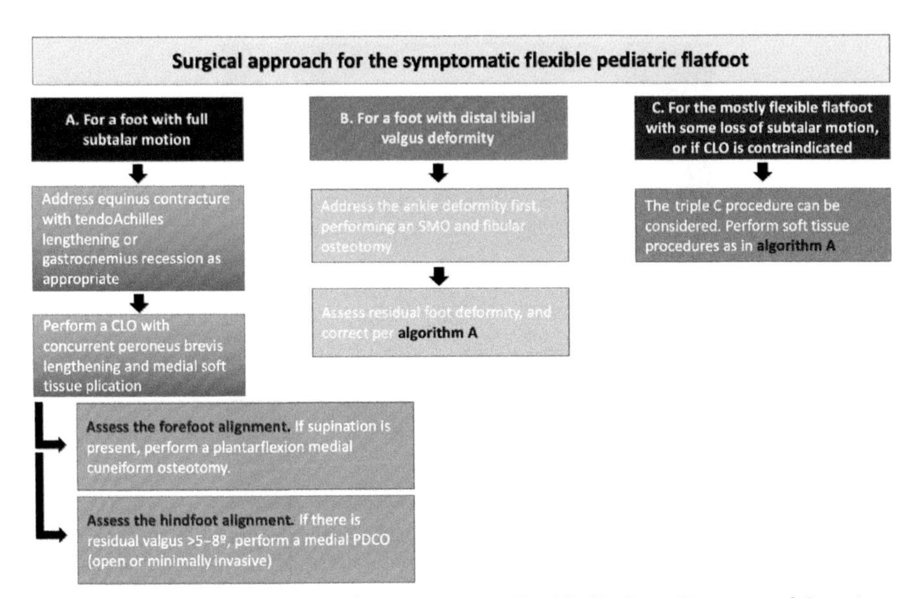

Fig. 19. Bony surgical procedures for symptomatic flexible flatfoot. (*Courtesy of* the private collection of Dr. M. Bouchard.)

longitudinal incision is made on the lateral border of the foot over the cuboid.[79] The peroneal tendons and sural nerve are protected.[79] The cuboid is exposed extraperiosteally.[6] The midpoint of the cuboid is confirmed from proximal to distal on fluoroscopy.[6] A lateral to medial cut is made at this site with a sagittal saw or osteotome.[6] The osteotomy is distracted laterally with an osteotome or lamina spreader and the medial cuneiform wedge is placed. If the graft is stable, no fixation is required, but the author notices the bone of the cuboid and the medial cuneiform graft are often soft and collapse without fixation. Any fixation method can be used for the cuneiform and cuboid. Rathjen and Mubarak[79] commonly used k-wires, but staple or plate and screw constructs are also options.

An algorithmic approach to selecting the optimal osteotomies in the pediatric flexible flatfoot is presented in **Fig. 19**.

Postoperative care

When osteotomies are performed, the author prefers immobilizing patients for 6 weeks in a non-weight-bearing short leg cast. If significant swelling is a concern, a bivalved cast or splint may be applied initially. Radiographs are obtained after cast removal at 6 weeks, and any percutaneous pins are removed. Generally, the patient is transitioned to a removable cast boot or walking short leg cast for 2 additional weeks, after which physiotherapy is initiated. Patients are counseled to avoid high-impact activities for 3 months and competitive sports for 6 months. An ankle-foot orthosis may be prescribed for children with underlying conditions causing excessive ligamentous laxity, such as Marfan syndrome.

SUMMARY

Bony procedures for the management of the symptomatic pediatric flexible flatfoot are effective techniques for correcting deformity and relieving pain, while maintaining supple joints.

CLINICS CARE POINTS

- Most pediatric flexible flatfeet are asymptomatic and do not require surgery.
- The calcaneal lengthening osteotomy effectively corrects hindfoot valgus, forefoot abduction, and talar head coverage.
- The PDCO is useful for correcting residual hindfoot valgus and can be combined with CLO or arthrodesis for additional correction.
- Intraoperative assessment for residual forefoot supination after hindfoot correction is critical and should be corrected with a plantarflexion osteotomy if present.
- Deformity arising from the distal tibia must be identified preoperatively, and if present, correction with hemiepiphyseodesis or an SMO should be considered.
- A concurrent gastrocnemius or Achilles contracture should always be evaluated for, and soft tissues should be addressed as needed.

ACKNOWLEDGMENTS

Thank you to Dr Bruce Sangeorzan for use of **Fig. 14**A–D and radiographs from his private collection.

DISCLOSURE

The authors have no commercial or financial conflicts of interest to disclose related to this work.

REFERENCES

1. Bouchard M, Mosca VS. Flatfoot deformity in children and adolescents: surgical indications and management. J Am Acad Orthop Surg 2014;22(10):623–32.
2. Bourgleh SM, Nemes RN, Hetaimish BM, et al. Prevalence of musculoskeletal normal variations of the lower limbs in pediatric orthopedic clinic. Saudi Med J 2019;40(9):930–5.
3. Uden H, Scharfbillig R, Causby R. The typically developing paediatric foot: how flat should it be? A systematic review. J Foot Ankle Res 2017;10:37.
4. Harris RI, Beath M. Army foot survey: an investigation of foot ailments in Canadian soldiers, vol. 1. National Research Council of Canada; 1947.
5. Mosca VS. Flexible flatfoot in children and adolescents. J Child Orthop 2010;4(2): 107–21.
6. Mosca VS. Principles and management of pediatric foot and ankle deformities and malformations. 1st edition. Wolters Kluwer Health; 2014.
7. Mosca VS, Bevan WP. Talocalcaneal tarsal coalitions and the calcaneal lengthening osteotomy: the role of deformity correction. J Bone Joint Surg Am 2012; 94(17):1584–94.
8. McKie J, Radomisli T. Congenital vertical talus: a review. Clin Podiatr Med Surg 2010;27(1):145–56.
9. Nahm NJ, Sohrweide SS, Wervey RA, et al. Surgical treatment of pes planovalgus in ambulatory children with cerebral palsy: static and dynamic changes as characterized by multi-segment foot modeling, physical examination and radiographs. Gait Posture 2020;76:168–74.
10. Mosca VS, Bouchard M. The foot. In: Flynn JMW S, Crawford H, editors. Lovell and winter's pediatric orthopaedics. 8th edition. Wolters Kluver; 2020. p. 1342–465, chapter 28.

11. Mosca VS. The child's foot: principles of management. J Pediatr Orthop 1998;18(3):281–2.
12. Reimers J, Pedersen B, Brodersen A. Foot deformity and the length of the triceps surae in Danish children between 3 and 17 years old. J Pediatr Orthop B 1995;4(1):71–3.
13. Evans AM, Rome K. A cochrane review of the evidence for non-surgical interventions for flexible pediatric flat feet. Eur J Phys Rehabil Med 2011;47(1):69–89.
14. Carr JB 2nd, Yang S, Lather LA. Pediatric pes planus: a state-of-the-art review. Pediatrics 2016;137(3):e20151230.
15. Pfeiffer M, Kotz R, Ledl T, et al. Prevalence of flat foot in preschool-aged children. Pediatrics 2006;118(2):634–9.
16. Golightly YM, Hannan MT, Dufour AB, et al. Racial differences in foot disorders and foot type. Arthritis Care Res (Hoboken) 2012;64(11):1756–9.
17. Shibuya N, Jupiter DC, Ciliberti LJ, et al. Characteristics of adult flatfoot in the United States. J Foot Ankle Surg 2010;49(4):363–8.
18. Sim-Fook L, Hodgson AR. A comparison of foot forms among the non-shoe and shoe-wearing Chinese population. J Bone Joint Surg Am 1958;40-A(5):1058–62.
19. Mann RA. Biomechanics of the foot and ankle. Surgery of the foot. Elsevier Inc.; 1986.
20. Dare DM, Dodwell ER. Pediatric flatfoot: cause, epidemiology, assessment, and treatment. Curr Opin Pediatr 2014;26(1):93–100.
21. Mosca VS. Calcaneal lengthening for valgus deformity of the hindfoot. Results in children who had severe, symptomatic flatfoot and skewfoot. J Bone Joint Surg Am 1995;77(4):500–12.
22. Davids JR, Gibson TW, Pugh LI. Quantitative segmental analysis of weight-bearing radiographs of the foot and ankle for children: normal alignment. J Pediatr Orthop 2005;25(6):769–76.
23. Choi JY, Hong WH, Suh JS, et al. The long-term structural effect of orthoses for pediatric flexible flat foot: a systematic review. Foot Ankle Surg 2020;26(2):181–8.
24. Akimau P, Flowers M. Medium term outcomes of planovalgus foot correction in children using a lateral column lengthening approach with additional procedures 'a la carte. Foot Ankle Surg 2014;20(1):26–9.
25. Baghdadi T, Mazoochy H, Guity M, et al. Evaluation of clinical and radiological results of calcaneal lengthening osteotomy in pediatric idiopathic flexible flatfoot. Arch Bone Jt Surg 2018;6(5):402–11.
26. Moraleda L, Salcedo M, Bastrom TP, et al. Comparison of the calcaneo-cuboid-cuneiform osteotomies and the calcaneal lengthening osteotomy in the surgical treatment of symptomatic flexible flatfoot. J Pediatr Orthop 2012;32(8):821–9.
27. Agashe MV, Sagade BS, Bansal AV. Functional and radiological outcomes following calcaneo-cuboid-cuneiform osteotomy for the treatment of planovalgus feet: a short-term analysis. Indian J Orthop 2021;55(Suppl 1):119–27.
28. Haeseker GA, Mureau MA, Faber FW. Lateral column lengthening for acquired adult flatfoot deformity caused by posterior tibial tendon dysfunction stage II: a retrospective comparison of calcaneus osteotomy with calcaneocuboid distraction arthrodesis. J Foot Ankle Surg 2010;49(4):380–4.
29. Suh DH, Park JH, Lee SH, et al. Lateral column lengthening versus subtalar arthroereisis for paediatric flatfeet: a systematic review. Int Orthop 2019;43(5):1179–92.
30. Mosca VS. Flexible flatfoot and skewfoot. Instr Course Lect 1996;45:347–54.

31. Yan GS, Yang Z, Lu M, et al. Relationship between symptoms and weight-bearing radiographic parameters of idiopathic flexible flatfoot in children. Chin Med J (Engl) 2013;126(11):2029–33.
32. Huang YC, Wang LY, Wang HC, et al. The relationship between the flexible flatfoot and plantar fasciitis: ultrasonographic evaluation. Chang Gung Med J 2004; 27(6):443–8.
33. Kalen V, Brecher A. Relationship between adolescent bunions and flatfeet. Foot Ankle 1988;8(6):331–6.
34. Iijima H, Ohi H, Isho T, et al. Association of bilateral flat feet with knee pain and disability in patients with knee osteoarthritis: a cross-sectional study. J Orthop Res 2017;35(11):2490–8.
35. Menz HB, Dufour AB, Riskowski JL, et al. Foot posture, foot function and low back pain: the Framingham Foot Study. Rheumatology (Oxford) 2013;52(12):2275–82.
36. Kothari A, Dixon PC, Stebbins J, et al. Are flexible flat feet associated with proximal joint problems in children? Gait Posture 2016;45:204–10.
37. Bresnahan PJ, Juanto MA. Pediatric Flatfeet-A disease entity that demands greater attention and treatment. Front Pediatr 2020;8:19.
38. Marengo L, Canavese F, Mansour M, et al. Clinical and radiological outcome of calcaneal lengthening osteotomy for flatfoot deformity in skeletally immature patients. Eur J Orthop Surg Traumatol 2017;27(7):989–96.
39. Ilfeld BM, Morey TE, Wang RD, et al. Continuous popliteal sciatic nerve block for postoperative pain control at home: a randomized, double-blinded, placebo-controlled study. Anesthesiology 2002;97(4):959–65.
40. Evans D. Calcaneo-valgus deformity. J Bone Joint Surg Br 1975;57(3):270–8.
41. Dumontier TA, Falicov A, Mosca V, et al. Calcaneal lengthening: investigation of deformity correction in a cadaver flatfoot model. Foot Ankle Int 2005;26(2): 166–70.
42. Anderson AF, Fowler SB. Anterior calcaneal osteotomy for symptomatic juvenile pes planus. Foot Ankle 1984;4(5):274–83.
43. Oeffinger DJ, Pectol RW Jr, Tylkowski CM. Foot pressure and radiographic outcome measures of lateral column lengthening for pes planovalgus deformity. Gait Posture 2000;12(3):189–95.
44. Zeifang F, Breusch SJ, Doderlein L. Evans calcaneal lengthening procedure for spastic flexible flatfoot in 32 patients (46 feet) with a followup of 3 to 9 years. Foot Ankle Int 2006;27(7):500–7.
45. Dolan CM, Henning JA, Anderson JG, et al. Randomized prospective study comparing tri-cortical iliac crest autograft to allograft in the lateral column lengthening component for operative correction of adult acquired flatfoot deformity. Foot Ankle Int 2007;28(1):8–12.
46. Templin D, Jones K, Weiner DS. The incorporation of allogeneic and autogenous bone graft in healing of lateral column lengthening of the calcaneus. J Foot Ankle Surg 2008;47(4):283–7.
47. Dayton P, Prins DB, Smith DE, et al. Effectiveness of a locking plate in preserving midcalcaneal length and positional outcome after Evans calcaneal osteotomy: a retrospective pilot study. J Foot Ankle Surg 2013;52(6):710–3.
48. Koutsogiannis E. Treatment of mobile flat foot by displacement osteotomy of the calcaneus. J Bone Joint Surg Br 1971;53(1):96–100.
49. Dwyer FC. Osteotomy of the calcaneum for pes cavus. J Bone Joint Surg Br 1959;41-B(1):80–6.

50. Niki H, Hirano T, Okada H, et al. Outcome of medial displacement calcaneal osteotomy for correction of adult-acquired flatfoot. Foot Ankle Int 2012;33(11): 940–6.
51. Kaplan JRM, Aiyer A, Cerrato RA, et al. Operative treatment of the cavovarus foot. Foot Ankle Int 2018;39(11):1370–82.
52. Gutteck N, Zeh A, Wohlrab D, et al. Comparative results of percutaneous calcaneal osteotomy in correction of hindfoot deformities. Foot Ankle Int 2019;40(3): 276–81.
53. Uglow MG. Percutaneous pediatric foot and ankle surgery. Foot Ankle Clin 2016; 21(3):577–94.
54. Mourkus H, Prem H. Double calcaneal osteotomy with minimally invasive surgery for the treatment of severe flexible flatfeet. Int Orthop 2018;42(9):2123–9.
55. Mendicino RW, Catanzariti AR, Reeves CL. Posterior calcaneal displacement osteotomy: a new percutaneous technique. J Foot Ankle Surg 2004;43(5):332–5.
56. Wills B, Lee SR, Hudson PW, et al. Calcaneal osteotomy safe zone to prevent neurological damage: fact or fiction? Foot Ankle Spec 2019;12(1):34–8.
57. Greffier J, Etard C, Mares O, et al. Patient dose reference levels in surgery: a multicenter study. Eur Radiol 2019;29(2):674–81.
58. Augustin G, Zigman T, Davila S, et al. Cortical bone drilling and thermal osteonecrosis. Clin Biomech (Bristol, Avon) 2012;27(4):313–25.
59. SahraNavard B, Hudson PW, de Cesar Netto C, et al. A comparison of union rates and complications between single screw and double screw fixation of sliding calcaneal osteotomy. Foot Ankle Surg 2019;25(1):84–9.
60. Malerba F, De Marchi F. Calcaneal osteotomies. Foot Ankle Clin 2005;10(3): 523–40, vii.
61. Demetracopoulos CA, Nair P, Malzberg A, et al. Outcomes of a stepcut lengthening calcaneal osteotomy for adult-acquired flatfoot deformity. Foot Ankle Int 2015;36(7):749–55.
62. Ebaugh MP, Larson DR, Reb CW, et al. Outcomes of the extended Z-cut osteotomy for correction of adult acquired flatfoot deformity. Foot Ankle Int 2019;40(8): 914–22.
63. Saunders SM, Ellis SJ, Demetracopoulos CA, et al. Comparative outcomes between step-cut lengthening calcaneal osteotomy vs traditional evans osteotomy for stage IIB adult-acquired flatfoot deformity. Foot Ankle Int 2018;39(1):18–27.
64. Mulhern JL, Protzman NM, Brigido SA, et al. Supramalleolar osteotomy: indications and surgical techniques. Clin Podiatr Med Surg 2015;32(3):445–61.
65. Paley D. Principles of deformity correction. 1st edition. New York: Springer-Verlag Berlin Heidelberg; 2002.
66. Stevens PM, Belle RM. Screw epiphysiodesis for ankle valgus. J Pediatr Orthop 1997;17(1):9–12.
67. Stevens PM, Kennedy JM, Hung M. Guided growth for ankle valgus. J Pediatr Orthop 2011;31(8):878–83.
68. Rupprecht M, Spiro AS, Breyer S, et al. Growth modulation with a medial malleolar screw for ankle valgus deformity. 79 children with 125 affected ankles followed until correction or physeal closure. Acta Orthop 2015;86(5):611–5.
69. Davids JR, Valadie AL, Ferguson RL, et al. Surgical management of ankle valgus in children: use of a transphyseal medial malleolar screw. J Pediatr Orthop 1997; 17(1):3–8.
70. Chopra V, Stone P, Ng A. Supramalleolar osteotomies. Clin Podiatr Med Surg 2017;34(4):445–60.

71. Becker AS, Myerson MS. The indications and technique of supramalleolar osteotomy. Foot Ankle Clin 2009;14(3):549–61.
72. Krahenbuhl N, Susdorf R, Barg A, et al. Supramalleolar osteotomy in post-traumatic valgus ankle osteoarthritis. Int Orthop 2020;44(3):535–43.
73. Krahenbuhl N, Zwicky L, Bolliger L, et al. Mid- to long-term results of supramalleolar osteotomy. Foot Ankle Int 2017;38(2):124–32.
74. Paley D, Tetsworth K. Mechanical axis deviation of the lower limbs. Preoperative planning of uniapical angular deformities of the tibia or femur. Clin Orthop Relat Res 1992;(280):48–64.
75. Cotton FJ. Foot statics and surgery. N Engl J Med 1936;214(8):353–62.
76. Conti MS, Garfinkel JH, Kunas GC, et al. Postoperative medial cuneiform position correlation with patient-reported outcomes following cotton osteotomy for reconstruction of the stage ii adult-acquired flatfoot deformity. Foot Ankle Int 2019; 40(5):491–8.
77. Romeo G, Bianchi A, Cerbone V, et al. Medial cuneiform opening wedge osteotomy for correction of flexible flatfoot deformity: trabecular titanium vs. bone allograft wedges. Biomed Res Int 2019;2019:1472471.
78. Mortimer JA, Bouchard M, Acosta A, et al. The biplanar effect of the medial cuneiform osteotomy. Foot Ankle Spec 2020;13(3):250–7.
79. Rathjen KE, Mubarak SJ. Calcaneal-cuboid-cuneiform osteotomy for the correction of valgus foot deformities in children. J Pediatr Orthop 1998;18(6):775–82.
80. El-Hilaly R, El-Sherbini MH, Abd-Ella MM, et al. Radiological outcome of calcaneo-cuboid-cuneiform osteotomies for planovalgus feet in cerebral palsy children: relationship with pedobarography. Foot Ankle Surg 2019;25(4):462–8.
81. Kim JR, Kim KB, Chong SW, et al. Treatment outcomes at skeletal maturity after calcaneo-cuboid-cuneiform osteotomy for symptomatic flatfoot deformity in children. Clin Orthop Surg 2020;12(2):252–7.

Management of Complex Tarsal Coalition in Children

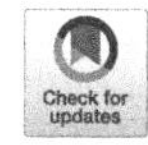

Shuyuan Li, MD, PhD[a,b,*], Mark S. Myerson, MD[a]

KEYWORDS

• Tarsal coalition • Complex coalition • Double coalition • Ball-and-socket ankle
• Osteotomy tibia

KEY POINTS

- Tarsal coalition is a congenital skeletal development disorder, with onset of symptoms typically occurring in early adolescence when the coalition starts to ossify. Complex tarsal coalition includes extensive talocalcaneal coalition, double or triple coalition, coalition with severe hindfoot deformities, or coalition with a ball-and-socket ankle deformity.
- The presence of severe rigidity associated with a double coalition, a ball-and-socket ankle, or a severe hindfoot deformity are factors that make correction complicated. A thorough physical examination combined with accurate imaging are essential to obtaining detailed information such as the location and size of the coalition, as well as alignment of both the ankle and the hindfoot.
- Hindfoot deformity present in most pediatric coalition cases can be corrected by an arthroereisis or calcaneus stop technique, calcaneus osteotomies, or hindfoot arthrodesis. In addition to a structural reconstruction, soft tissue and muscle balancing also need to be considered in particular to address any peroneus brevis contracture caused by long-term hindfoot valgus.
- The ankle joint must be involved in preoperative planning in every case. By doing so, a solid foundation is laid for further surgical planning, which includes coalition resection, stabilization of the foot and ankle, and correcting alignment with osteotomies, arthrodesis, and soft tissue balancing.

Tarsal coalition is a congenital condition caused by failure of differentiation and segmentation of the mesenchyme, which leads to partial or complete fusion between 2 bones.[1–3] This kind of intertarsal bridge can be osseous, cartilaginous, or fibrous. Owing to lack of complete joint formation, the movement of the involved joints is somehow limited, which affects the function of the hindfoot and causes overloading and stress on adjacent joints.[4] The most common tarsal coalitions are calcaneonavicular (CN) and talocalcaneal (TC) coalitions, which make up about 90% of the tarsal

[a] Department of Orthopaedic Surgery, University of Colorado, Denver, CO, USA; [b] Steps2Walk, Denver, CO, USA
* Corresponding author. 4950 S Yosemite Street, F2-392, Greenwood Village, CO 80111, USA
E-mail address: drshuyuanli@gmail.com

Foot Ankle Clin N Am 26 (2021) 941–954
https://doi.org/10.1016/j.fcl.2021.07.012

coalitions,[4,5] but this article focuses on less commonly treated coalitions including the posterior facet, talonavicular (TN) joint, calcaneocuboid (CC), or naviculocuboid coalitions and a double or triple coalition. The purpose of this article is not to introduce concepts of treatment of common tarsal coalitions but to share the authors' experience in managing more complex tarsal coalitions as outlined earlier. The challenge with these complex cases is to accurately diagnose the extent of the deformity and base clinical decision making accordingly.

DIAGNOSTIC ALGORITHM

A tarsal coalition is usually asymptomatic at a young age and begins to be troublesome with ossification of the coalition and gradual loss of movement of the involved joints. Ossification usually occurs at the age of 12 to 16 years in TC coalitions, and at the age of 8 to 12 years in CN coalitions.[1,6] These symptoms can include pain of the foot and leg, associated with instability of the ankle, etc. The location of pain varies in different kinds of tarsal coalitions, for example, posteriorly extended middle facet coalition and posterior facet TC coalitions are not only likely to cause pain in the subtalar joint, easily diagnosed by palpation over the sinus tarsi, but also are the result of compression and tension below the medial malleolus or even over the tibial nerve, which manifests as tarsal tunnel syndrome.[7–9] CN coalitions are more typically associated with lateral foot pain and a rigid flatfoot deformity. Most osseous coalitions regardless of the type present with a fixed flatfoot deformity,[10] and if caused by a TN, a more extensive, or rigid coalition, instability of the ankle with or without an associated ball-and-socket ankle joint.[4,11,12] Rarely, a severe tarsal coalition can be found in patients with a congenital cavovarus or clubfoot deformity.[13,14] In all patients with a tarsal coalition, careful clinical and radiographic examination of the ankle is essential because inversion and eversion may be present through the ankle and not the hindfoot, which confuses the clinical picture.

Regardless of the magnitude of the coalition, we always ask the patient to sit on the examination table with both legs and feet hanging down naturally, and in this position, it is easy to make the diagnosis because the foot does not assume a normal plantarflexed and inverted resting position and is always slightly dorsiflexed and abducted due to hindfoot rigidity.[15] The examination should include the alignment and range of motion of both the ankle and the hindfoot, stability of the ankle, tenderness, and the strength of different muscle groups. In these complex deformities it is essential to understand the extent of the rigidity of the hindfoot, particularly when caused by constant peroneus brevis muscle contraction and not rigidity of the joint itself.[16,17] We find it helpful in the child with a rigid flatfoot deformity, to differentiate peroneal muscle contracture from true joint rigidity by injecting the common peroneal nerve at the fibular neck with 5 to 10 mL 1% xylocaine. This procedure immediately temporarily paralyzes the peroneal (and of course the muscles of dorsiflexion) and is helpful to identify the presence of motion in the hindfoot. This procedure is important in the older child when one is considering an arthrodesis for treatment.

In addition to weight-bearing anteroposterior and lateral views of the foot, hindfoot alignment view and oblique views of the foot are also necessary. It is rare that we would resort to an MRI for the diagnosis of a complex coalition; however, a computed tomographic (CT) scan is essential. CT scan not only determines the location and size of the coalition but also is most important when a double coalition is present. The worst potential for error is when a CN coalition is clear on radiographs, and treatment is initiated only to subsequently find that a TC coalition is also present, and treatment fails. Although studies report that MRI has a higher sensitivity and specificity than CT scan,[18,19] we do not use MRI for diagnosis of complex coalitions because the extent of the deformity is more clearly visible and delineated on CT. For those readers who have access to a weight-bearing CT, this has shown tremendous capacity to assess both alignment and structure in 3 dimensions, giving us a much clearer picture of the foot and ankle.[20–22] One can precisely locate the coalition and track its boundaries on 3-dimensional reconstructed images.[23] Two-dimensional images in any specific view can also be reconstructed using the weight-bearing CT data, so that physicians who are used to conventional radiological images could obtain even more information. Last but not least the very low radiation dose enables weight-bearing CT to be used safely in pediatric patients.[24]

TREATING COMPLEX TARSAL COALITION

After making the diagnosis, we base treatment of these complex coalitions on the type, location, size, flexibility or rigidity of the involved joints, stability of the hindfoot and ankle, alignment of the hindfoot and ankle, and the age of the child. As stated earlier, a complex coalition includes a double or triple coalition, coalition with severe hindfoot deformities, those associated with a ball-and-socket ankle deformity, or those that are associated with severe rigidity. These very rigid deformities require special attention because resection rarely succeeds and even arthrodesis must be carefully planned to realign the foot correctly. The goal for surgery should be to maximize movement and function, but this is only possible in these complex cases when associated with a double or a posterior facet coalition. Perhaps the most important aspect of treatment is to realign the foot and ankle regardless of the type of treatment initiated.

DOUBLE AND POSTERIOR FACET COALITION RESECTION

Resection applies to most pediatric isolated TC or CN coalitions but is also indicated for a double coalition (TC and CN) and in particular a posterior facet coalition.[25–28] The key point here is not whether a coalition is resectable, but whether the joint function is reversible after resection, implying both a healthy and stable articulation. We will not go into the details of resection versus arthrodesis here with the isolated coalition but focus more specifically on a double and posterior facet coalition resection technique. We have not found that a double coalition is a contraindication to resection; however, in most cases, the subtalar joint becomes very unstable and stability with realignment of the hindfoot becomes imperative.

For resection of a middle facet TC coalition, our approach is similar to that described in another article in this issue, with one additional technique tip in which we described how to find and open the middle facet quite easily by inserting a dilator through the sinus tarsi, pushing it medially, which always exits just posterior to the coalition and anterior to the posterior facet.[25] This approach pops open the TC joint and makes the margins of the coalition easy to identify and remove without worrying about inadvertent injury to the posterior facet. A posterior facet coalition is usually located on the posteromedial aspect of the joint, and a simple excision of the coalition is adequate and will not cause any significant joint defect. The approach to the resection is no different than that for a middle facet coalition, by extending the incision more posteriorly. We still use a dilator technique through the sinus tarsi to identify and open the joint, but then insert a laminar spreader just anterior to the posterior facet and adjacent to the middle facet to distract open the joint and visualize the coalition, which is easily removed with an osteotome. **Fig. 1** demonstrates an

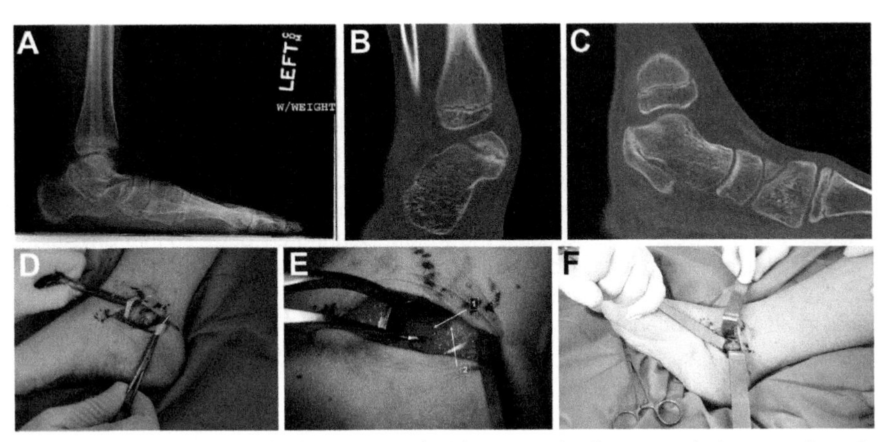

Fig. 1. This is an 11-year-old who presented with a posterior facet correlation noted on the lateral radiograph and CT scan (*A–C*). A standard posteromedial approach was used (*D*), and a laminar spreader was inserted behind the TC to distract open the joint (*E*). The undersurface of the talus is noted (1), and the posterior facet coalition is now visible (2). The coalition is then easily removed with an osteotome (*F*).

example of a posterior facet coalition, and the lateral radiograph can be quite confusing until a CT scan is obtained because for practical purposes this looks similar to a severe middle facet coalition.

We have never been concerned about the size of a TC coalition in children, despite a few studies proposing that coalitions involving more than 50% of the TC area will have a poorer prognosis[29–32]; this is all anecdotal,[33] and in most of these double coalitions we will remove both in children regardless of the size and base the decision more on rigidity preoperatively (this is where blocking the common peroneal nerve becomes useful). The one aspect of resection of a double coalition is that it creates a very unstable hindfoot, and following resection we then decide which adjunctive procedure such as a calcaneus stop, calcaneus osteotomy, or arthroereisis should be added to stabilize the hindfoot.[25] Our experience is that an arthroereisis is not stable enough because it tends to fall out of the tarsal canal following the coalition removal, and we use either a calcaneal stop or a calcaneus osteotomy or both in combination. After reducing the subtalar joint to neutral, if this produces mild forefoot supination, we will add a medial cuneiform opening wedge osteotomy to create a more plantigrade forefoot.

When managing CN as part of a double coalition, the approach is quite straightforward and does not require much elaboration here. We would like to emphasize that the key to success is complete excision of the bone bridge comprising the zone of the calcaneal-cuboid-navicular talus. For adequate resection, the lateral edge of the navicular should be flush with the lateral margin of the talar neck, and this also applies to the superomedial margin of the calcaneus and cuboid.[15] We begin the double coalition resection medially and then go laterally to remove the CN complex. **Fig. 2** emphasizes an important aspect of a double coalition associated with an extremely rigid hindfoot in a 9-year-old. Although one recognizes that an arthrodesis at this age is far from ideal, it is hard to imagine just how unstable and flexible the hindfoot became at the completion of resecting the double coalition. Despite the goal of attaining mobility, there was profound instability following resection with the hindfoot in valgus and which would have caused subfibular

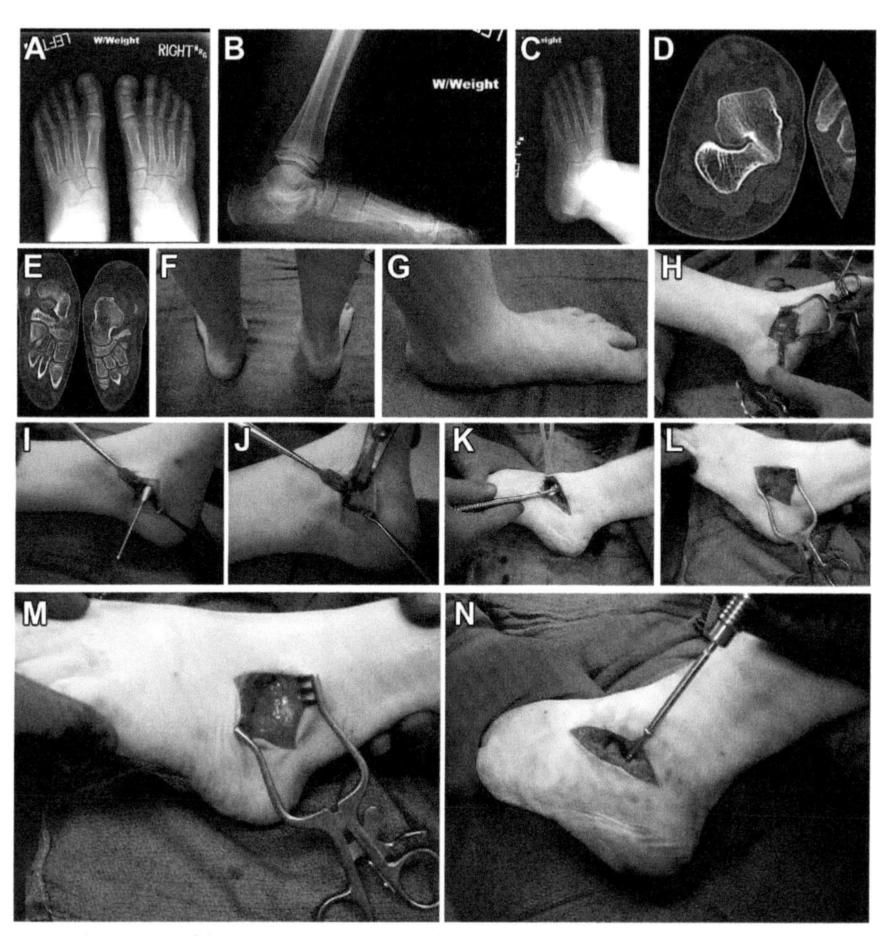

Fig. 2. This 9-year-old presented with severe flatfoot deformity and bilateral foot pain associated with a double coalition. The extent of the correlation is visible on radiographs (*A–C*), on CT scan (*D, E*), and in clinical images (*F, G*); this presented as an extremely rigid deformity. A standard medial approach was used for resection of the TC, using a dilator technique and a laminar spreader to open up the coalition as previously described (*H–J*). A second incision was made laterally for removal of the CN coalition (*K*). The foot was now extraordinarily flexible and mobile noting opening of the subtalar joint on inversion (*L*) and subfibular impingement with eversion of the hindfoot (*M*), corrected with a calcaneal stop screw procedure (*N*).

impingement if left unaddressed. An arthroereisis was inserted, but it fell out of the foot medially, and a calcaneal stop screw was used successfully to correct the deformity. We have used alternative techniques for insertion of the calcaneal stop screw. The screw can be inserted either vertically in the sinus tarsi or obliquely through the lateral process of the talus into the body of the talus to block calcaneal eversion. Either of these procedures seems to be adequate and has been equally successful in our hands. If following the use of an arthroereisis or a calcaneal stop screw persistent valgus is present, we recommend adding a medial translational osteotomy of the calcaneus.

SUBTALAR ARTHRODESIS FOR SEVERE RIGID DEFORMITY

It is difficult to know when in the child an arthrodesis is required, but we have noted that for a very rigid deformity, and in those following resection if the hindfoot remains rigid, a subtalar arthrodesis and rarely a triple arthrodesis is required. One key technical point to make when performing a subtalar arthrodesis is to correct the flatfoot deformity and in particular the hindfoot valgus simultaneously. It is difficult to take out a medially-based wedge from the subtalar joint from a lateral approach, and if the latter is used, then the easiest method to use is to internally rotate the subtalar joint. This method automatically corrects the hindfoot valgus but will also supinate the forefoot, which can then be corrected with a cuneiform osteotomy.

MULTIPLANAR DEFORMITY CORRECTION

In some feet with severe rigidity there are multiple apices of deformity, and this can effectively be approached as if one were performing a revision hindfoot arthrodesis with a goal of obtaining a plantigrade foot. Most cases of TN coalition that we have treated have all been associated with a ball-and-socket ankle that must be stabilized, generally with a medial closing wedge supramalleolar osteotomy to correct the valgus deformity in the ankle and hindfoot.[12] Occasionally the foot is so rigid that the only approach to take would be to correct the deformity by performing an osteotomy through the TN coalition and converting the rigid deformed hindfoot into a stable well-aligned triple arthrodesis (**Fig. 3**). In the latter case one notes a severe rocker bottom deformity, equinus of the hindfoot, a negative calcaneal pitch angle, and the obvious and extensive TC coalition associated with a TN coalition. The easiest method to approach this deformity is to correct both the TN and subtalar joints on the medial side of the foot. As already noted, it is difficult to realign the subtalar joint that is fixed in valgus from a lateral approach. Following removal of the TC

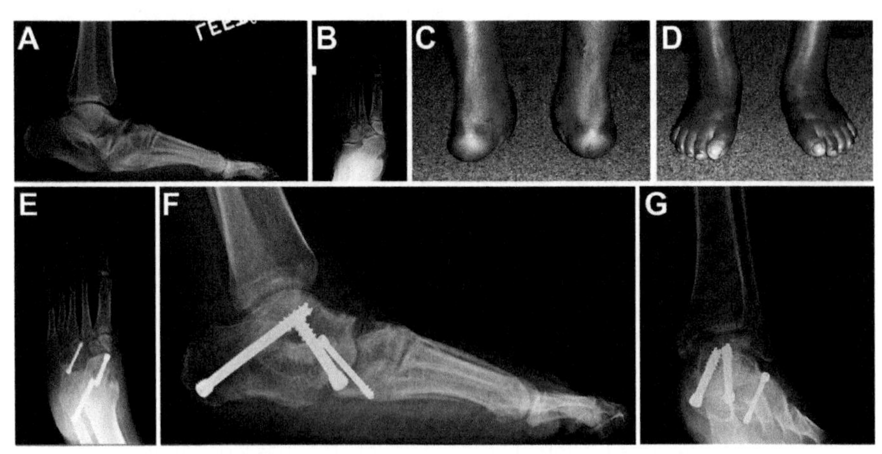

Fig. 3. This is a 15-year-old who presented with severe hindfoot pain, stiffness, and subfibular impingement, associated with this TN coalition. A rocker bottom deformity of the hindfoot was present with the calcaneus in equinus, and a mild ball-and-socket ankle was deformity noted (*A–D*). Because the ankle was quite stable despite the mild ball-and-socket deformity, a tibial osteotomy did not need to be performed, and the deformity was corrected by converting the coalition into a triple arthrodesis with an osteotomy across the TN joint, which adducted and plantarflexed the medial column (*E–G*).

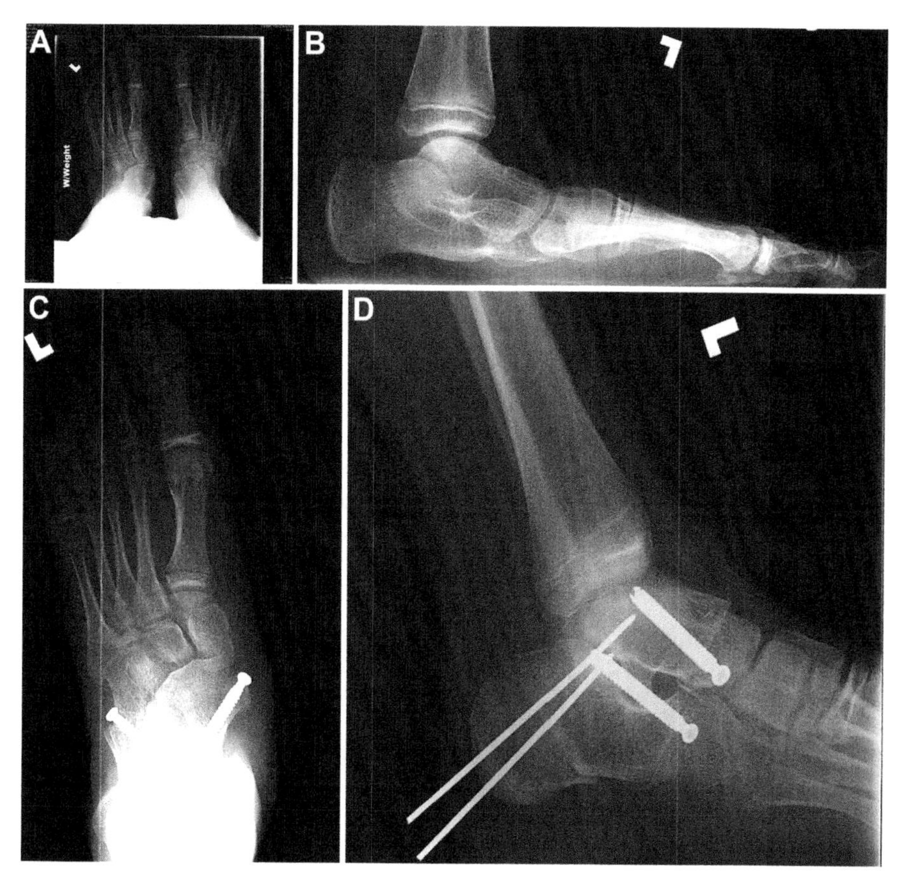

Fig. 4. This 12-year-old presented with severe hindfoot deformity and pain but with a stable ankle associated with a CC and TN coalition, in addition to a rocker bottom hindfoot deformity (*A, B*). This condition was corrected with an osteotomy across Chopart joint, which pronated, adducted, and plantarflexed the medial column, in combination with a medial translational osteotomy of the calcaneus (*C, D*).

coalition and exposure of the subtalar joint it was easier to remove a medial wedge from the subtalar joint as well as a biplanar wedge from the TN coalition (medial and plantar) followed by a small lateral incision to perform the CC arthrodesis (see **Fig. 3**). **Fig. 4** demonstrates a similar deformity but in a younger child, also with a TN and CC double coalition. Again, note the abduction of the Chopart joint, equinus of the hindfoot associated with a rocker bottom deformity, and the abnormal subtalar joint. Because of the age of the child, as an alternative to a subtalar arthrodesis, a calcaneus osteotomy was performed in conjunction with a biplanar osteotomy across the TN and CC coalition.

USING SUPRAMALLEOLAR OSTEOTOMY IN TREATING THE BALL-AND-SOCKET ANKLE

A ball-and-socket ankle deformity is often seen in some patients with tarsal coalition and a severe flatfoot deformity, particularly with the more complex coalitions.[11,13] Instead of being a hinge joint with movement only in the sagittal plane, a ball-and-socket ankle is a spherical articulation between the tibial plafond and the talus, which has potential movement in multiple planes. There are different theories about this phenomenon, some thinking that the ball-and-socket ankle is a consequence of the hindfoot valgus deformity and overstress on the lateral side of epiphysis of the distal tibial epiphysis. Others believe that both the ball-and-socket ankle and the coalition are part of a congenital development problem.[34–40] Regardless of the cause, the epiphysis of the distal tibia becomes hemispherical, which causes the distal articular surface of the tibia to develop into a concave shape, and subsequently reshapes the top of the talus into a convex surface. Moreover, the distal fibular articular surface becomes wider and more concave. Therefore, it is not difficult to understand that patients with a ball-and-socket ankle deformity present with severe hindfoot valgus deformity, subfibular impingement, and ankle instability.

A ball-and-socket ankle is easily missed in cases of tarsal coalition because most of the focus is on the foot. Regardless of the cause of the flatfoot deformity, we routinely obtain an anteroposterior radiograph of the ankle joint and where necessary a CT scan to evaluate the ankle. In a case with a ball-and-socket ankle, the valgus deformity of the hindfoot cannot be successfully corrected if the ankle deformity is not addressed because the hindfoot will always drift back into valgus (**Figs. 5** and **6**). Ellington and

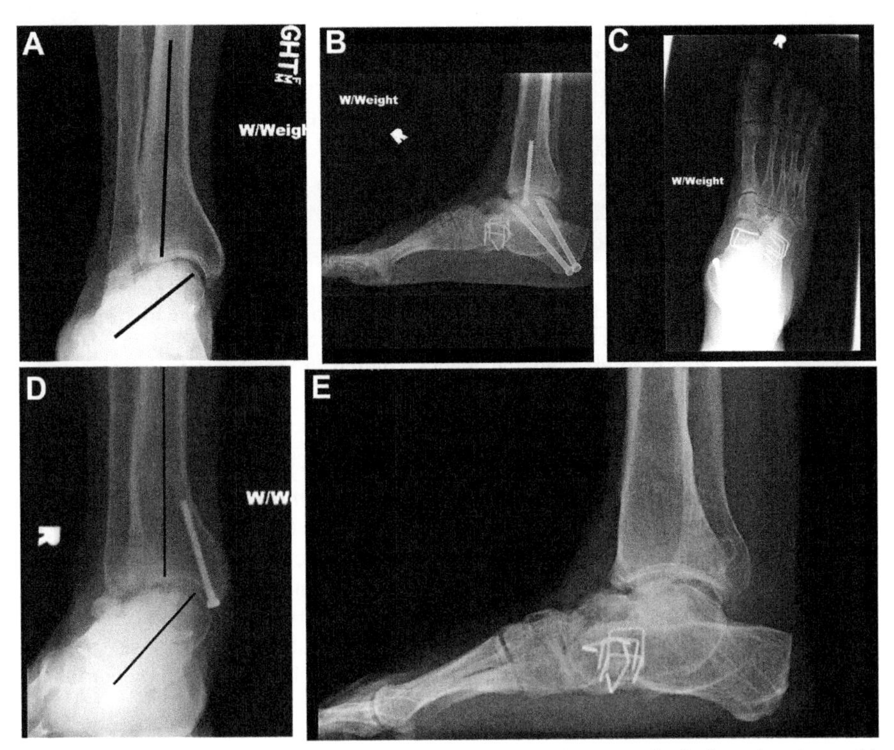

Fig. 5. This is a 15-year-old who presented with a TN coalition and a ball-and-socket ankle with severe valgus deformity associated with subfibular impingement despite a hypoplastic fibula (*A*). A hindfoot arthrodesis that was performed in this adolescent was destined to fail because it cannot correct the biomechanical alignment of the limb (*B, C*). Note the worsening valgus deformity of the ankle (*D*); this was followed 3 years later by severe degenerative arthritis of the ankle (*E*).

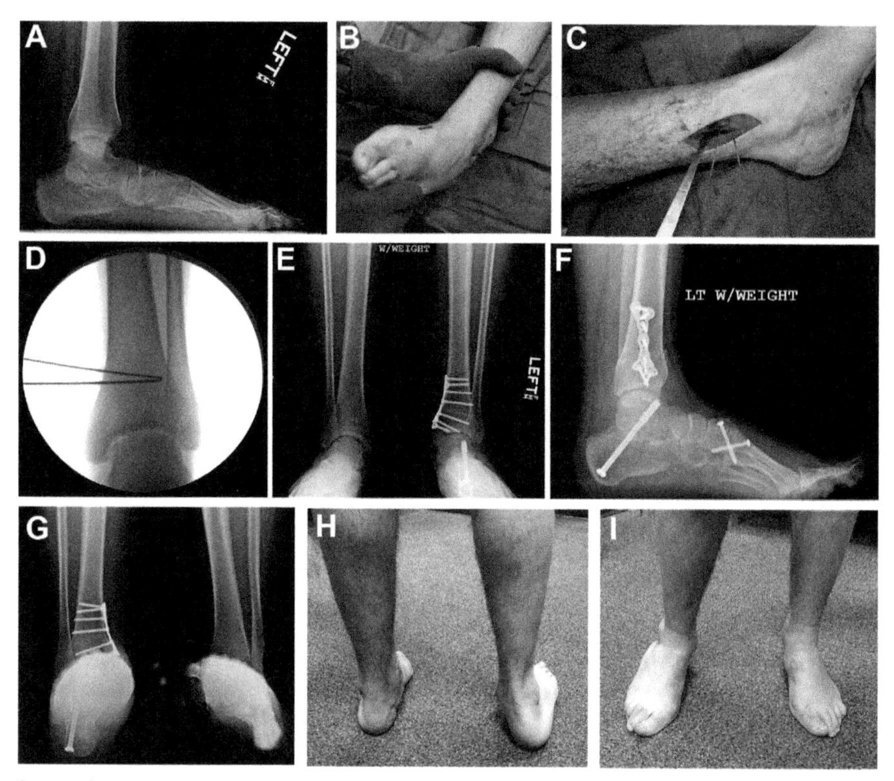

Fig. 6. This is a 14-year-old with an extensive hindfoot coalition, associated with a ball-and-socket ankle. He had previously undergone an attempted extra-articular subtalar arthrodesis with persistence of pain associated with subfibular impingement (*A*). Note the position of the hindfoot with the 4 foot supinated to reduce the hindfoot and ankle into a neutral position associated with a fixed supination deformity (*B*). The most important aspect of correction included a closing wedge supramalleolar osteotomy (*C, D*). The final result on the left foot following the supramalleolar osteotomy and arthrodesis of the subtalar and first tarsometatarsal joints is presented (*F–I*).

Myerson[12] reported on 13 adult patients with ball-and-socket ankle cases associated with a TN tarsal coalition, using a medial closing wedge supramalleolar osteotomy in 9 cases and arthrodesis in 4 patients, combining where necessary with additional hindfoot reconstruction procedures. Of the patients undergoing a supramalleolar osteotomy, 5 patients reported good and 4 reported fair results. Good results were obtained in all 4 patients treated with arthrodesis (2 with a tibiotalocalcaneal arthrodesis and 2 with a pantalar arthrodesis). The investigators noted that not all patients required a medial column procedure following either the supramalleolar osteotomy or the arthrodesis; this depended on the extent of the fixed forefoot supination that was present following the more proximal correction of the valgus deformity. The criteria for deciding between a supramalleolar osteotomy and an arthrodesis were determined by the presence of arthritis and whether the ankle deformity was manually correctable under fluoroscopy (**Figs. 7** and **8**).

In correcting a ball-and-socket ankle deformity with a medial closing wedge supramalleolar osteotomy, a 10-cm medial incision is centered at the level of the

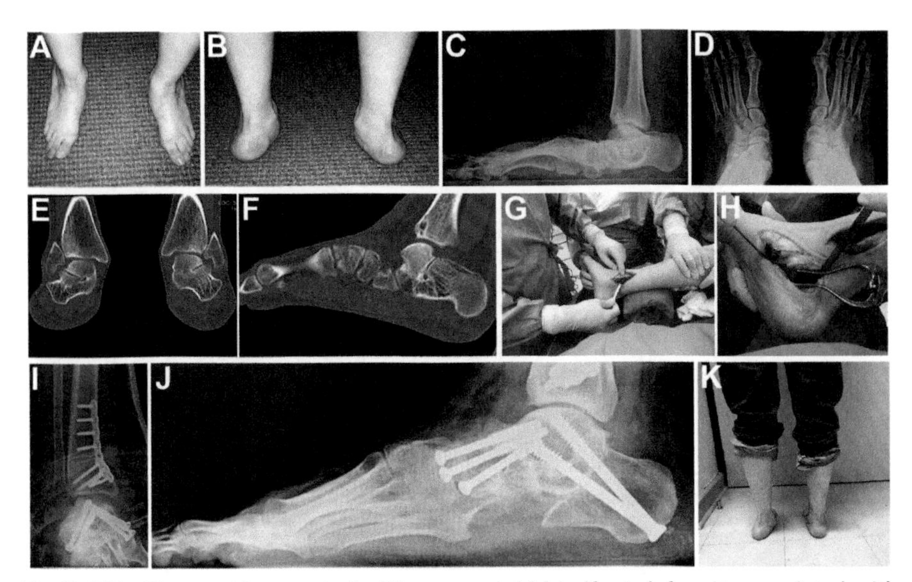

Fig. 7. This 15-year-old presented with severe rigid hindfoot deformity associated with subluxation of the subtalar and TN joints and a rigid oblique talus. The ball-and-socket configuration of the ankle associated with the coalition is easily visible (*A–F*). The treatment commenced with closing wedge supramalleolar osteotomy (*G*), followed by an extensive medial incision through which a subtalar and closing wedge TN arthrodesis was performed (*H*). The immediate postoperative and final radiographic and clinical result is presented (*I–K*).

osteotomy, which is usually 2 cm proximal to the growth plate of the distal tibia. It is not necessary to incise the periosteum or to elevate it in children, and unnecessary stripping should be avoided. An electrocautery should be used to mark the location of the proximal and distal osteotomy, which is determined by the angulation of the ankle and apex of the deformity. The size of the wedge is usually around 4 to 5 mm without including the thickness of the saw blade. Two 2.0-mm K-wires are inserted under fluoroscopy to delineate the osteotomy in a converging fashion so that they will meet at the lateral cortex of the tibia. A closing wedge osteotomy is then performed along but within the boundary of the K-wires. The lateral cortex should be kept intact to facilitate closing the osteotomy as a hinge and stabilizing the afterward fixation, because a fibula osteotomy is not often required. If the lateral cortex is penetrated and opens when closing the tibia medially, one can use a small 3-hole plate at the apex of the wedge either before or after performing the osteotomy. In some cases with a more severe ankle deformity, if adequate correction cannot be obtained after the tibial osteotomy, then the lateral cortex of the tibia is perforated and an oblique fibular osteotomy is added through a separate lateral incision to facilitate sufficient medial angulation of the distal ankle. In a child with an open growth plate, 3-mm pins can be used to fix the supramalleolar osteotomy. Once the ankle is realigned and stabilized, the associated tarsal coalitions can be addressed, in addition to correcting any hindfoot deformities as described in earlier discussion. It is important to reevaluate the forefoot to see if a Cotton osteotomy is needed to correct any residual forefoot supination.

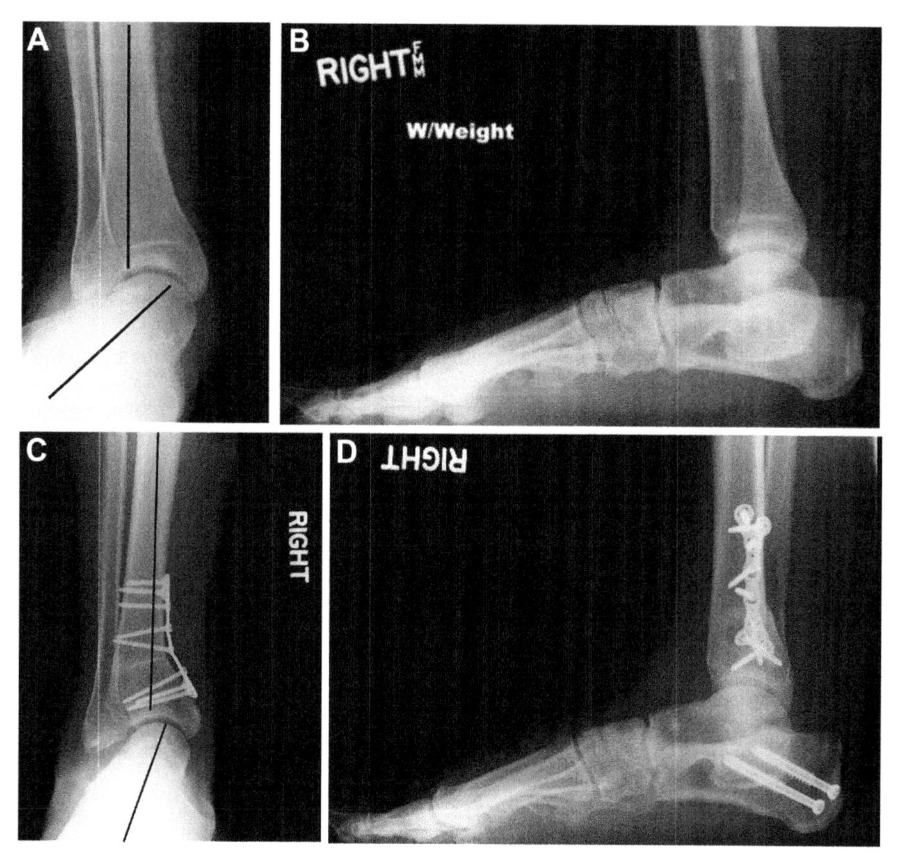

Fig. 8. This is a 16-year-old who presented with a TN and CC coalition associated with a ball-and-socket ankle, a hypoplastic fibula, and severe valgus deformity of the ankle (*A, B*). Note the marked improvement in the alignment of the ankle and foot following a medial closing wedge supramalleolar osteotomy and a medial translational osteotomy of the calcaneus (*C, D*).

SUMMARY

Tarsal coalition is a congenital skeletal development disorder, which can present with pain, deformity, instability in hindfoot and ankle, and eventually arthritis due to restricted movement and subsequent uneven stress in the involved tarsal joints. Onset of symptoms typically occurs in early adolescence when the coalition starts to ossify. Hindfoot deformity presents in most pediatric coalition cases. Depending on the severity, it can be corrected by an arthroereisis or calcaneus stop technique, calcaneus osteotomies, or hindfoot arthrodesis. Soft tissue and muscle balancing also need to be considered in cases with a hindfoot deformity, in particular to address any peroneus brevis contracture caused by long-term hindfoot valgus. There is no consensus on whether a peroneus brevis release should be added to structural reconstruction.

The presence of severe rigidity associated with a double coalition, a ball-and-socket ankle, or a severe hindfoot deformity are factors that make correction complicated. A thorough physical examination combined with accurate imaging are essential to obtaining detailed information such as the location and size of the coalition, as well as alignment of both the ankle and the hindfoot. The ankle joint must be involved in preoperative planning in every case. By doing so, a solid foundation is laid for further surgical planning, which includes coalition resection, stabilization of the foot and ankle, and correcting alignment with osteotomies, arthrodesis, and soft tissue balancing.

CLINICS CARE POINTS

- Careful preoperative physical examination including diagnostic injection is important in treatment planning for complex tarsal coalitions.
- Both radiographic examination and computed tomographic scan that involve not only the foot but also the ankle are necessary to analyze the location and size of the coalitions, determining the presence of arthritis in the involved or adjacent joints, and if there are any deformities including a ball-and-socket ankle, which is frequently associated with complex tarsal coalitions.

DISCLOSURE

The authors have nothing to disclose.

REFERENCES

1. Downey MS. Tarsal coalition. In: Banks AS, Downey MS, Martin DE, et al, editors. McGlamry's comprehensive textbook of foot and ankle surgery. 3rd edition. Philadelphia: Lippincott Williams & Wilkins; 2001. p. 993–1031.
2. Leonard MA. The inheritance of tarsal coalition and it relationship to spastic flat foot. J Bone Joint Surg Br 1974;56B(3):520–6.
3. Harris BJ. Anomalous structures in the developing human foot. Anat Rec 1955; 121:399.
4. Tachdjian Mihran O. The Child's foot. Philadelphia: W.B. Saunders Company; 1985. p. 261–85. Tarsal Coalition.
5. Camasta CA, Graeser TA. Pediatric tarsal coalition and pes planovalgus. In: Butterworth ML, Marcoux JT, editors. The pediatric foot and ankle. Switzerland AG: Springer Nature; 2020. p. 191.
6. Katayama T, Tanaka Y, Kadono K, et al. Talocalcaneal coalition: a case showing the ossification process. Foot Ankle Int 2005;26(6):490–3.
7. Hong CH, Lee HS, Lee WS, et al. Tarsal tunnel syndrome caused by posterior facet talocalcaneal coalition: a case report. Medicine (Baltimore) 2020;99(26): e20893.
8. Bixby SD, Jarrett DY, Johnston P, et al. Posteromedial subtalar coalitions: prevalence and associated morphological alterations of the sustentaculum tali. Pediatr Radiol 2016;46(8):1142–9.
9. Alaia EF, Rosenberg ZS, Bencardino JT, et al. Tarsal tunnel disease and talocalcaneal coalition: MRI features. Skeletal Radiol 2016;45(11):1507–14.
10. Blakemore LC, Cooperman DR, Thompson GH. The rigid flatfoot: tarsal coalitions. Clin Podiatr Med Surg 2000;17(3):531–55.
11. Lamb D. The ball-and-socket ankle joint. J Bone Joint Surg 1958;40-B:240.
12. Ellington JK, Myerson MS. Surgical correction of the ball and socket ankle joint in the adult associated with a talonavicular tarsal coalition. Foot Ankle Int 2013; 34(10):1381–8.

13. Charles YP, Louahem D, Diméglio A. Cavovarus foot deformity with multiple tarsal coalitions: functional and three-dimensional preoperative assessment. J Foot Ankle Surg 2006;45(2):118–26.
14. Stuecker RD, Bennett JT. Tarsal coalition presenting as a pes cavo-varus deformity: report of three cases and review of the literature. Foot Ankle 1993;14(9):540–4.
15. Myerson MS, Kadakia AR. Resection of a middle facet coalition. In: Reconstructive foot and ankle surgery: management of complications. 3rd edition. Philadelphia: Elsevier; 2018. p. 366–70.
16. Lyon R, Liu X, Cho S. Effect of tarsal coalition resection on dynamic plantar pressures and electromyography of lower extremity muscles. J Foot Ankle Surg 2005;44(4):252–8.
17. Blair J, Perdios A, Reilly C. Peroneal spastic flatfoot caused by a talar osteochondral lesion: a case report. Foot Ankle Int 2007;28(6):724–6.
18. Emery KH, Bisset GS 3rd, Johnson ND, et al. Tarsal coalition: a blinded comparison of MRI and CT. Pediatr Radiol 1998;28(8):612–6.
19. Guignand D, Journeau P, Mainard-Simard L, et al. Child calcaneonavicular coalitions: MRI diagnostic value in a 19-case series. Orthop Traumatol Surg Res 2011;97(1):67–72.
20. Hirschmann A, Pfirrmann CW, Klammer G, et al. Upright cone CT of the hindfoot: comparison of the non-weight-bearing with the upright weight-bearing position. Eur Radiol 2014;24(3):553–8.
21. Burssens A, Peeters J, Buedts K, et al. Measuring hindfoot alignment in weight bearing CT: a novel clinical relevant measurement method. Foot Ankle Surg 2016;22(4):233–8.
22. Lee KM, Chung CY, Park MS, et al. Analysis of three-dimensional computed tomography talar morphology in relation to pediatric pes planovalgus deformity. J Pediatr Orthop B 2019;28(6):591–7.
23. Iehl C, Auch E, Vivtcharenko V, et al. Talocalcaneal coalition resection and bone block subtalar joint arthrodesis: a techinical tip. J Foot Ankle 2020;14(2):211–8.
24. Godoy-Santos AL, Netto CC, Weight-bearing CT International Study Group. Weight-bearing computed tomography of the foot and ankle: an update and future directions. Acta Ortop Bras 2018;26(2):135–9.
25. Li S, Myerson MS. Excision of a middle facet tarsal coalition. JBJS Essent Surg Tech 2020;10(1):e0114, 1-14.
26. Hamel J. Die Resektion der talokalkanearen Coalitio im Kindes und Adoleszentenalter ohne und mit Stellungskorrektur [Resection of talocalcaneal coalition in children and adolescents without and with osteotomy of the calcaneus]. Oper Orthop Traumatol 2009;21(2):180–92.
27. Scott AT, Tuten HR. Calcaneonavicular coalition resection with extensor digitorum brevis interposition in adults. Foot Ankle Int 2007;28(8):890–5.
28. Masquijo JJ, Jarvis J. Associated talocalcaneal and calcaneonavicular coalitions in the same foot. J Pediatr Orthop B 2010;19(6):507–10.
29. Luhmann SJ, Schonecker PL. Symptomatic talocalcaneal resection: indications and results. J Pediatr Orthop 1998;18:748–54.
30. Wilde PH, Torode IP, Dickens DR, et al. Resection for symptomatic talocalcaneal coalition. J Bone Joint Surg Br 1994;76:797–801.
31. Scranton PE. Treatment of symptomatic talocalcaneal coalition. J Bone Joint Surg Am 1987;69:533–9.
32. Comfort TK, Johnson LO. Resection for symptomatic talocalcaneal coalition. J Pediatr Orthopp 1998;18:283–8.

33. Khosbin A, Law PL, Caspi L, et al. Long term functional outcomes of resected tarsal coalitions. Foot Ankle Int 2013;34:1370–5.
34. Channon GM, Brotherton BJ. The ball and socket ankle joint. J Bone Joint Surg 1979;61:85–9.
35. Dieter B, Karbowski A, Ludwig S. Congenital ball and socket anomaly of the ankle. J Pediatr Orthop 1996;16:492–6.
36. Santiago FR, Moreno CP, Barea LC, et al. Ball and socket ankle joint with hypoplastic sustentaculum tali. Eur Radiol 2002;12:S48–50.
37. Stevens PM, Aoki S, Olson P. Ball and socket ankle. J Pediatr Orthop 2006;26: 427–31.
38. Takakura Y, Tamai S, Masuhara K. Genesis of the ball and socket ankle. J Bone Joint Surg 1986;68:834–7.
39. Takakura Y, Tanaka Y, Kumai T, et al. Development of the ball and socket ankle as assessed by radiography and arthrography. J Bone Joint Surg Br 1999;81: 1001–4.
40. Tarr RR, Resnick CT, Wagner KS, et al. Changes in tibiotalar joint contact areas following experimentally induced tibial angular deformities. Clin Orthop Relat Res 1985;199:72–80.

UNITED STATES POSTAL SERVICE®

Statement of Ownership, Management, and Circulation (All Periodicals Publications Except Requester Publications)

1. Publication Title: FOOT AND ANKLE CLINICS OF NORTH AMERICA
2. Publication Number: 016 – 368
3. Filing Date: 9/18/2021
4. Issue Frequency: MAR, JUN, SEP, DEC
5. Number of Issues Published Annually: 4
6. Annual Subscription Price: $344.00
7. Complete Mailing Address of Known Office of Publication (*Not printer*) (*Street, city, county, state, and ZIP+4®*)
ELSEVIER INC.
230 Park Avenue, Suite 800
New York, NY 10169

Contact Person: Malathi Samayan
Telephone (*Include area code*): 91-44-4299-4507

8. Complete Mailing Address of Headquarters or General Business Office of Publisher (*Not printer*)
ELSEVIER INC.
230 Park Avenue, Suite 800
New York, NY 10169

9. Full Names and Complete Mailing Addresses of Publisher, Editor, and Managing Editor (*Do not leave blank*)

Publisher (*Name and complete mailing address*)
DOLORES MELONI, ELSEVIER INC.
1600 JOHN F KENNEDY BLVD. SUITE 1800
PHILADELPHIA, PA 19103-2899

Editor (*Name and complete mailing address*)
LAUREN BOYLE, ELSEVIER INC.
1600 JOHN F KENNEDY BLVD. SUITE 1800
PHILADELPHIA, PA 19103-2899

Managing Editor (*Name and complete mailing address*)
PATRICK MANLEY, ELSEVIER INC.
1600 JOHN F KENNEDY BLVD. SUITE 1800
PHILADELPHIA, PA 19103-2899

10. Owner (*Do not leave blank. If the publication is owned by a corporation, give the name and address of the corporation immediately followed by the names and addresses of all stockholders owning or holding 1 percent or more of the total amount of stock. If not owned by a corporation, give the names and addresses of the individual owners. If owned by a partnership or other unincorporated firm, give its name and address as well as those of each individual owner. If the publication is published by a nonprofit organization, give its name and address.*)

Full Name	Complete Mailing Address
WHOLLY OWNED SUBSIDIARY OF REED/ELSEVIER, US HOLDINGS	1600 JOHN F KENNEDY BLVD. SUITE 1800 PHILADELPHIA, PA 19103-2899

11. Known Bondholders, Mortgagees, and Other Security Holders Owning or Holding 1 Percent or More of Total Amount of Bonds, Mortgages, or Other Securities. If none, check box → ☐ None

Full Name	Complete Mailing Address
N/A	

12. Tax Status (*For completion by nonprofit organizations authorized to mail at nonprofit rates*) (*Check one*)
The purpose, function, and nonprofit status of this organization and the exempt status for federal income tax purposes:
☒ Has Not Changed During Preceding 12 Months
☐ Has Changed During Preceding 12 Months (*Publisher must submit explanation of change with this statement*)

13. Publication Title: FOOT AND ANKLE CLINICS OF NORTH AMERICA
14. Issue Date for Circulation Data Below: JUNE 2021

15. Extent and Nature of Circulation		Average No. Copies Each Issue During Preceding 12 Months	No. Copies of Single Issue Published Nearest to Filing Date
a. Total Number of Copies (*Net press run*)		266	232
b. Paid Circulation (*By Mail and Outside the Mail*)	(1) Mailed Outside-County Paid Subscriptions Stated on PS Form 3541 (Include paid distribution above nominal rate, advertiser's proof copies, and exchange copies)	160	150
	(2) Mailed In-County Paid Subscriptions Stated on PS Form 3541 (Include paid distribution above nominal rate, advertiser's proof copies, and exchange copies)	0	0
	(3) Paid Distribution Outside the Mails Including Sales Through Dealers and Carriers, Street Vendors, Counter Sales, and Other Paid Distribution Outside USPS®	78	65
	(4) Paid Distribution by Other Classes of Mail Through the USPS (e.g., First-Class Mail®)	0	0
c. Total Paid Distribution [*Sum of 15b (1), (2), (3), and (4)*] ▶		238	215
d. Free or Nominal Rate Distribution (*By Mail and Outside the Mail*)	(1) Free or Nominal Rate Outside-County Copies included on PS Form 3541	13	3
	(2) Free or Nominal Rate In-County Copies Included on PS Form 3541	0	0
	(3) Free or Nominal Rate Copies Mailed at Other Classes Through the USPS (e.g., First-Class Mail)	0	0
	(4) Free or Nominal Rate Distribution Outside the Mail (Carriers or other means)	0	0
e. Total Free or Nominal Rate Distribution (*Sum of 15d (1), (2), (3) and (4)*)		13	3
f. Total Distribution (*Sum of 15c and 15e*) ▶		251	218
g. Copies not Distributed (*See Instructions to Publishers #4 (page #3)*) ▶		15	14
h. Total (*Sum of 15f and g*)		266	232
i. Percent Paid (*15c divided by 15f times 100*) ▶		94.82%	98.62%

* If you are claiming electronic copies, go to line 16 on page 3. If you are not claiming electronic copies, skip to line 17 on page 3.

16. Electronic Copy Circulation	Average No. Copies Each Issue During Preceding 12 Months	No. Copies of Single Issue Published Nearest to Filing Date
a. Paid Electronic Copies ▶		
b. Total Paid Print Copies (Line 15c) + Paid Electronic Copies (Line 16a) ▶		
c. Total Print Distribution (Line 15f) + Paid Electronic Copies (Line 16a) ▶		
d. Percent Paid (Both Print & Electronic Copies) (16b divided by 16c × 100) ▶		

☒ **I certify that 50% of all my distributed copies (electronic and print) are paid above a nominal price.**

17. Publication of Statement of Ownership
☒ If the publication is a general publication, publication of this statement is required. Will be printed in the DECEMBER 2021 issue of this publication. ☐ Publication not required.

18. Signature and Title of Editor, Publisher, Business Manager, or Owner
Malathi Samayan - Distribution Controller — Malathi Samayan — Date: 9/18/2021

I certify that all information furnished on this form is true and complete. I understand that anyone who furnishes false or misleading information on this form or who omits material or information requested on the form may be subject to criminal sanctions (including fines and imprisonment) and/or civil sanctions (including civil penalties).

Moving?

Make sure your subscription moves with you!

To notify us of your new address, find your **Clinics Account Number** (located on your mailing label above your name), and contact customer service at:

Email: journalscustomerservice-usa@elsevier.com

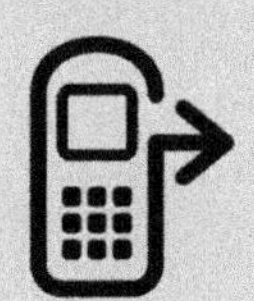

800-654-2452 **(subscribers in the U.S. & Canada)**
314-447-8871 **(subscribers outside of the U.S. & Canada)**

Fax number: 314-447-8029

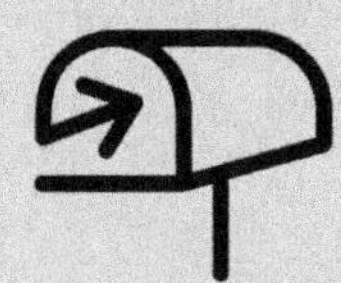

Elsevier Health Sciences Division
Subscription Customer Service
3251 Riverport Lane
Maryland Heights, MO 63043

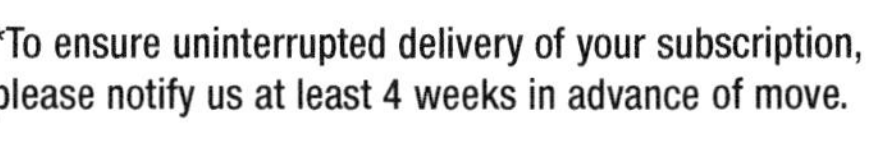

*To ensure uninterrupted delivery of your subscription, please notify us at least 4 weeks in advance of move.

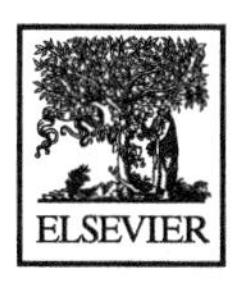

Printed and bound by CPI Group (UK) Ltd, Croydon, CR0 4YY
08/05/2025
01864704-0003